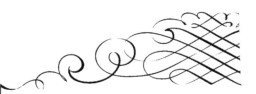
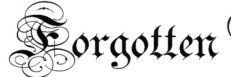
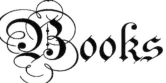

ISBN 978-0-243-26128-4
PIBN 10790733

For support please visit www.forgottenbooks.com

1 MONTH OF
FREE
READING

at
www.ForgottenBooks.com

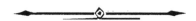

By purchasing this book you are eligible for one month membership to ForgottenBooks.com, giving you unlimited access to our entire collection of over 1,000,000 titles via our web site and mobile apps.

To claim your free month visit:
www.forgottenbooks.com/free790733

TRANSACTIONS

OF THE

National Dental Association

AT THE

THIRTEENTH ANNUAL MEETING

HELD AT

Birmingham, Ala., March 30—April 2, 1909

PHILADELPHIA
PRESS OF THE "DENTAL COSMOS"
The S. S. White Dental Mfg. Co.
1910

DISCLAIMER.

CONTENTS.

GENERAL SESSIONS.

PAGE

First General Session... 1
    Meeting called to order by the president, Dr. V. E. TURNER............. 1
    Welcome extended to the Association on behalf of the city of Birmingham
        and the dental profession of Alabama 1
    President reads his annual address....................,..................... 1
    Paper—Reading of Dr. E. C. KIRK's paper.......................... 2

Second General Session 2
    Paper—Reading of Dr. JAMES McMANUS' paper..................... 2
    Election of Officers 2

Third General Session 3
    Discussion of Dr. McMANUS' paper.............................. 3

Fourth General Session.. 3
    Vote of thanks extended to Drs. Donnally and Bryant for assistance given
        the Committee on Legislation 3
    Resolution setting forth that no other than the regularly appointed com-
        mittee is authorized to speak for the Association with regard to
        army and navy dental legislation 3
    Report of the Committee on President's Address 3
    Paper—Reading of Dr. L. G. NOEL's paper 4
    Paper—Dr. W. STORER How's paper read by title 4
    Installation of the new president, Dr. B. L. THORPE 4
    Vote of thanks to the retiring president, Dr. V. E. TURNER, and other
        officers of the Association................................ 4
    Vote of thanks to the Local Committee of Arrangements 4
    Adjournment 4

SECTION III.

ORAL SURGERY, ANATOMY, PHYSIOLOGY, HISTOLOGY, PATHOL-OGY, ETIOLOGY, HYGIENE, PROPHYLAXIS, MATERIA MEDICA, AND ALLIED SUBJECTS.

PAGE

Proceedings 169
   Paper—"Recent Progress in Oral Surgery." By Dr. TRUMAN W. BROPHY 169
   Discussion 176
   Paper—"The Evolution of Tools." By Dr. A. H. THOMPSON 183
   Discussion 190
   Report of Committee on Oral Hygiene. By Dr. J. P. CORLEY 193
   Paper—"Oral Hygiene in Alabama." By Dr. F. A. JOHNSTON 194
   Paper—"What We Have to Give." By Dr. PAUL GARDINER WHITE 197
   Joint discussion of the three foregoing papers on oral hygiene 202
   Paper—"Dentistry, Past and Present, as Seen by a Modern Hygienist."
      By Dr. L. C. TAYLOR 205
   Joint discussion continued 209
   Resolution carried to place 5000 copies of the N. D. A. pamphlet "The Mouth and the Teeth" in the hands of the Committee on Oral Hygiene for distribution 213

CLINICS.

[*See note on page 218.*]

Appendix.

Organization of the N. D. A. 221
  OFFICERS 221
  EXECUTIVE COUNCIL 221
  EXECUTIVE COMMITTEE 221
  ORGANIZATION OF SECTIONS 222

PAGE

COMMITTEE ON HISTORY 222
      "   ON STATE AND LOCAL SOCIETIES 223
      "   ON DENTAL JOURNAL 223
      "   ON NATIONAL DENTAL MUSEUM AND LIBRARY 223
      "   ON ORAL HYGIENE 223
      "   ON NECROLOGY 224
      "   ON LEGISLATION 224
      "   ON SCIENTIFIC RESEARCH 224
      "   ON PUBLICATION 224
      "   ON CLINICS 224
LOCAL COMMITTEE OF ARRANGEMENTS 225
SPECIAL COMMITTEE ON PHARMACOPEIAL CONVENTION 225
List of Members.. 226
PERMANENT MEMBERS WITHOUT DUES 237
SURVIVING CHARTER MEMBERS SOUTHERN DENTAL ASSOCIATION 237
Past Presiding Officers:
Prior to Consolidation—
    EX-PRESIDENTS AMERICAN DENTAL ASSOCIATION 238
    EX-PRESIDENTS SOUTHERN DENTAL ASSOCIATION 238
EX-PRESIDENTS OF THE NATIONAL DENTAL ASSOCIATION 239
Constitution... 240
ORDER OF BUSINESS 248
STANDING RESOLUTIONS 249
RULES OF ORDER 250
Code of Ethics 251

THIRTEENTH ANNUAL MEETING

OF THE

National Dental Association,

HELD AT

BIRMINGHAM, ALA., MARCH 30 TO APRIL 2, 1909.

TUESDAY—First General Session.

THE first general session of the thirteenth annual meeting of the National Dental Association was called to order at 10 o'clock Tuesday morning, March 30th, by the president, Dr. V. E. Turner, Raleigh, N. C.

The President introduced the Rev. Sterling Foster, D.D., of Birmingham, who invoked the divine blessing on the deliberations of the association.

The President then presented Mr. J. R. Copeland, who welcomed the association to Birmingham on behalf of the city authorities.

Dr. L. F. LUCKIE, chairman of the Local Committee of Arrangements, welcomed the association on behalf of the dental profession of Alabama.

Dr. J. Y. CRAWFORD, on behalf of the National Dental Association, responded to the addresses of welcome.

Dr. WM. CRENSHAW, vice-president from the South, was called to the chair, and the president, Dr. V. E. TURNER, read his annual address. (See page 14.)

On motion Dr. Crenshaw appointed the following Committee on the President's Address: Dr. B. Holly Smith, Dr. William Carr, and Dr. Burton Lee Thorpe.

Dr. H. J. BURKHART, chairman of the Executive Council, reported as follows:

A paper by Dr. E. C. Kirk, entitled "The Dental Relationships of Arthritism," with the discussion, after which the general session would adjourn until 12 M. Wednesday, March 31st.

At 2.30 P.M. Section II would be called, with the section officers in charge; at 8 P.M. Section III, and at 9.30 Wednesday morning Section I.

On motion the report was received and adopted.

The President, Dr. Turner, resumed the chair and announced the reading of a paper by Dr. E. C. KIRK, entitled "The Dental Relationships of Arthritism." (See page 20.)

Adjourned until Wednesday at 12 o'clock.

WEDNESDAY—Second General Session.

The general session was called to order by the president, Dr. Turner, at 12 o'clock. The order of business was the reading of a paper by Dr. JAMES McMANUS, entitled, "A Side-light on Professional Interest." (See page 41.)

The time for the election of officers as fixed in the by-laws having arrived, the discussion of Dr. McManus' paper was deferred until 2.30 o'clock.

ELECTION OF OFFICERS.

The President appointed Drs. J. D. Patterson, Chas. McManus, and Geo. S Vann as tellers.

The following officers were elected for the ensuing year:

President—Burton Lee Thorpe, St. Louis, Mo.

Vice-president from the West—W. T. Chambers, Denver, Colo.

Vice-president from the East—C. W. Rodgers, Dorchester, Mass.

Vice-president from the South—T. P. Hinman, Atlanta, Ga.

Corresponding Secretary—H. C. Brown, Columbus, Ohio.

Recording Secretary—C. S. Butler, Buffalo, N. Y.

Treasurer—A. R. Melendy, Knoxville, Tenn.

Executive Council—H. J. Burkhart, Batavia, N. Y.; A. H. Peck, Chicago. Ill.; B. Holly Smith, Baltimore, Md.; Waldo E. Boardman, Boston, Mass.; C. L. Alexander, Charlotte, N. C.

Members of Executive Committee for Three Years—C. M. Work. Ottumwa, Iowa; V. H. Jackson, New York, N. Y.; W. G. Mason, Tampa, Fla.

Denver, Colo., was selected as the place for holding the next annual meeting. and the third Tuesday in July 1910 as the date.

On motion the President and Executive Council were empowered to meet and appoint section officers and the regular committees for the ensuing year.

The general session then adjourned until 2.30 P.M.

WEDNESDAY—Third General Session.

The third general session was called to order Wednesday afternoon at 2.30 o'clock by the president, Dr. V. E. Turner, and the discussion of Dr. James McManus' paper was then taken up (see page 51), after which the association adjourned until Thursday morning, April 1st, at 12 o'clock.

THURSDAY—Fourth General Session.

The fourth general session was called to order by the president, Dr. Turner, at 12 o'clock Thursday, April 1st.

The first order of business was the report of the Executive Council, by the chairman, Dr. BURKHART, as follows:

The Executive Council recommends that the thanks of the association be extended to Drs. Donnally and Bryant of Washington, for the able and conscientious assistance given the Committee on Legislation during the past year.

RESOLVED, That the National Dental Association desires it to be distinctly understood that no other committees or individuals are authorized to speak for this association with respect to army and navy legislation, other than the regularly appointed committee, and any member of the association interfering with the purpose of this committee shall be held responsible to the association.

On motion the report was adopted.

Dr. B. HOLLY SMITH presented the report of the Committee on the President's Address, as follows:

REPORT OF COMMITTEE ON PRESIDENT'S ADDRESS.

Mr. President and Members of the National Dental Association,—Your committee appointed for the consideration of the President's address congratulate the association upon the conservative, timely, and masterful character of the address.

Many of the suggestions of the president must be received by the members of this association as paternal advice or recommendation, and we feel sure that they will contribute to a general uplift of the welfare of our associates. Some of the recommendations, however, deserve to give birth to legislative enactments which will presumably secure for the association and our beloved calling, everywhere, abundant fruit.

The suggestion of the president that some definite time be set for the establishment of a journal has already borne fruit in the passage today by the Executive Council of a resolution fixing a time for the publication of the first issue.

The "clean and dignified campaign for the development of the membership of our association" recommended by the president already gives great promise of success, as twelve or fifteen states today indicate through their representatives or letters from their officers that they will join the National in a body. We, your committee, urge the necessity of a consecutive and consistent effort on the part of the officers and members of this association to establish a loyal relation between our National body and the various state dental associations throughout the country, and that especially the corresponding secretary who is elected this year shall undertake a systematic correspondence with the officers of said state societies, and where possible visit them as a representative of this association and present the claims and advocate the interests of our National body.

We further urge that the Committee on Oral Hygiene constitute itself a bureau for the dissemination of information and literature upon the subject, and that the members, by letter and by every other means, such as publication, carry on a propaganda for clean mouths. We believe that what has been written or accomplished on this line in one state should be made known through our officers in every state in the Union.

We further recommend the encouragement of every effort for dental inspection in our schools, public and private, and for the delivery by well-equipped members of our association of public lectures before guilds and associations upon the subject of oral hygiene.

We further recommend that $250 of interest on a relief fund in possession of this association be appropriated to the Miller International Memorial fund.

B. HOLLY SMITH, *ch'man*,
WM. CARR,
B. L. THORPE,
Committee.

Dr. H. J. BURKHART, chairman of the Council, moved that the paper by Dr. W. STORER HOW, entitled "Doctor of Dental Science," be read by title, the author not being present.

The motion was carried and the paper ordered published in the Transactions. (See page 72.)

The next order of business was a paper by Dr. L. G. NOEL, entitled "The Management of the Teeth and Mouth from the Age of Six to Adolescence." (See page 62.)

The next order of business was the installation of officers, and the newly elected president, Dr. B. L. Thorpe, was presented by Dr. Turner, and addressed the association, thanking the members for the honor conferred upon him by his election as presiding officer.

Dr. J. Y. CRAWFORD moved that the thanks of the association be extended to the retiring president and the other officers of the association for their efforts in making the meeting a success.

Motion carried.

Dr. BURKHART moved that a vote of thanks be extended to the Local Committee of Arrangements for their untiring efforts on behalf of the association.

Motion carried.

There being no further business before the meeting, on motion the association adjourned to meet in Denver, Colo., on the third Tuesday in July 1910.

MINUTES

OF THE

EXECUTIVE COUNCIL.

PURSUANT to the by-laws, the Executive Council convened in the Council chamber of City Hall, Birmingham, at 9 A.M., March 30, 1909, with the following members present: Drs. H. J. Burkhart, chairman, C. S. Butler, secretary, Turner, Smith, Hetrick, Boardman, and Peck.

The program as prepared and published by the committee was on motion adopted as the official program of the meeting, and the order for the opening general session was made the President's address and the paper by Dr. E. C. Kirk on "The Dental Relationships of Arthritism." At 2.30 P.M. Section II would convene, with the section officers in charge, at 8 P.M. Section III, and at 9 A.M. Wednesday Section I.

The first general session to adjourn at 12 M.

The usual bills of the secretary for printing, stationery, and postage were received and referred to the Auditing Committee. Bills from the treasurer, Clinic Committee, and section officers were re-received and referred to the Auditing Committee. Dr. J. D. Patterson, chairman of the committee to print the pamphlet "The Mouth and the Teeth,"

presented a bill, which on motion was ordered paid.

Dr. H. L. WHEELER, chairman of the Journal Committee, presented the following report:

REPORT OF THE COMMITTEE ON DENTAL JOURNAL.

BIRMINGHAM, ALA., March 30, 1909.

To the National Dental Association:

Your Committee on Dental Journal offers the following report:

Prior to calling a meeting of the committee, the chairman, Dr. H. L. Wheeler, and the undersigned visited, on December 19, 1908, the printing and publishing establishment of the *Journal of the American Medical Association* in Chicago, and thus obtained much valuable data applicable to the needs of our journal.

On January 30th a regular meeting was held at Dr. Wheeler's office, 12 W. 46th st., New York. All the members of the committee were present, namely, Dr. Wheeler, Dr. C. S. Butler of Buffalo, Dr. Frank Taylor of Boston, Dr. F. W. Stiff of Richmond, and Dr. Dunning of New York.

After full discussion, the following motions were made and carried:

(1) To send a circular letter to members of state societies, announcing the proposed publication of the journal, and calling for individual pledges to subscribe—two hundred dollars of the committee's expense fund to be allotted for this purpose.

(2) Drs. Wheeler and Taylor to procure
from the organization comprising the Allied
Societies a statement of the terms upon which
they would be willing to make over to the
National Dental Association the journal now
published by them, having in view the future
publication of their transactions by the N.
D. A.

(3) That all members of the committee
endeavor to secure from public-spirited men
in the profession pledges to support the enterprise to the extent of certain amounts, to
form a guarantee fund, 'payable *pro rata*, to
meet any deficit during the first two years of
the journal's existence.

(4) To keep the editorial management of
the journal, for the present, within the committee.

The meeting then adjourned at the call of
the chair.

A circular letter, with return postal, appended hereto, was prepared by the committee
and sent to 4000 members of the state societies who are not members of the N. D. A.
At this writing 469 conditional agreements
to subscribe have been received in reply.

Upon Dr. Stiff's suggestion, about three
hundred circulars have been sent to as many
secretaries of state and local societies, a separate letter being inclosed with each, request-
ing that the circular be read at the next
meeting of each society. A number of agreement slips were inclosed with each communication. Many favorable replies have been received from these secretaries and other individuals promising to co-operate in the work
of securing subscriptions.

In reply to the inquiries of Drs. Wheeler
and Taylor, the following societies, known as
the Allied Societies, have agreed to merge
their journal into the National journal, provided that the latter shall at all times publish their transactions as arranged by their
editors, and provided that the ethical standards which have governed the Allied Societies shall be maintained by the National
dental journal: The New York Institute of
Stomatology; the American Academy of Dental Science; the Harvard Odontological Society; the Metropolitan District of Massachusetts Dental Society, and the Boston and
Tufts Dental Alumni Association.

The work of securing pledges for the guar-

antee fund has progressed rather slowly to
date. A list of these pledges is appended.

W. B. DUNNING, *Secretary.*

(The foregoing is from the secretary of
the committee.)

There having been received upward of five
hundred pledges from individual dentists at
$2 each, and from secretaries of societies
twenty-five—of which three are non-commit-
tal, one announces that the whole state society has voted to subscribe to the journal,
and twenty-one of the secretaries personally
favor the project and will bring it before their
societies when they meet;—

Therefore we are prepared to immediately
publish a journal; this being made possible,
first, by 500 individual pledges of $2, the
subscription of the National for its membership, $750, and private pledges of $400;
by the eventual support of the societies publishing the *Journal of the Allied Societies*,
$1500, and by the pledge of a public-spirited
member of the profession to make good any
deficiency. We are therefore now prepared to
publish the journal.

We recommend that your committee be authorized to solicit and receive subscriptions
from all sources for the National dental journal.

RESOLVED, That the committee be continued,
that it be authorized to make all necessary
arrangements for publishing, and that it issue
the first *Journal of the National Dental Association* on October 1, 1910.

Respectfully submitted,
HERBERT L. WHEELER, *Chairman.*

The report was received, and after an
informal discussion by the members of
the Council and others present the committee was continued, and the resolution
to begin the publication of the journal
with October 1910 was adopted.

The bill of expenses of the committee
was received and referred to the Auditing Committee.

Dr. T. W. BROPHY, chairman of the
Miller Memorial Fund, presented the following report:

REPORT OF COMMITTEE ON MILLER MEMORIAL FUND.

BIRMINGHAM, ALA., April 1, 1909.

To the National Dental Association:

Your committee on the W. D. Miller Memorial Fund most respectfully submits the subjoined report:

A circular letter has been mailed to the officers of every state dental society in the United States, and also to many of the larger local societies.

The Dental Society of the State of New York has pledged $1000, and the Illinois State Dental Society has also pledged $1000. No further pledges have been made. Inquiry, however, has shown us that other states will join in this movement, and our country will contribute to the fund in a most substantial manner.

The societies will be again appealed to, and the funds secured will be placed in the hands of the chairman of the International Fund at the time of the meeting of the Fifth International Dental Congress, Berlin, Germany, August 1909.

Respectfully submitted,

TRUMAN W. BROPHY,
B. HOLLY SMITH,
For the Committee.

The report was received, and on motion the accrued interest on the San Francisco Relief Fund, to the amount of $250, was contributed to the fund.

Dr. EDWARD C. MILLS of Columbus, Ohio, presented the following:

To the National Dental Association:

At a meeting of the Columbus Dental Society of Columbus, Ohio, held Tuesday, March 23, 1909, the following resolutions were adopted:

Whereas, The late Dr. Willoughby D. Miller, who devoted his life to untiring research for the benefit of dental science, was an American and an Ohioan by birth; and

Whereas, It is desired to obtain an expression of opinion from the various dental societies and associations meeting during the interval pending the next meeting of the Ohio

State Dental Society (December 1909); therefore be it

RESOLVED, That the Columbus Dental Society, Columbus, Ohio, suggest the advisability of raising a fund for a suitable memorial, by the dental profession of America, to commemorate the life and work of the said Dr. Willoughby D. Miller; said memorial to take such form as may be determined by the consensus of opinion of the various dental organizations of this country; and be it further

RESOLVED, That the Ohio State Dental Society, at its next annual meeting, be requested to take charge of the Miller American Memorial matter and of such correspondence as may be received pertaining to the same.

H. V. COTTRELL, *President,*
GILLETTE HAYDEN, *Secretary.*

On motion the communication was received and the movement indorsed, with the stipulation that no funds should be solicited before September 1909, on the ground that prior solicitations might interfere with the international movement.

The committee on the Fifth International Dental Congress presented the following report, which on motion was received and adopted:

REPORT OF COMMITTEE ON FIFTH INTERNATIONAL DENTAL CONGRESS.

BIRMINGHAM, ALA., March 30, 1909.

To the National Dental Association:

The American National Committee of the Fifth International Dental Congress herewith submit the following report:

A meeting of the committee was held Tuesday afternoon, March 30, 1909, in the Hotel Florence. The following members were present: Drs. Chas. McManus, Wm. Carr, G. V. I. Brown, F. E. Ball, Burton Lee Thorpe, and the chairman.

A communication from Dr. Schaeffer-Stuckert, the secretary-general of the Fifth International Dental Congress, was read by the chairman, in which it was explained that the American National Committee was officially vested with power by the Committee of Organization of the Fifth International Dental Congress to decide upon the eligibility of all applicants for membership of the congress coming from the United States of America.

The American National Committee is further informed that by decision of the Committee of Organization of the congress, all reputable holders of the national degree of their respective countries will be entitled to membership in the congress.

In furtherance of the work of the committee in so far as it relates to determining the ethical standing and eligibility of American applicants for membership in the congress, the American National Committee has by resolution authorized those of its members who shall be in attendance at the congress to act for the whole committee in determining questions of eligibility as they may arise at the time of the congress.

The Committee of Organization having authorized the American National Committee to nominate an honorary president of the congress on behalf of the United States of America, your committee has pleasure in announcing that it has nominated Prof. Truman W. Brophy of Chicago for that office. Similarly at the request of the Committee of Organization, your committee has nominated Prof. M. H. Cryer to prepare an address upon a scientific subject of general interest, to be read upon behalf of the dental profession of America at the opening of the general session of the congress.

As honorary presidents of sections, your committee nominates the following:

Section I: Anatomy, Physiology, and Histology—M. H. Cryer, Philadelphia, Pa.

Section II: Pathology and Bacteriology—J. D. Patterson, Kansas City, Mo.

Section III: Chemistry, Physics, and Mettallurgy—L. E. Custer, Dayton, Ohio.

Section IV: Diagnosis and Special Therapeutics—J. Howard Gaskill, Philadelphia, Pa.

Section V: Oral Surgery and Surgical Prosthesis—G. V. I. Brown, Milwaukee, Wis.

Section VI: General and Local Anesthesia—M. C. Smith, Lynn, Mass.

Section VII: Operative Dentistry—S. H. Guilford, Philadelphia, Pa.

Section VIII: Artificial Teeth, including Crowns—D. O. M. LeCron, St. Louis, Mo.

Section IX: Orthodontia—Victor H. Jackson, New York, N. Y.

Section X: Hygiene of the Mouth and Teeth—Wm. H. Potter, Boston, Mass.

Section XI: Education and Legislation—Wm. Carr, New York, N. Y.

Section XII: History and Literature—Chas. McManus, Hartford, Conn.

Your committee has deemed it advisable to suggest that delegates officially appointed to represent the United States Government at the congress be nominated for such office, and in that connection the following names are proposed: H. J. Burkhart, Batavia, N. Y.; Truman W. Brophy, Chicago, Ill.; M. H. Cryer, Philadelphia; William Carr, New York; Burton Lee Thorpe, St. Louis, Mo.; J. D. Patterson, Kansas City, Mo.; F. E. Ball, Fargo, N. D.; L. E. Custer, Dayton, Ohio; J. Y. Crawford, Nashville, Tenn.; B. Holly Smith, Baltimore, Md.; G. E. Savage, Worcester, Mass.; E. R. Warner, Denver, Colo.; L. L. Barber, Toledo, Ohio; Jas. W. Hull, Kansas City, Mo.; Geo. E. Warner, Grand Junction, Colo.; A. R. Melendy, Knoxville, Tenn.; Waldo E. Boardman, Boston, Mass.; G. V. I. Brown, Milwaukee, Wis.; David Stern, Cincinnati, Ohio; Stanley Rich, Nashville, Tenn.; Celia Rich, Nashville, Tenn.

Your committee has been solicited by the chairman of the several sections of the congress to report to them the names of colleagues who will participate in the work of the sections, either by the presentation of papers, by demonstrations, by clinics, or by exhibits.

Your committee has been unable to give a satisfactory response to those requests, owing to the fact that it has been without sufficient information as to the *personnel* of those who are likely to attend the congress, and therefore requests that all who expect to attend the congress will, as promptly as possibly, notify the secretary of the committee of their intention, so that the chairmen of the sections may be officially informed thereof, and proper places may be reserved for American delegates upon the program of the congress.

Your committee desires to make a special minute expressing the sense of great loss which they, in common with the whole dental profession, have sustained in the death of one of our number, Dr. Alison Wright Harlan of New York. In his long and active career, and as a result of his intense interest and enthusiasm in all that pertained to the progress and welfare of our profession, he had familiarized himself thoroughly with the local conditions surrounding the practice of dentistry in practically all the civilized countries of the globe, and we feel that it is quite within bounds to say that no man of his time had a more comprehensive grasp of the international relationships of our calling. The many close personal friendships which in the course of his travels he had built up among the representative men in dentistry of all nations made him as much at home among the profession of foreign lands as he was among those of his native land, and to-day his loss is mourned thoughout the world of dentistry with a sincerity and depth of feeling not second to that which we ourselves feel.

To fill the vacancy caused by the death of Dr. Harlan, your committee has appointed Dr. S. H. Guilford of Philadelphia.

Respectfully submitted,

EDWARD C. KIRK, *Chairman,*
BURTON LEE THORPE, *Sec'y.*

The bill for expenses of the committee was received and referred to the Auditing Committee.

Dr. J. D. PATTERSON, chairman of the Committee on Revision, presented its report, which was on motion received and the committee instructed to print in pamphlet form the proposed revision of the constitution, and to send a copy to each of the members.

On motion the proceedings of the thirteenth annual session were awarded to the *Dental Cosmos,* on the same terms as heretofore.

The report of the Treasurer was received. (See next page.)

On motion the report and the books of the treasurer were referred to the Auditing Committee.

Dr. W. F. LITCH, chairman of the Necrology Committee, presented the following report:

REPORT OF THE NECROLOGY COMMITTEE.

The Necrology Committee report that the National Dental Association has since its last meeting in 1908 lost by death the following: Dr. Luis Lane Dunbar and Dr. A. W. Harlan, both distinguished as teachers and practitioners; also Dr. Wm. H. Fundenberg.

The leading facts regarding the life and professional career of Dr. Dunbar are given in the following obituary notice from the *Pacific Dental Gazette* of February 1909:

Dr. Luis Lane Dunbar.

LUIS LANE DUNBAR died at his home in Belvedere, Cal., on Wednesday morning, December 30, 1908. He had spent most of his life in San Francisco, having been in dental practice there for about thirty-five years. By long-continued labor and a great devotion to this calling he early took a leading place in the profession, and for many years past was in the enjoyment of a following and practice of which anyone would be proud, but which few are privileged to experience. Some months past he was stricken down with a severe illness, but regained his health to such an extent as to permit him to return to his practice, in which he remained busy up to the day before his death. Even then he did not show any unusual condition, but early the next morning was taken with heart failure, and the end came as a great surprise and almost instantly.

For years past he had been an earnest worker in the interest of the dental profession, having been a member of several dental societies, and from time to time offering contributions to its literature. He took an active part in furthering the first state dental law, and ever since its organization was deeply interested in the welfare of the dental department of the University of California. He served it in different positions, first as clinical instructor in 1882-83-84; in 1885 as professor of pathology and therapeutics; from 1889 to 1899, as professor of operative dentistry and dental histology, at which time he retired from active work in the department and was appointed to the honorary position of emeritus professor of operative dentistry. He also served the University of California as dean of the dental department for ten years, from 1889 to 1899.

REPORT OF THE TREASURER.

RECEIPTS.

1908.

July 16th—

Balance incidental fund, last settlement	$1780.52
Received—Dues to March 26, 1909	1810.00
" Southern Branch to March 26, 1909	308.00
	$3898.52

DISBURSEMENTS.

July 20th—

A. H. Peck, exp. Executive Council meeting	$55.00

July 30th—

A. R. ——, exp. Treasurer's office	92.92
S. S. White Dental Mfg. Co., postage, mailing Trans.	75.21
Matthews-Northrup Co., printing	270.34
Chs. S. Butler, exp. Secretary's office	33.20
B. L. Thorpe, exp. Corresponding Secretary's office	26.91
A. R. Melendy, salary as Treasurer	200.00
Chas. S. Butler, sby as Secretary	400.00
E. P. Dameron, exp. Section I	26.30
Geo. E. Savage, exp. Clinic	181.63
W. E. Boardman, exp. to New York on meet'g	17.90
F. W. Stiff, exp. Clinic	5.28
J. P. Corley, exp. Committee on	20.50
Chas. McManus, exp. Committee on History	38.25
Wms. Donnally, xp. Legislation Committee	57.40

October—

H. J. Burkhart, exp. Council m't'g Pitt-b'g	40.25
14th. Chas. S. Butler, " " "	45.25
19th. V. E. Turner, " " "	55.00
26th. W. E. Boardman, " " "	76.32

November—

25th. F. O. Hetrick, " " "	75.00
" B. Holly Smith, " " "	30.00

December—

Bro't forward	$1822.66 $3898.52
3d. Geo. E. Savage, exp. Clinic Committee	44.28
14th. A. H. Peck, exp. Executive Council meeting, Pittsburg	30.00
22d. Geo. W. Davis, engrossing Fillebrown memorial letter	30.00
26th. Chas. S. Butler, exp. Legisl't'n Com., Wash.	64.75
28th. H. C. Brown, " " "	46.60

February—1909.

2d. Chas. S. Butler, " " "	66.00
3d. H. C. Brown, " " "	44.85
" V. E. Turner, " " "	39.50
8th. Wm. Crenshaw, " " "	120.40
" " " "	75.00
	$2384.04
Balance incidental fund, March 26, 1909	$1514.48

SPECIAL FUNDS.

Special Relief Fund, with interest to January 1, 1909	$4150.85
Special Journal Fund, July 1, 1908	$483.92

October 14, 1908—

Received of Local Committee on Arrangements, Boston (for Journal fund)	275.61
Interest to January 1, 1909	11.12
	$770.65

January 31, 1909—

Chas. S. Butler, exp. Journal Com, New York	$15.75

February 4th—

Fr. T. Taylor, " " "	20.50
F. W. Stiff, " " "	25.70
	$61.95
Balance Journal Fund, March 26, 1909	$708.70

Respectfully submitted,

A. R. MELENDY, *Treasurer.*

Approved: { V. H. JACKSON, M. F. FINLEY, H. B. McFADDEN, *Auditing Committee.*

Dr. Dunbar was born in Evansville, Ind., September 1, 1849, and died in his sixtieth year. He first came to San Francisco in 1863, where he attended the public schools and later St. Mary's College; he then went to Ohio and was graduated in dentistry from the Ohio College of Dentistry in 1874, after which he returned to San Francisco, where he has since been located.

He was a member of the California State Dental Association, the Delta Sigma Delta Fraternity, and the Order of Masons.

He was married in 1874, and his wife and son survive him.

The Necrology Committee are indebted to Dr. Burton Lee Thorpe for the following account of the life and work of Dr. A. W. Harlan:

Dr. Alison W. Harlan.

ALISON W. HARLAN, D.D.S., M.D., A.M., died March 6, 1909, of hernia brought about by a fall in a bath-tub while on a visit to Boston, February 21st. This required operative procedure. He was taken to the hospital and operated on by Dr. Dawbarn, a New York surgeon, the operation lasting four hours. His death followed the operation.

His death was a shock to his many friends, and dental surgery has suffered a distinct loss in his passing. Few men in the profession have been more prominent or contributed more to the science than A. W. Harlan. From his entrance into dentistry to his demise he has occupied a commanding position in the profession, and has been the recipient of nearly all the honors his associates could bestow upon him.

Dr. Harlan was a man of most studious habits and an indefatigable worker. He was an enthusiast in his profession, and nature singularly and felicitously adapted him to the exceptional requirements of his profession. His ideals were high, and his courage and purposes were fitly exemplified in his achievements. His amiability, coupled with his mastery of every subject coming within the reach of his work, brought him the respect, esteem, and friendship of those who had the good fortune of his acquaintance.

He was born November 15, 1851, in Indianapolis, Ind. His parents were Austin B. (who is still living, aged eighty-two years)

and Elizabeth L. Harlan, old residents of that city. He was educated in the public schools of his native state, and in 1867 entered the dental offices of Drs. Kilgore and Helms, prominent dentists at that time of that city, where he prosecuted his studies for more than two years. In 1869, when a little more than eighteen years of age, he located in Chicago, opening an office for himself early in 1869. He built up a practice rapidly. He matriculated in the Ohio College of Dental Surgery at Cincinnati and was graduated as D.D.S. from that institution in 1880; he was graduated from the Rush Medical College as M.D., and Dartmouth College conferred the A.M. degree upon him. He was an unusually skilled practitioner and had the widest knowledge of the principles and practice of his profession. He was an incessant worker and student, and an enthusiast in anything he undertook. Possessing as he did the widest knowledge of dental surgery, and being an expert diagnostician of dental disorders as well as an expert therapeutist, his opinions were widely sought as a consultant by members of his profession, who sent patients to him from all parts of the world. He was esteemed and respected by all those who had the good fortune of his friendship.

Dr. Harlan was an enthusiastic dental society attendant and contributed much to the success of the meetings he attended. He occupied many responsible offices in the various societies with which he was connected. He was president of the Illinois State Dental Society in 1882, president of the Chicago Dental Society from April 1, 1884, to April 1885. He was a member of the first State Board of Dental Examiners of Illinois, being associated in the same with Drs. Judd, Cushing, Black, and Kitchen. He founded the Odontological Society of Chicago, which held its twenty-fifth anniversary in November 1908, when he served as its president. He was corresponding secretary of the American Dental Association 1882-86; first vice-president 1888-89, and was elected president in 1890, serving in this capacity at the thirty-first annual session at Saratoga Springs, August 4, 1891. He also was president of the Mississippi Valley Association of Dental Surgeons. He was one of the organizers, a member of the general executive committee, and secretary-general of the Columbian Dental Congress, Chicago, August 14 to 19, 1893; was prominent in the Third International Dental Congress at Paris, and in the Fourth at St. Louis, and had he lived he would have been equally prominent in the Fifth at Berlin 1909. He was one of the organizers of the Fédération Dentaire Internationale, and had attended each annual session of that body since its organization. He was a great traveler, not only in the United States, but he had crossed to Europe some twenty times. He was a member of the American Medical Association, the American Dental Society of Europe, the Central Dental Association of New Jersey, the Odontological Society of New York, the First District Dental Society of New York, the National Dental Association, the Supreme Chapter Delta Sigma Delta Fraternity, the Interstate Dental Fraternity, the Illinois Society of New York, the Indiana Society of New York, the Manhattan Club of New York, the New York Athletic Club and the Siwanoy Club, honorary member of the St. Louis Society of Dental Science, and the St. Louis Auxiliary Chapter Delta Sigma Delta.

Dr. Harlan contributed very largely to the literature of dental surgery. He wrote and read many papers before dental societies. He was editor of the *Dental Review* from its beginning in 1886 to 1901, except for the year 1894, when it was edited by Dr. C. N. Johnson.

He was one of the organizers of the Chicago College of Dental Surgery in 1882, and its professor of materia medica and therapeutics until his removal to New York city in 1904. He also was professor of dental surgery in the College of Physicians and Surgeons of Chicago. He had a large and wealthy *clientèle* both in Chicago and in New York. In the latter city his residence was at Mt. Vernon.

Dr. Harlan was married January 4, 1871, to Miss Bessie M. Nurison of Rock Island, Ill. They reared a family of nine children. His second marriage took place in 1903, to Miss Mary E. Gallup of Boston, who survives him.

The funeral took place on Tuesday, March 9th, from the church of the Transfiguration, when Rev. Dr. Houghton preached a most impressive sermon. The interment was in

Kensico Cemetery, about thirty miles above New York city. Several of his old friends acted as pallbearers, viz, Dr. Allen W. Haight (formerly of Chicago), Dr. Archibald Campbell, his family physician at Mt. Vernon, Dr. Robert Oliver of West Point, Dr. Wm. Carr of New York, Dr. Louis C. LeRoy of New York, Dr. Chas. A. Meeker of Newark, Dr. C. F. Holbrook of Newark.

Many of his professional friends and friends of the family were in attendance.

Dr. William F. Fundenberg.

Wm. F. Fundenberg was born in Chambersberg, Pa., November 25, 1827. He was the son of Dr. Daniel Fundenberg of Lewiston, Md., who was descended from Freiherr [Baron] Walter von der Burg, whose descendants settled in Maryland in 1627. Dr. Fundenberg's mother was Rebecca Fahnestock, also of an old Maryland family.

After having graduated in medicine Dr. Fundenberg studied dentistry with Dr. S. P. Hullihen of Wheeling, W. Va., and in 1852 began dental practice in Pittsburg, Pa., in which city he was for many years the leading dental practitioner. His genial and kindly nature endeared him to hosts of friends.

In 1855 he was appointed aide-de-camp, with the rank of lieutenant-colonel, to Gov. James Pollock. Later in the same year he received the appointment of surgeon from the Czar, but on his way to the Crimea he learned in Paris that peace between Russia and the allies was declared. Dr. Fundenberg served in the civil war as surgeon of the 136th and 176th Pennsylvania regiments, and was a member of the Order of the Loyal Legion. He was a member of the American Medical Association, of the Allegheny County Medical Society, of the National Dental Association, the Pennsylvania State Dental Society, and other kindred organizations.

Dr. Fundenberg's death occurred at Atlantic City, N. J., on Sunday, November 22, 1908.

Four children survive him, two, Dr. Walter H. Fundenberg and Dr. Edwin C. Fundenberg, continue in Pittsburg the practice of their father's profession.

Respectfully submitted,
Wilbur F. Litch, *Chairman.*

The Auditing Committee reported that the books and accounts of the treasurer had been examined and found correct; also the bills of the various officers and committees, and recommended that they be paid.

On motion the report was received and the recommendation adopted.

The Membership Committee reported that the following had presented proper credentials and had been admitted to membership in the Association:

REPORT OF THE MEMBERSHIP COMMITTEE.

G. E. Whitmore, Mann bldg., Little Rock, Arkansas.

Chas. A. Thatcher, Ashtabula, Ohio.

C. C. Prentiss, Hartford, Conn.

Oscar Carrabine (First District Dental Society), New York, N. Y.

T. P. Donelan, Odd Fellows bldg., Springfield, Ill.

Hugo Franz, Chicago, Ill.

Henry H. Schuhmann, Chicago, Ill.

T. C. Hutchinson, Decorah, Iowa.

John Oppie McCall, Binghamton, N. Y.

Chas. A. Bradshaw, Syracuse, N. Y.

Thos. C. Swift, Mt. Vernon, N. Y.

Chas. D. Wright, New York, N. Y.

Arthur L. Swift, New York, N. Y.

Chas. F. Jones, New York. N. Y.

Stephen Palmer, Poughkeepsie, N. Y.

J. R. Callahan, Cincinnati, Ohio.

S. Marshall Weaver, Cleveland, Ohio.

. E. C. Mills, Columbus, Ohio.

S. D. Ruggles, Portsmouth, Ohio.

Chas. W. Myers, Montpelier, Ohio.

Axel N. Bruzelius, Lima, Ohio.

Forrest G. Eddy, Providence, R. I.

There being no further business, the Council adjourned.

CHARLES S. BUTLER, *Secretary.*

President's Address.

By V. E. TURNER, D.D.S.

I AM deeply sensible of the distinguished honor which you so generously conferred upon me at our last meeting. In making my acknowledgment for your courtesy words are inadequate to express my grateful thanks for this, the highest honor within the gift of this national body of scientific and progressive men. It is especially gratifying to me to have this opportunity to round out my professional career under such honorable circumstances.

During my term of office I have received from the officers and members of this association only the kindest and most courteous treatment, and I take this occasion to express my sincere appreciation of all that this means. I am proud to be your presiding officer, but to be entirely frank, I have many misgivings as to your wisdom in this choice; still I know that I can rely upon your patient forbearance and co-operative support in the discharge of the responsible duties which lie before me.

THE DATE OF THIS MEETING.

The Executive Council considered very carefully the matter of fixing the time of this meeting. As has been stated before, this date was selected out of consideration for the expressed wish of many members that the meeting should not be held during a period of the year which would interfere with their vacation, and because of the fact that the association at Boston voted that the meeting should not be held in Birmingham during the month of July or August, and furthermore because it was believed that many who might go to Europe this year to attend the Fifth International Dental Congress would not return in time for a meeting in September.

Under all of the circumstances it was decided to hold this session in the spring, when the South would present a more inviting climate to those coming from the North and West, and when it would be equally pleasant for the southern members. Whatever criticism may have been made by those who hold a different opinion, it cannot be truthfully said that the Council was influenced by any motive other than that of conserving the best interest of the association. and of pleasing the greatest number of its members. It was at first suggested that this date would be too early to secure a full and satisfactory report from the committees and sections, but the Council claimed that most of this work is usually done within the last three months preceding the meeting; this has, generally speaking, proved to be the case.

The chairmen of the sections were promptly urged to commence actively the work of securing papers of interest, and I venture the assertion that never before in the history of this association has there been a more responsive, painstaking, or obliging set of gentlemen occupying these positions of trust. The splendid results of their activities are shown in the program. There are four papers from distinguished members to be read before the general sessions.

All of the sections are filled with papers of a high order from eminent men, which will undoubtedly invite interesting discussions, and I can but feel that many important steps in real progress will be taken at this meeting.

As we were promised a most hearty co-operation by these southern gentlemen, I wrote personal letters to the presidents of each of the southern state societies urging prompt action on their part in securing a good attendance, and I believe they have done all that could be expected of them.

BIRMINGHAM.

We accepted in the spirit in which it was extended the cordial invitation of the Southern Branch to meet in this city, which is one of the new cities of the South. Only a few years ago it was a mere village, and we cannot fail to admire the pluck and enterprise of a people who have made such marvelous and substantial progress in so short a time. Their warm and hearty hospitality is a most delightful incident of this meeting.

The state of Alabama is a grand old commonwealth, her people are typical southern gentlefolk, generous, broad-minded, and progressive. They have been foremost in the endeavor to promote progress in dental surgery, and are especially notable in that they were the first to secure by legislative enactment a statute requiring a definite qualification for a dental practitioner.

THE MILLER MEMORIAL FUND.

It is with no disposition to be censorious that I express sincere regret that this fund has not increased more rapidly. Last year it was thought that on account of the financial disturbances many were slow to contribute to this most worthy cause, but it is a reflection upon our profession that up to this time we have been so unmindful of the great achievements of our departed brother.

When one not only spends his whole life for the cause of humanity, but when he has accomplished so much in revealing the hidden forces of nature, and when he has given an impetus to exact scientific investigation from which we have great reason to hope that a new era may dawn upon dentistry in the near future, is it right that we should accept this legacy, and forget from whom it came?

Such ingratitude to our *confrère* is not in keeping with the traditions of a learned and cultured profession, and we should honor the memory of this man who has been a blessing to mankind.

When a state or a country fails to remember the eminent services of those citizens who as statesmen or soldiers have been prominent in achieving the liberty and happiness of the people, it is recreant in its duty. So let us in a united effort swell the fund until it shall reach an amount worthy of the man and his achievements, and show to the world who has been its benefactor.

REVISION OF THE CONSTITUTION.

It would seem out of place to present here any thought upon the question of the revision of the constitution, as the committee appointed at Boston to consider this matter will doubtless make a report at this meeting, when all will have a chance to discuss such changes as may be proposed. The necessity for increasing our membership, however, is becoming a most serious problem, and prompt action should be inaugurated to induce the young members of the profession to join us. We need them to aid us in pushing forward the car of progress, and we can compensate them by affording them excellent facilities for the acquisition of useful knowledge, which this national body offers to all who will become actively identified with it.

Generally speaking, the more recent graduates have entered upon the study of their profession with better preliminary preparation than was formerly the case, and on this account are better equipped to master the curricula of the dental school of the present.

Many are ripe for association work when they leave college, and for the future of our science it behooves us to cultivate these young men, and to encourage them to identify themselves promptly with this society, in order that they may keep in touch with this body, which stands so firmly for the advancement of our calling. We should meet them with great cordiality and endeavor to invite their interest and induce them to become workers.

From our own standpoint it is essential that this association should be representative in numbers as well as in its *personnel,* and we should not only make it easier for men to enter it but should begin an active but dignified campaign to enlarge our membership.

This should apply not only to the newer members of the profession but also to the great class of desirable and influential practitioners who, either through indifference to its importance or from real or fancied obstacles to their induction into its membership, have already passed a number of years of their professional life without affiliation with our National Association.

DENTAL LEGISLATION.

At our meeting in Boston last year it was decided that the bill as passed by the Senate (No. 4432) should be advocated before the House committee having this in charge, and that every possible effort should be made to influence its passage by the House. When the question of appointing a committee for this service was considered by the Executive Council, many letters were read containing various suggestions as to the *personnel* of the committee. It was pretty generally known that the former members would not serve if re-appointed, so it was decided that the officers of the association —except the president—would be acceptable to all parties, and these were constituted the Legislative Committee. It was believed that they could convince the committee of the House of Representatives that the National Dental Association, being the representative national body and the highest organized authority on dentistry in the United States, was fully authorized to act for the profession in the country, and that it could state officially that all interests were united and harmonized in a desire to have enacted the Senate bill No. 4432. This committee was new at this work but has labored most earnestly, availing itself of the assistance of all who have been sufficiently interested to devote any time to the matter or to use their influence to accomplish the object. While it was predicted by many that there was only a small chance for success, still the committee determined to leave no stone unturned to comply with the mandate of the association.

The chairman of this committee and our two secretaries have labored with unremitting energy to induce the House committee to report the bill. It is believed that if the bill could have been gotten before the House it would have passed with a good majority.

STATE OF THE PROFESSION.

I congratulate the profession upon the growing impetus which the influence of this body has given to all departments of dental activity. At no period of the history of the world has there been a more earnest and determined effort to solve the problems which confront us in affording relief to human suffering and in prolonging human life itself.

. But besides this investigation into the causes of morbid conditions in order that they may be remedied, it is especially gratifying to note the development of research into the causes of immunity from these conditions. How much nobler it is to be able to prevent disease than to be able to cure it after it has begun! The dental world is contributing its share to this great movement in all branches of the healing art. A deeper study of the saliva and the significance of its various constituents, a further investigation of the bacterial inhabitants of the mouth, and a more extended knowledge of the food elements and their behavior in the environment of the teeth, should in course of time yield to us a knowledge of the means of preventing dental caries, which is the most widely occurring of all human disorders.

The subject of the mastication of food has in the last few years been brought forcibly to our attention, and the question of the preparation of the food in the mouth for its subsequent passage into the succeeding portions of the alimentary tract, and the influence of this upon the body economy, offers a fruitful field for further understanding. Oral hygiene, one of the most important branches of our professional work, is now not only attracting greater interest on the part of dentists, but also the consideration of the medical profession, the lawmakers, and philanthropists. Under the auspices of the Massachusetts Council of Dental Hygiene there was held in Boston a most notable meeting in January, which had for its object a conference and an open discussion upon dental and oral hygiene and its relation to the public health. The purpose of this meeting was to bring before parents, the school board, and educators in general the importance of this subject. The character and attainments of those participating in these discussions would indicate an interest so strong and so broad that it is hoped that before long legislation may be enacted which will secure a suitable fund to provide efficient dental service for the children in the schools and factories. Already the dentists themselves are doing an altruistic work in this direction in some localities, especially in the cities of New Haven, Conn., Reading, Pa., and other places, and these unselfish and humanitarian deeds deserve the highest praise and commendation at our hands.

Recognizing that health is our most

important asset, and that the oral cavity is capable of almost unlimited influence for good or evil upon the human economy, we of the dental profession, having more especially in charge this portion of the body, must put our shoulders to the wheel and work more actively to establish with the public an intelligent conception of the evils which commonly prevail in the care of the mouth, and must prescribe the remedy and assist in carrying it into effect. The committee of the National Dental Association having in charge this department has been seriously embarrassed by the lack of sufficient funds to prosecute this work. It is our duty and responsibility to maintain and encourage in every way the services of this committee. The small pamphlet authorized by the association for distribution among the laity has been highly complimented, and will doubtless be productive of much good.

It should be a matter of congratulation to this society that its members and the profession in general are establishing themselves as a worthy influence in the communities of this country. This has been expected as a matter of course as the profession has increased in age and in attainments. While its members as individuals and as representatives of an honorable and dignified calling have, by force of right, established themselves in this position, yet considering the profession as a whole, it is an undoubted fact that each year the standard of the men entering its ranks has steadily become higher.

Men of better preliminary attainment are applying for admission to our colleges, and our examining boards are providing with licenses men who are possessed of greater qualifications for professional life than has been the average heretofore.

OUR JOURNAL.

The committee appointed to formulate some plan for the publishing of a dental journal under the authority of this body have been quite active and earnest in the effort to solve this problem, and have made some progress in maturing plans for its publication.

It is believed that in the near future there will be a realization of our most ardent hopes in this direction. The publication of an official organ would serve to extend the usefulness of our society enormously.

FIFTH INTERNATIONAL DENTAL CONGRESS.

In the light of the cordial support given to the last dental congress held in this country by the profession of other nations, it behooves us not to fall behind in representation at the congress to be held in Berlin in the summer. The part taken by American dentists during the last century in the development of our profession should be maintained in this international gathering, and it is earnestly hoped that this body may officially take such further steps in this direction as may be in accord with the wishes of the Committee on Organization already appointed.

I take this opportunity to commend in the highest term our worthy recording secretary for his most prompt and efficient aid in the management of the affairs of the association; he has shown great ability in the difficult task. The chairman and the Executive Council have at all times been most responsive and helpful, and have always been willing to share in the responsibilities of the management.

Since our last meeting I have necessarily been thrown much in contact with and in communication with the members of the National Dental Association, and I have been greatly impressed and gratified at their uniform kindness and courtesy. Their attitude has been one of great interest in the broadening of the functions of this association and the harmonizing of all of its elements for progress. Many of my personal friends in this society, with whom I have had for years the most delightful relations, have become dearer to me than ever, and have exhibited a degree of loyalty most touching. In fact, I can conscientiously apply to each one of them the beautiful tribute, "He bore without reproach the grand old name of gentleman."

The Dental Relationships of Arthritism.

By EDWARD C. KIRK, D.D.S., Sc.D.

IN the study of disease phenomena there is an ever-increasing tendency to investigate more deeply into the underlying causes of the many departures from normality which constitute "the ills that flesh is heir to." At no time in the history of the healing art has the search for the remote causes of disease been more active than at present, and as a result of this persistent investigation the prospect of a rational solution of many of the graver pathological problems grows continually brighter.

The era of bacteriological investigation inaugurated three decades ago by the studies of Koch and Pasteur has been fruitful in explaining the mechanism of infection and in isolating the *materies morbi* of a long category of disorders, besides throwing a flood of light upon the biological activities of a vast number of pathogenic bacteria. The mode of action of disease-producing organisms has been made out with such clearness in so many specific instances that the major principles governing the processes of infection and of tissue reaction toward the infecting organism may be said to have been scientifically demonstrated. The varying resistance of individuals to the invasion of infectious organisms has, however, driven the inquiry beyond the part or rôle played by bacteria as factors in disease production, into the study of the defensive forces of the organism against bacterial invasion, a problem which must necessarily be solved before the science of pathology can furnish a full answer to the question of disease causation—or, indeed, before we can clearly understand what disease is, in a strictly scientific sense.

It has long been recognized that the susceptibility to disease is more pronounced in certain individuals than it is in others, and from very early times this peculiar tendency has given rise to various theories as to its origin. It has been referred to as a dyscrasia or as a diathesis, acquired or inherited, and much of the old humoral pathology involved the same conception. Modern investigation is slowly evolving the solution of the problem by studying the nature of the defensive forces of the organism, and results thus far attained justify the belief that certain definite substances in the blood and body juices of immune individuals constitute the means upon which the defensive mechanism is based. These defensive bodies—as antitoxins, agglutinins, bacteriolysins, and opsonins, as they are variously described —appear to be coincident with that condition of sound bodily health which is the result of a normal physiological equilibrium, and are absent or less active when the normal physiological equilibrium is disturbed. In proportion as the study of bacterial invasion has developed the underlying principles which upon the one hand determine how invasion takes place, and upon the other hand how the invasion is combated by the normal defensive mechanism of the body, the attitude of medical science toward the problem of disease has tended to focus itself more strongly upon the prophylactic side, and to address its efforts to disease prevention by building up the natural defensive forces of the organism to their highest efficiency. The crusade against the spread of tuberculosis by enforcing better hygienic conditions, both personal and environmental, the successful warfare against yellow fever by destruction of the breeding-places of the mosquito, and similar efforts to eradicate the unhygienic conditions that harbor the common house-fly, the house-rat, and similar carriers of disease germs are common and familiar examples.

RELATION OF FOOD HABITS TO SYSTEMIC VULNERABILITY.

A more recent crusade, and, while less dramatic, a by no means less important one for the reinforcement of the bodily defenses against disease invasion, is the dietetic propaganda inaugurated by Mr. Horace Fletcher, who has demonstrated by many practical examples and by various series of carefully conducted scientific tests that human efficiency, measured either as units of potential, as intellectual effort, or as resistance to disease invasion, is directly related to the question of nutrition, and he has incidentally

shown that our conceptions of the standards of normality in the nutritional process, in so far as they relate to intake of food in relation to output of work, have heretofore been wrong. Mr. Fletcher has shown that we have not only eaten too much, but that we have eaten badly, and that in thus overfeeding ourselves we have invited disease from without by creating it from within.

The dietetic question in relation to health is a very ancient one; indeed, the consideration of some of its aspects must, in the nature of the case, have been coincident with man's earliest attempts to feed himself. Like all other intricate physical problems, whatever knowledge was attained in relation to it was derived wholly from empirical observation until quite recent times, when this vital question, like all other phenomena of nature, was brought under the exacting scrutiny of precise scientific study. It had been observed for years that excessive feeders died, as a rule, earlier than the more abstemious, and it further became known that certain types of disease were more common among the overfed, indeed were characteristic of the so-called "high liver," and still later it was noted that these over-nourished individuals were actually manufacturing within their own bodies, as an output or waste product of their disordered nutritional processes, certain substances that were poisonous in character and which exerted a toxic effect upon the entire organism, this effect becoming intensified until it became fatal to the individual, or so reduced the natural defenses of the body that he was carried off by an acute disease due to a bacterial invasion from without.

The development of the idea of a diathetic state or condition due to faulty nutrition and culminating in auto-intoxication or self-poisoning, with reduction of the defensive forces against bacterial invasion, has had its principal growth and most pronounced expression in France, and it is due to the devoted labors of certain eminent investigators of that country that this important view of disease production has attained scientific prominence and is gaining a wider practical significance.

Prof. Dr. Van Noorden of Frankfurt a. M., in his monograph on "Diseases of Metabolism and Nutrition," says: "Within recent years the idea has become firmly established in the minds of physicians that a variety of morbid phenomena are due to auto-intoxication—are, in other words, attributable to certain poisonous metabolic products. This view, it is true, is not new, for it was familiar to the physicians of past generations, and was part of the teachings of the medical folk-lore of long ago. It was not, however, until Bouchard and his pupils published their investigations on the subject of auto-intoxication that this theory attained the dignity of a scientific doctrine. At first we German physicians were by no means inclined to accept the theory of auto-intoxication that was being so enthusiastically proclaimed. Of late years, however, our attitude has become more friendly to the doctrine; this change of front is due to the fact that a number of toxic products of metabolism have actually been isolated, and their mode of origin in the organism and their pathologic effect determined to the satisfaction of the former critics of the doctrine. We do not, of course, know all that we should properly know about the poisonous metabolic products that we incriminate in so many morbid states; but in a large group of important symptom-complexes we are fortunately in possession of a number

of facts that suffice to ground the doctrine of auto-intoxication on a solid chemical basis."

I have made the foregoing quotation from an eminent exponent of German scientific conservatism to emphasize the fact that the doctrine of auto-intoxication as a factor in disease causation and as a prodromal state of bacterial invasion rests upon an accepted scientific foundation. It is also to be understood that the phase of auto-intoxication here under consideration is that which is due to faulty metabolism the result of disordered nutrition, and is exclusive of intoxication resulting from the absorption of putrefactive toxins produced by intestinal bacteria.

"ARTHRITISM."

The subject of malnutrition and its effects is quite too extensive for consideration in a brief paper, but there are certain general features of the subject that confront us in our special work as dental practitioners to which I desire to ask your attention, namely, the class of cases exhibiting that type of malnutrition which the French students of the general question designate as arthritism.

Dr. L. Pascault of Paris, in his brochure entitled "Arthritism the Disease of Civilization," has given a most graphic picture of the general aspects and mode of development of the complexus of disorders which are characteristic of the arthritic state, and I cannot do better than briefly epitomize some of the main features of his essay.

The typical arthritic, according to Pascault, is rarely developed in a single generation; he is generally a product of several generations of bad dietetic habits. The ancestor of the arthritic—a grandfather, perhaps, or some more remote relative in direct line—was strong, vigorous, active, and generally endowed with the qualities that assure success in life; a great worker, either physically or mentally, he died in old age after a useful life, leaving a numerous progeny. As in the case of well-balanced individuals the intake of food is usually proportioned to the daily expenditure of energy, we may conclude *a priori* that this hearty and vigorous ancestor was also a great eater, and from that fact we may note certain consequences, among which according to Pascault are the following: His digestive apparatus, put to work upon a bountiful food supply, becomes developed in all of its constituent parts, his stomach acquires the habit of no longer feeling satisfied until it has reached a maximum distension, and all his tissues are obliged to accelerate their metabolic processes in order to utilize it, and thus lose the habit of functioning economically, hence the constantly recurring need which, transmitted to the nervous centers and perceived by consciousness, translates itself into an exaggeration of the appetite, inducing him to eat more than is really necessary for him. This is not all, for of the foods thus unwisely taken, while the carbohydrates (starches, sugars, and fats) are easy of combustion and leave in the economy after their destruction only liquid or gaseous waste products easy of elimination, it is not the same in the case of the nitrogenized foods, which are broken up with difficulty and require from the liver and kidneys a very complicated work of rehandling before their waste products are thrown out. In the case of this pre-arthritic ancestor, he has had not only muscular or cerebral activity, but all his organs, all his tissues, all of his cells without exception, func-

tionate with abnormal activity. No machine can endure being continually overdriven, no matter how well it may be constructed; it becomes fatigued and worn out in the long run, and so in the case of the particular type of human machine under consideration we may say that the exuberance of health and activity which characterized the pre-arthritic ancestor was the real promoter of the morbid troubles from which his descendants suffer.

The representatives of the second generation are handicapped by an inheritance which if uncorrected will cause them to develop into true arthritics. They have, in spite of a robust appearance, inherited a diminished vigor, an exaggeration of appetite which they do not recognize, or which, on the other hand, they may regard as a virtue of health rather than an abnormality, and above all they have inherited a cellular impress characterized by rapidity of metabolic activity readily recognized by the appearance in the urine, not of abnormal morphological elements, for destructive changes have not as yet begun to appear in the tissues, but there is a pronounced augmentation of all the normal waste products—urea, uric acid, phosphoric acid—and notably of the total acidity of the urine. The incessant effort demanded of the stomach, the intestines, and the large glands, the liver and pancreas, concerned in the disposition of this excess of food involves a corresponding excitement of the vascular system and the induction sooner or later of a passive, even permanent congestion of the digestive viscera, leading to plethora and later to obesity as middle life is reached, or even earlier. Thus the arthritic transforms his excess of carbohydrate food into fat, or he may expel through his urine the sugars which

have not found a place in his muscles or
his liver, developing thus a glycosuria or
diabetes, or he may accumulate his re-
sidual proteids at those points of his
economy or in those tissues where the
circulation is sluggish, as in the articu-
lar tissues, developing gout, or may eliminate them through his mucous membranes, producing catarrh. To these results must be added all those morbid
manifestations of a disordered over-nutrition grouped under the general term
lithiasis—that is to say, gravel and stone
of the bladder, kidney, and liver, together with their corollaries, cystitis and
hepatic and nephritic colic.

There yet remains to be considered the
degenerative effect of this over-stimula-
tion of cell function by an excess of food,
with the corresponding production and
retention of the irritative waste products
of nutrition, upon the cells themselves.

The secreting cells, those of sensation,
motion, and special sense, act differently
in the presence of an excess of pabulum
to the supporting or connective tissue
group of cell elements. The latter, according to Pascault, appear to be endowed with a considerable power of attraction and absorb nutriment with avid-
ity; they assimilate it, hypertrophy, mul-
tiply with extreme rapidity, then shortly
they undergo fibrous change, and shrinking like a cicatricial tissue they strangle
the secreting cells, or those of sensation,
motion, or special sense, as the case may
be, which under normal conditions it was
their mission to support. Or, on the
other hand, if the nutrient material is
rich in calcareous salts, the cells become
saturated or calcified, thus cutting off
their supply of blood and lymph and inducing the condition broadly described
as sclerosis.

VARIOUS PATHOLOGICAL EXPRESSIONS OF
NUTRITIONAL IMBALANCE — ALVEOLAR
PYORRHEA.

Time will not permit a more extended
recital of the progressive phases or detailed phenomena portrayed by the author
from whose graphic picture of arthritism
I have drawn these few examples of its
varied expressions. Indeed, so manifold
are the clinical manifestations of the underlying morbid state of nutrition induced by an ill-balanced food habit with
respect to the needs of the individual,
that any description must needs be but
schematic and general in character.
What I do hope to emphasize is that
there is such a state as a physiological
nutritional equilibrium which when over-
balanced upon the side of nutritional excess develops a condition of disease within
the economy itself which may have a variety of local as well as general manifestations, and which further becomes a pre-
cursor of other disease phenomena by
lessening vital resistance so that invasion
of pathogenic bacteria becomes possible.
The secondary pathological expressions
of over-nutrition which characterize the
arthritic state may manifest themselves
in widely different ways from a clinical
standpoint, depending upon the character of the organs or tissues which
are most prominently involved; thus
the groups of symptom complexes may
be such as arise from liver complications, with structural as well as functional disturbances of that organ and of
the pancreas, and produce the type of
individual designated by Pascault as the
hepatique, or the kidney may become the
seat of lesions with a corresponding train
of disturbances creating the *type rénal* of
the French, and similarly the disorder

may have its dominating expression as the nervous or catarrhal, according as the corresponding structures and tissues are most prominently involved; but in all these classes the underlying fault or aberration from physiological normality appears to be a lack of nutritional balance characterized in its beginnings and through its formative period by an over-nutrition, due to the intake of an excess of pabulum which is beyond the power of the organism to properly utilize.

It is in precisely the group of morbid states here under consideration that we find the majority of those disorders which affect the tissues constituting the retentive apparatus of the teeth, and which we collectively designate as interstitial gingivitis, pyorrhea alveolaris, etc., as well as that other disorder the etiology of which has so long been shrouded in mystery, viz, chemical erosion of the teeth. Medical literature abounds in reports of the coincidence of destructive necrotic inflammations of the alveolar structures with the various nutritional disturbances due to the arthritic condition. The whole of the major work of Talbot on "Interstitial Gingivitis" is a research which by any candid and intelligent reasoner should be accepted as a demonstration that the auto-intoxication resulting from malnutrition is the principal factor which leads to bacterial invasion of the alveolar structures, causing destructive inflammation of the supporting tissues of the teeth. M. L. Rhein, in a paper on the "Oral Expressions of Malnutrition," read before the Odontological Society of New York in March 1896, and again in a paper on "Pyorrhea Alveolaris," read before the Chicago Dental Society in February 1899, has clearly related the alveolar disease to malnutrition as its general predisposing cause. C. N.

Peirce, H. H. Burchard, and others too numerous to mention, have advocated the same view, and it is at least worthy of note that in the majority of instances those who have held to the malnutritional theory have based their convictions upon the results of scientific research as well as upon careful clinical observation.

In several communications, notably in a paper read before the Maryland State and District of Columbia Dental Societies in June 1908, on "The Constitutional Element in Certain Dental Disorders," I endeavored to show, among other things, the method by which the physiological equilibrium of nutrition is disturbed in cases of over-nutrition, and how insufficiency of oxidizing power leads to the production of certain abnormal waste products, causing auto-intoxication, and that the poisoning and irritation of the alveolar tissues in that manner renders them susceptible to bacterial invasion. I furthermore called attention to the fact that the character as well as the total quantity of food was an important factor in determining the nature of the subsequent auto-intoxication; that where the totality of food was in excess of the total oxygen-carrying capacity of the blood as measured by its hemoglobin content, and where the carbohydrate factor of the food supply was excessive, there resulted not only a carbonic acid toxemia, with high urinary acidity, but because of the selective affinity of the carbohydrates for the oxygen supply the proteids were incompletely oxidized and a consequent increase of formation of the purin bases occurs instead of the normal output of nitrogen surplus as urea—a point of view confirmed by the chemical study of the urine in arthritic cases.

We are yet lacking a careful study of the opsonin content of the tissues of the pre-arthritic individual—that is to say, before the stage when distinct lesions of the secretory apparatus are recognizable; but because of the known toxemia resulting from excessive carbonic acid formation and the suboxidation of proteids in the primary arthritic stages on the one hand, and on the other hand the susceptibility of these subjects to bacterial invasion, as evidenced by the prevalence of pyorrhea alveolaris among them, and their proneness to attacks of influenza and of rheumatism, which latter has now come to be classed as a bacterial infection, we are justified, upon *a priori* grounds at least, in suspecting that even in the earlier stages the arthritic subject has a diminished resistance to bacterial invasion, and would therefore show a lowering of the defensive bodies below that of the normally healthy individual.

With respect to the effect of a dietetic habit or regimen low in nitrogen and excessive on the carbohydrate side, the prevalent conditions among the Hindus furnish an interesting example. All American and European dentists practicing in India bear testimony to the prevalence of pyorrhea alveolaris in that country among Hindus and Europeans alike. Dr. H. B. Osborn of Rangoon, Burmah, writing to me from Chittagong in December 1908, says, concerning pyorrhea: "When one thinks that every native and almost every European mouth in India is in somewhat the same condition (*i.e.* suffering from a 'shaky' condition of the teeth) it makes one wish one knew more about it. While I did not learn very much about it in college, I think I am right in saying that I was taught that pyorrhea was curable. With all respect to the authors of that statement, I would like to see a case cured in India. I am strongly of the opinion (I am very humble regarding the worth of my opinions) that local treatment is of only slight temporary value, and systemic treatment is something in regard to which I am in dark ignorance." The observations of Dr. Osborn as to the prevalence of pyorrhea alveolaris in India are borne out by many other competent observers. The Hindus are almost wholly vegetarians. Recently the question of the diet of the Hindu in relation to his physical condition and development has been the subject of governmental investigation. Prof. D. McCay has made a report to the Indian government which is reviewed in *Nature* for November 12, 1908. He finds from his study of Hindu physique that while the native Bengali maintains his nitrogenous equilibrium on his vegetable diet, nevertheless the low nitrogen intake acts deleteriously, reduces the blood protein, and tends to produce degenerative changes, especially in the kidneys. He is not only physically incapable, as compared with the European, but he also becomes more easily exhausted; his blood pressure is below normal, and his lack of stamina makes him an easy prey to infectious diseases. Professor McCay further suggests the probability of dangerous decomposition products being formed from the large fat and carbohydrate intake rendered necessary by a poor nitrogen diet (auto-intoxication). Professor McCay, commenting upon the prevalence of diabetes in its worst form among the Bengal natives, attributes it to the carbohydrate excess in their dietary, and asserts that it proves conclusively that the evils from this cause may be more real than those attributed to an excess of protein in the diet. The vigorous African savage has been generally a meat-eater, and if whites make their homes successfully in the tropics it is probable that the protein intake in their diet will not be radically changed to meet the climatic conditions.

The foregoing observations as to the relationships of malnutrition to alveolar infection have been already pointed out by other writers, and the coincidence of diabetes mellitus and alveolar pyorrhea has been specifically referred to by Rhein in the paper already quoted. In my own communications I have endeavored to trace the relationship of improper feeding to the condition of malnutrition which precedes the alveolar infection or other tissual or organic changes—notably the renal involvement—as the case may be. The diabetic factor is a striking and important one. As I have shown in several papers, a condition simulating diabetes mellitus often occurs as a functional disturbance before any tissual lesion is observable, or at least before glycosuria is manifest. This functional disturbance is the phosphatic diabetes of Ralfe and Tessier, and corresponds to that stage of arthritism described by L. Pascault in which the inherited cellular impress of a high rate of metabolic activity produces under the further stimulation of an excess of pabulum a pronounced augmentation of all the normal waste products, and which in the phosphate diabetic expresses itself as an abnormal phosphatic loss through the urine, with corresponding symptoms of general nutritional disturbance. The mechanism of this phosphatic loss I have elsewhere described in detail. Diabetic glycosuria occurs at a later stage of arthritism, and the susceptibility of diabetics to bacterial invasion has been generally noted and carefully studied. Rhein has found the pyorrheal condition so prevalent and so characteristic among diabetics that he has proposed for the alveolar disorder in these cases a distinctive designation. Wm. Martin Richards of New York, in the *Journal of the American Medical Association* for January 23d of this year, writes to the editor as follows: "I have lately been impressed by the coincidence of pyorrhea alveolaris (pus coming up over the gums from the roots of the teeth) and sugar and albumin in the urine, and the disappearance of these symptoms when the teeth were cured. I am collecting two hundred cases of pyorrhea alveolaris with urine examinations before and after the pyorrhea is cured. I wish to ask other practitioners who are interested in this subject to kindly send me any results which they have in the same line—that is, when they find sugar and albumin in the urine, will they have the teeth investigated and find out how many of such patients have pyorrhea alveolaris? This is a subject of interest to all of us, and I am sure that the results will amply repay us for the trouble involved."

In carrying out such an investigation it would be of the utmost importance to determine to what extent the oral condition and the state of the kidneys were interchangeably influenced by treatment of either morbid state. The communication of Dr. Richards seems to imply that in the case which he had under observation the cure of the alveolar pyorrhea wrought a cure of the kidney trouble. In the absence of positive data this would seem doubtful, for reasons which will appear later.

The susceptibility of diabetics to bacterial infection, especially to pus infections, has long been recognized and is well known. Recently various scientific studies of the altered defensive mechanism of diabetics has been made, so that we are in possession of considerable data of a practical character with respect at least to the degree of increased susceptibility which diabetics manifest toward pus-producing organisms as compared with the resistance of the normal individual. In an elaborate research made by Drs. John C. Da Costa and E. J. G. Beardsley, published in the *American Journal of the Medical Sciences* for September 1908, it is shown from an average of fifty cases of diabetes mellitus that the opsonic index varied considerably with respect to streptococcus, to staphylococcus, and to tubercle bacillus, the three organisms employed in the tests. The average index of all the cases for each organism named was as follows: Staphylococcus 0.65, streptococcus 0.56, and tubercle bacillus 0.73. That is to say, the index was only a little more than half normal for the ordinary pus-forming bacteria, while it was scarcely three-fourths normal for tubercle bacillus. It is regrettable that for our present purposes the opsonic reaction to the pneumococcus was not also tested, that organism being so constantly concerned in invasions of the alveolar tissues.

I have called attention to the work of Da Costa and Beardsley in order to emphasize the fact that in diabetes mellitus the resistance to bacterial invasion of the pus-producing variety is greatly reduced below the normal standard, which fact, in connection with the data I have brought forward to show the prevalence of alveolar pyorrhea among diabetics and the prevalence of diabetes mellitus among those of arthritic type due to the effects of defective food habits and prolonged overfeeding, is of much significance. It serves to indicate that the phenomenon of bacterial invasion is to a degree conditioned by the extent of the internal resistance of the tissues and body fluids

of the organism, and as resistance is lowered by the abnormal nutritional state which I have in general terms expressed here as arthritism, the invasion of disease-producing bacteria is not only more likely to take place in the first instance, but it is likely to become more grave and extensive when it does occur.

AN ILLUSTRATIVE CASE.

The following history of a case will illustrate my contention: On January 21, 1909, Mr. J. E. was brought to my office by his dentist, Dr. Frederick Sauers of Philadelphia, for consultation. Dr. Sauers' history of the case is here given in his own words:

Mr. J. E., a man of about thirty-eight years of age, married, called at my office January 7th with the lower left central and lateral incisor teeth very sore. The case seemed to me like an abscessed condition, the lateral being the more painful of the two. I drilled into it with the expectation of finding a dead pulp, but I found it alive and in good condition. I then advised the patient to poultice the inside of the mouth, take a mustard foot-bath and six grains of quinin and go to bed.

The following day he called again, in great pain. I found conditions reversed, the central being more sore than the lateral. Thinking I had drilled the wrong tooth I drilled into the central, but found the pulp in healthy condition. The next day his physician was called; he prescribed a tonic and also treated for neuralgia, with no relief to the patient.

On January 11th I was called again, and found the patient in much worse condition, the two affected teeth very loose, gums swollen in front and back. I lanced the gums inside and outside; found but little pus. This gave the patient relief for a short time. The following day I was called and the patient requested me to extract the teeth. I extracted the central incisor, hoping that would give him relief, but without much success. The following day I extracted the lateral. The other teeth up to this time did not seem to be affected. Two days later, however, I found the two right incisors in precisely the same condition as the ones extracted had been. In the meantime the pain became so severe at times that his physician resorted to the use of hypodermic injections of morphin. I extracted the remaining incisors without any relief. A few days later I found the rest of the teeth in the lower jaw affected exactly the same as the ones I had extracted. The lower part of the face had been swollen since the third day of the trouble.

This completes the dental history of the case up to January 21st, the date when Dr. Sauers brought the patient to my office.

Upon examination of the patient I found considerable swelling of the tissues covering the outer aspect of the body of the mandible, and that the patient could open the mouth only with difficulty. Around the entire alveolar border of the mandible the gum tissue was swollen from an accumulation of pus, and all of the remaining teeth were loose in their sockets. They were all otherwise sound. Near the internal angle of the jaw between the last molar and the ramus there was a determination of pus, and before evacuating the contents I requested Dr. Nathaniel Gildersleeve of the bacteriological laboratory of the University of Pennsylvania to see the case and come prepared to take cultures of the abscess contents. This was done at once with all precautions against contamination from the bacteria of the oral cavity. The abscess cavity was freely evacuated and afterward washed out with dilute antiseptic washes and a ten per cent. argyrol solution injected through the abscess tract, which extended from the socket of the lateral incisor to the third molar.

An inquiry was made into the general health status of the patient, and I learned from his wife that for several years he had had sugar in his urine, for which at different times he had been given treatment. I endeavored to get into telephonic communication with his physician but was unable to do so; I, however, reached the chemist who had been making the urinary analyses, and

learned from him that his examinations had extended over a period of four or five years, and that they had showed from one to one and a half per cent. of sugar, some albumin, and occasionally a few casts, during that time. In view of this unfavorable history I insisted that the patient be placed at once in the hospital for treatment as to his diabetic condition and for appropriate care as to his local difficulty.

After some delay he was admitted to the University Hospital under the care of Dr. David L. Edsall as to his general condition and under the care of Dr. Cryer from the oral surgical standpoint. Notwithstanding the skilled and constant care to which he was subjected the patient became rapidly worse and died at 9 o'clock P.M. on February 7th, just thirty-one days after the date of the initial alveolar infection.

The urine records in this case present a typical picture of diabetes mellitus, with sugar, acetone, and diacetic acid. During the ten days while the patient was under observation in the hospital the fluctuation in the sugar content of the urine ranged from below 1 per cent. to 5 per cent. On January 27th and 28th it was but a trace. On February 1st it rose to 5 per cent., dropped the next day to a trace, then rose slowly to 1 per cent., later to 3.75 per cent., dropped to 3.5 per cent. the day before death, and to 3 per cent. on the day of death.

Dr. Cryer informs me that there was a marked fluctuation in the flow of pus from the inflamed territory about the mandible corresponding synchronously with the fluctuations in the sugar content of the urine.

Dr. Gildersleeve's report on the bacteriological examination of the pus exudate is as follows:

Character of pus: Yellowish, creamy consistence, odor not offensive; contains some small caseous masses.

Microscopic examination: Appearance of pus as found in acute suppurative processes.

Contains the following organisms: Streptococci, pneumococci, other micrococci appearing like the pyogenic cocci, and long slender spirochetæ. No tubercle bacilli could be found.

Cultures were made on agar and blood serum and the following organisms isolated: Pneumococcus. Streptococcus pyogenes. Bacillus mesentericus (of no significance).

The opsonic index of this patient was not taken, for the reason that the fact that diabetes mellitus causes a lowering of the opsonic index is already established.

We have here the record of an infection by ordinary mouth bacteria through the alveolar tissues upon a ground in which the internal resistance to invasion was lowered by systemic disease, viz, diabetes mellitus, a disorder which in our present knowledge of its etiology must be classified as belonging to the malnutritional diseases, as this paper has already endeavored to set forth. We must conclude that but for the lowered resistance of this case the invasion would have been but superficial or would not have occurred at all. Had it been but superficial and exhibited the clinical features which it possessed when first observed by Dr. Sauers it would have been quickly diagnosed as a simple case of pyorrhea alveolaris. As it was, however, the infection of the whole mandibular periosteum ensued, the pyorrhea developed into a case of necrosis of the jaw, and terminated fatally.

From the mass of data now at our command with respect to the systemic relationships of these alveolar infections it would appear to be unsafe, as it is certainly unwise, to continue to ignore them and to regard alveolar pyorrhea wholly as a local disorder amenable wholly to local treatment. · ·

Discussion.

Dr. G. V. I. BROWN, Milwaukee, Wis. I am grateful for this opportunity to say how much I appreciate the paper. In the first place, one of the valuable points which impressed me was the fact that Dr. Kirk has laid such a complete, systematic, and of course orderly foundation based upon facts that are undisputed among investigators not only in this country, but in other countries as well, so that we might be prepared to understand the statements which follow. I think a great deal of the trouble that we have had in the past has been that men who have studied the subject extensively have brought the developments and results of their investigations, and expected our minds to receive them as they themselves understand them after years of thought, and therefore what they have given us has not been properly digested in more senses than one.

The second feature of the paper that impressed me as valuable was the fact that Dr. Kirk has endeavored to bring the light of medical and pathological research of a general character before us in such a manner as to focus it upon our own field of investigation, so that one in studying the work and results that have been obtained in this division is at once put in touch with the great investigators and the vast amount of research that is developing other branches of pathological science.

I should like to ask Dr. Kirk to tell us whether he tested the individual whose case he described with regard to other portions of his body than those mentioned, and whether he has sections of the different vital organs? I have a report from one patient who had very much the same difficulty, with some such condition as described by Dr. Kirk, who appeared to have pyorrhea alveolaris or at least ulcerative stomatitis or some similar disease affecting the structures around his teeth, and we found upon post-mortem examination of tissue with the microscope the same round-celled infiltration, and a similar destructive process going on in every vital organ of the body, just as we found in the alveolar structures and mucous membrane of the mouth. I am inclined to believe that the individual Dr. Kirk cited would have shown similar infiltration of the different organs of the body. In the case I speak of, we had a well-defined leukemia, as indicated by the blood count. I know that in Dr. Kirk's case all these matters must undoubtedly have been considered by those in charge, and had there been any great abnormality in the number of red and white corpuscles or notable factors especially indicated in the blood examination, such facts would have been included in his description.

There is one point, however, that is still of interest to us in this matter, which was referred to by the essayist, and that is the question of opsonic index. He calls our attention to this, and with due consideration we must consider that in addition to the question of imperfect metabolism and all that Dr. Kirk has included in the term arthritism, there is yet to be developed another factor which bears upon the question of immunity, and the best example that I can give is shown in the treatment of tuberculosis. Tuberculosis, aside from its well understood bacteriologic factor, is definitely recognized as a disease of malnutrition, and the chief consideration in its modern general treatment is in the direction of more air, in order that there may be better oxygenation, therefore more perfect

metabolism, and an increased amount of carefully selected food for the purpose of changing the food element which is so needed in these cases. I have recently had the opportunity of having under observation in hospitals quite a number of patients who were being treated from time to time with tuberculin injections for the purpose of creating an immunity to the disease, and the evidence borne by these patients is very important for us in consideration of our present subject, because patients being treated may have tubercular necrosis in any or various parts of the body. Some of these patients were affected by hip-joint disease, others had abdominal abscess, others still, affections of the bones of the feet, the hands, etc. All bore evidence of extensive destruction of the affected tissues, but all were, or seemed to be, in course of recovery under approved general treatment supplemented by injections of tuberculin.

I believe that before we can fully solve the problems of the subject now so ably spread before us we shall be required to go somewhat beyond this question of metabolism and search a little farther for the full and complete answer to that which may, for the present, be termed immunity to disease, in other words, lessened susceptibility of the tissues in this region to those pathologic affections which are favored by the constitutional conditions referred to. I am, as you all know, a very firm believer in the constitutional relationship of the oral cavity, and I have carefully followed the work of Dr. Talbot, which has been so plain to me for years that I have often wondered how anyone ever questioned its importance. Nevertheless, there are local factors that require our attention, because the reason why these conditions are manifested so frequently in the mouth are: First, we have structures which are somewhat less resistant by reason of their transitory character and by reason of the peculiar vascular supply of the parts—therefore all disorders are manifested quickly in the gingival region and in the alveolar structures; secondly, there is always an opportunity for bacteria to gain entrance, and thirdly, there is an ever-present opportunity for local irritation. Therefore, if I take the view correctly from Dr. Kirk's paper as I understand it from hearing it read—not having had an opportunity to study it in advance—the lesson is, that whatever our treatment be, we must direct our extreme efforts toward overcoming the constitutional conditions, and then must supplement that with the best local treatment our utmost skill may devise, in order that there may be less tendency for excursion of disease in this region.

I believe this paper will do a great deal of good.

Dr. M. L. RHEIN, New York, N. Y. What I shall have to say will chiefly serve the purpose of emphasizing some of the points which the essayist has made in his very valuable paper.

A more logical analysis of the etiology of this phase of malnutrition has never been presented to any association, nor has any more logical analysis of the subject ever been published. We were very fortunate last year to receive a magnificent contribution on this theme from Professor Leary of Boston, and this particular paper is a worthy addition to the same. I want, as I did last year, to point with special emphasis to the fact that the subject-matter with which the essayist dealt yesterday was entirely upon one phase of the symptoms we meet as dentists in the condition generally spoken of as pyorrhea alveolaris, interstitial gingivitis, Riggs' disease, or by whatever name you choose to call it. Practically the same condition existed last year—for the essayist at that time, Professor Leary, simply dwelt upon one etiological factor, just as Professor Kirk yesterday devoted his attention to one etiological factor, and it is this point that is of special importance. These are the class of contributions we have wanted for some time. This condition of the diseased pericemental tissues, surrounded perhaps by a purulent discharge, has generally been considered and discussed as a whole, and I wish here to emphasize the importance of taking up and considering this pathological subject in its different phases, as was so beautifully demonstrated last year at Boston, just as yesterday by the essayist. Attention was devoted yesterday especially to the study of the effects of intestinal auto-intoxication, or intestinal intoxication, take it as you will, and the forms of malnutrition resulting therefrom and showing themselves to us in a diseased condition of the pericemental tissues.

I do not believe that anyone who listened to the paper yesterday can fail to be convinced or see the corollary there presented, that these disease conditions that we meet so often are symptoms of the malnutrition produced by the initial toxic condition that eventually brought about the various diseases there enumerated. The essayist devoted considerable time to one particular condition, the diabetic condition, hoping, I have no doubt, by concentrating his thought on this point to show more conclusively the story of cause and effect.

In the course of his paper he spoke of a communication published by Dr. Richards of New York, asking for our aid in presenting to him such cases of pyorrhea alveolaris, if you choose to call it such, where the diabetic condition existed, and the effect of the cure of the pyorrhea upon the diabetic condition. I received a similar communication from Dr. Richards, and my reply was that it was impossible to reply intelligently to his proposition, because he was placing the cart before the horse; that the symptoms such as we meet are the results of the diabetic condition and that the diabetic condition would have to be brought under control before any work on our part would have any material result. It has been frequently asserted by dentists who have taken this erroneous, illogical, pathological hypothesis in the same manner as Dr. Richards, that the swallowing of ordinary bacteria was sufficient to produce such poisons and toxic conditions as to bring about that general condition. The careful study, however, of the recognized scientific pathology of to-day shows the fallacy of such a conclusion so completely that in view of the time allotted to the discussion of this paper it is unnecessary to go into this feature. The essayist definitely pointed out the fallacy of any such conclusion. The ordinary bacteria that are swallowed, whether with the food or otherwise, are thoroughly taken care of in the intestinal tract, if the system is in proper condition. It is granted that where a severe pyorrheal condition exists, there is no doubt at all that the swallowing of large amounts of purulent matter aggravates the toxic conditions of this tract, but that it is the initial factor in producing such a diseased condition is contrary to every physiologic fact that we have at our command. The one point that I wish to make in the discussion of this subject is to draw attention strongly to the fact that the teachings which have been given to us by some men, namely, that the time to clean the mouth is before eating, so that people shall not swallow their food filled with bacteria, are simply not only illogical but at variance with the best results which have been determined prophylactically. Such remains of food should be removed after the meal, not allowing it to remain in the mouth until the next meal.

Dr. EMORY A. BRYANT, Washington, D. C. Being merely a practical man, it is with a great deal of temerity that I rise to discuss this paper, and the only reason I have for discussing it is a practical one.

When I read the title of the paper, "Dental Relationships of Arthritism," I tried to understand what the subject-matter would be, judging from its title, and judging from results it was a lamentable failure, and as a practical illustration I venture to say that there are not five men in the house who can give the definition of arthritism. There are some members of our profession who have a great tendency to take up high-sounding names and use them, while the terminology used could be more practical and such with which we are familiar and which is in general use. As this was evidently a medical term, I asked several of the leading physicians in Washington if they could tell me from the title of the paper what the subject-matter might cover, but not one could tell me. My conversation with one medical specialist brought out the fact that he had never heard of the term arthritism, but that the word evidently is derived from or has connection with arthritis, and refers to the gouty diathesis. I then went to the medical dictionaries, and after wandering through two and finding nothing

3

to enlighten me, finally obtained a copy of the latest editions and there found the word itself.

I refer to this because the practical man, or the man who does not obtain advance copies of a paper, has to figure out what the essayist means to cover by the title alone. Judging from what I have heard and remember of the paper, it is a magnificent paper upon the subjects of malnutrition, auto-intoxication, diabetes, pyorrhea alveolaris, and the gouty diathesis. The term "arthritis" is generally used to signify any disease whatever involving a joint. It is also employed to designate inflammation of all the structures forming the joint, as distinguished from mere synovitis: "The causes of joint disease in general are connected either with disordered nutrition, in which case it assumes the inflammatory type, or with disordered function; the latter may depend upon the former or be unconnected with it, or again the cause may be local in its origin or arise from a constitutional defect."

Again, when we refer to the medical works under the head of "joints," we find that the word refers more especially to one which admits of more or less motion in one or both bones. Taking this fact, and considering that all of the diseases referred to under the term of arthritis pertain only to joints of this description, naturally we should infer from the title of the paper that it covers subject-matter pertaining to a joint of this description, which takes us to the articulation of the inferior with the superior maxillary, the only joint composed of tissues in which disease of the malnutrition or auto-intoxication type may be supposed to arise; but as I understand the paper, it does not refer to this joint at all. I fail to observe as a practical man anything in the paper that relates to a joint in the generally accepted meaning of that word. Perhaps I fail to grasp the situation, and that may be because my practical ideas are not educated up to the standard of the scientist. You know the story of the boy who asked his father what a scientist was, and the father answered, "A scientist, my son, is a man who can tell you the things you already know, in such unfamiliar language that you regard it as something new."

The case which the essayist mentioned. where death occurred was, if I may judge upon its face, simply necrosis caused by external infection and not auto-intoxication. I may be mistaken, but I do not think so, and perhaps if I had had the opportunity to inspect the paper before the discussion, I might have come closer to what the essayist has in mind as well as to the probable cause, but not having had a copy, I can only make conjectures.

Regarding some matter referred to by the essayist I have to say something that may be of interest, perhaps of information to you. We have for several years been entertained by articles on gouty diathesis, faulty metabolism, etc., with a special emphasis upon uric acid in the blood as being the cause of pyorrhea alveolaris, etc. I want to at least correct an impression that seems to have become fastened upon the mind of the dental profession with regard to uric acid and the dire results which it is supposed to incur in the field of our work, and to that end I will read an extract from "Osler's Modern Medicine," by Thomas B. Futcher, M.B., of Johns Hopkins Hospital, vol. i, page 811:

From the clinical standpoint, the etiology of gout is closely connected with nitrogen metabolism, and with the formation and excretion of certain compounds of which nitrogen is a component.

There is a steadily growing conviction among the best students of this disease at the present day that uric acid plays little or no part in the actual etiology of gout. Although an excess of uric acid in the blood and of its salts in the tissues dominates the picture in well-marked cases, this excess of uric acid is held to play a secondary part and to be a mere weapon of the disease. There is no experimental proof showing that an excess of uric acid causes any special toxic symptoms. The growing belief is that gout is really a disease of the intermediary metabolism. Origin of the uric acid of the blood: Possibilities are three—(1) The diminished destruction of oxidation. (2) Increased formation. (3) Diminished excretion by the kidneys.

There is an unfortunate tendency on the part of many physicians to ascribe certain obscure symptoms to a so-called uric acid diathesis, especially if they find a deposit of uric acid or urates in the urine, although there is often not a vestige of evidence to justify this view. There are certain health resorts in this country from which nearly every patient comes away imbued with a firm conviction that his blood is filled with uric acid, and that this is responsible for his various nervous features. The patients are usually pleased with the explanation, and it is a difficult task to disabuse their minds of the fallacy. We know now that by far the largest proportion of uric acid is derived from "endogenous" purins of the body and in much smaller proportion from the "exogenous" purins of the food. It was also claimed that red meats and game were specially to be avoided, but recent investigations by Kaufmann and Mohr show there is no greater uric acid output when a person is fed on red and dark meats than when he is given white meats in the same amounts. If the former are in any way more injurious, this is probably referrable largely to the fact that they are less easily digested. The balance of evidence at the present day is against the exclusion of meats and in favor of their being allowed in moderate amounts.

Dr. Futcher mentions as food to be avoided: Meat extracts, owing to their nitrogenous extracts and salt. Salt fish, fish roe, and caviar, and all highly seasoned foods are forbidden; pepper, paprika, and mustard should not be allowed in dressing, cucumbers and tomatoes, alcoholic drinks, wines, liquors, etc.; but he allows eggs, fresh fish in moderation, milk, starchy foods freely, vegetables, fruit, fats such as butter freely, and plenty of water before breakfast. I bring this out because patients, as well as the members of our own profession, continually refer to the uric acid bugaboo in connection with the treatment of pyorrhea alveolaris, claiming that it must be gotten rid of before we can hope for a successful outcome of our local treatments. It would appear to me as a practical man that it might be well for our profession to allow the medical profession to at least agree upon constitutional cause and effect before we adopt their ideas as facts. I never have believed and I have yet to be shown where there is any constitutional connection which affects pyorrhea alveolaris one way or another, except in the indirect manner in which all disease which tends to lower the tone of the whole system may also affect the tissues surrounding the teeth. From my practical observations pyorrhea appears very strongly to be directly due to inability to properly clean the teeth at the gum margins, owing to whatever cause, and that the deposit of tartar resulting therefrom is a chemical one produced by the affected fluids from the parotid and sublingual and maxillary glands.

Frequently these glands leave a calcic deposit before their fluids meet the fluids of the mouth; why not afterward? We not only cure this condition by local treatment, but in many instances the simple expedient of making the patients change their mastication of food from one side of the mouth to the other immediately changes the calcic deposits to the unused side of the mouth, and eliminates it from the used side. These are merely the observations of every man who attempts to handle pyorrheal cases, and who has more or less success with local treatments. If those who believe pyorrhea to be a constitutional disease will take some practical cases, treat them only systemically after one removal of the calcic deposits, and prove that there is no return of the trouble under such treatment, or will show practically that with systemic treatment they can obtain as good or even better results than do the advocates of local treatment, I for one shall be pleased to acknowledge that I have been wrong, and to adopt the right.

I have no further criticism to make, but in closing I wish to say that I hope that our scientific men when they propose to read a paper on a so-called scientific subject will at least give the paper a title by which the practical man may know what the subject-matter will be, so that we may read up enough to be able to comprehend what the essayists are driving at.

Dr. RHEIN. In making a motion that Dr. Kirk be allowed the privilege of closing the discussion on his paper, if he so desires, I wish to add a word. The quotation which was read by Dr. Bryant is a very valuable one to insert in this discussion, as it conforms precisely with every point that was brought out by the essayist. It is unfortunate that Dr. Bryant was unable to appreciate what Dr. Kirk said yesterday, because it forces him to argue against a theory that he is in accord with, and a careful reading of the paper will thoroughly demonstrate that fact.

Dr. J. D. PATTERSON, Kansas City,

Mo. This subject is one of great interest to me, but I should not have risen to discuss it had it not been for the statement made by Dr. Rhein that in the treatment of this distressing disease no material result toward success can be assured until the diabetic condition is cured. With all emphasis, I wish to say that the experience of those who are daily treating this distressing disease is directly contrary to such an opinion. We know that whatever the predisposing condition or the systemic condition may be, if local surgical treatment and sanitation is used there comes at once a remarkable improvement. Nevertheless Dr. Rhein says that there is no material improvement until the systemic condition is corrected.

Dr. RHEIN. What disease are you speaking of?

Dr. PATTERSON. You made the statement that in the disease commonly called pyorrhea alveolaris no material result toward success could be assured until the systemic condition is corrected.

Dr. RHEIN. I said that in the diabetic cases, the diabetic condition should be under control.

Dr. PATTERSON. Let it be so. The fact of the matter is that none of us deny the predisposing influence in this disease. The consideration of systemic conditions which result from nutritional disturbances and which effect pathological conditions in the oral cavity should receive careful study from the members of the dental profession, and the therapy that will correct such predisposition to the loss of the investing membranes of the dental organs should be diligently sought, whether in pyorrhea or in other pathological conditions of the dermal structures. It may be said, however, that the aid of drugs in correcting these systemic conditions must ever be secondary to the surgical treatment.

Dr. Kirk yesterday—and perhaps, as Dr. Rhein says, he was only discussing one phase, and he did it in a well-founded, magnificent and scientific manner—entered the speculative field when he said that nutritional disturbances resulting in faulty metabolism coupled with bacterial invasion caused the disease that we denominate pyorrhea alveolaris, leading us to the fair assumption that the bacteria had some method of entering that tissue through the nutritional disturbance, faulty metabolism, or auto-intoxication. Now, my claim is that bacterial invasion is not present until there is some solution of the continuity of the gingival border of the gum around the cervix of the tooth, and that these nutritional disturbances never cause that lesion at the gum margin by which the bacteria gain entrance.

I am very much interested in this subject, and I am interested in another thing. I know that the teachings of Dr. Rhein and Dr. Kirk, Dr. Peirce, Dr. Burchard, and others have prevented hundreds and hundreds of competent men all through the West, where I know them best, from interfering with and trying to correct this disease, because they have been taught, as a fair conclusion from all the articles that have appeared from these men, that little or nothing can be done until the systemic condition is corrected; thus, because the disease is one that is hard to control—it is hard for the patient and hard for the operator—and requires more skill and more care than ordinary operations in dentistry, and because they do not like the work, this has given them an excuse not to try to do anything for the relief of sufferers. I know that this is so, and I

know that injury has been done in that way, and I wish to protest against it and say that whatever the systemic conditions, the proper surgical local treatment gives immediate and prompt relief; then let it be reinforced with the correction of the systemic condition in whatever way best suits the patient. The best means, as you and I should know, is not therapy, not vaccines, but vigorous exercise, fresh air, good food, sunshine, and good sleep. In this way good blood is gained to enable the tissue to throw off any kind of irritation. Dr. Kirk and others would make you believe, because they say little or nothing about the factor of local irritation, that these conditions are due wholly to nutritional disturbances. I never saw one case, and I have seen hundreds of them, in which I could not say that local irritation was the initiative cause, whatever the systemic condition was. I have records of hundreds of cases, and have carefully gone into the clinical history of these cases and have published the reports, and I tell you that the people coming to me for treatment of pyorrhea—and my opinion is indorsed by a great many practical men working in this field every day—exhibit no greater percentage of constitutional disturbances than those who come to us for ordinary operations of filling teeth, making plates, crowns, and bridges; a record of several years shows just about ten to fifteen per cent. of such cases. The fact of the matter is that the great majority of people who come for treatment of pyorrhea are remarkably vigorous and healthy. I do not say that without careful observation and inquiry, often consulting the patients' physician to find out if they have any faulty metabolism. People who come to me for pyorrhea treatment show no evidence of faulty nutrition and are not tottering on the brink of the grave from faulty metabolism and auto-intoxications, but they are healthy, vigorous, strong people. When they are asked what their ailment is, they say that there is nothing the matter with them; they are healthy and strong as can be—men and women tell me that same thing—and I assure you that this is true with the vast majority of cases that present in my practice. Keep a record as I have done and see what the result will be.

That reminds me—I am not criticizing anybody, but would emphasize what I am trying to say—disabuse your minds of the idea that you cannot relieve these patients, and by that I mean relieve them from pain, from inflammation, from exudations, from pus; comfort in every way can be restored to these teeth merely with local treatment and sanitation. I know this to be so, and I know it is so because hundreds of practitioners all over the country are successful with local treatment every day; at the same time I do not deny the effect of nutritional disturbances upon the progress of the disease, and that we should join hands with the physician to whom we refer the patient for the correction of that faulty metabolism. I am reminded that the man who read the paper is a friend of mine, and I believe that the most scientific man we have, and whom I admire very much, is doing injury on account of the fact that he avoids or says little or nothing in all the papers which he has written—and hé has written many others ou the same line—about the local surgical treatment; and that he is doing that injury by giving to men, to you and me, an excuse not to touch the disease because it is such hard work. I am also reminded that in the same city

from which he comes, years ago there were two men of high repute and great attainments who did much for the dental profession, but at the same time did more to injure the dental profession than any two men that ever lived on account of their advocating the filling of root-canals with cotton.

Dr. RHEIN. Just one word of reply to Dr. Patterson. There is nothing in the papers of Dr. Kirk nor in any of mine that does not conform precisely with the position of Dr. Patterson, namely, that surgical treatment should be commenced at the start in every form of this disease, except in cases of diabetes. Modern scientific surgery teaches that surgical interference is not warranted until the diabetic condition is under control, and in all the treatises that I have published on this subject I have excepted this one form of malnutrition. I have warned the profession not to commence local treatment in this particular form of malnutrition until the diabetic condition is under control.

Dr. PATTERSON. Why?

Dr. RHEIN. It would take more time than I have the right to consume to go into the pathology of diabetes, and I am sure that there are many men within the sound of my voice who recognize the correctness of this practice as pertaining to this particular form of disease.*

Dr. KIRK (closing the discussion). Answering the inquiry made by Dr. Brown, I have to say that no examina-

* At the request of Dr. Rhein, we add the following to clarify his statement of position: "It has been found that when diabetes is not under control, injuries to the tissues are not followed by regeneration but by necrosis. Furthermore, in those diabetics in whom acetone is found to be present, fatal results may be at any moment expected after any form of traumatism."

tion was made of the other tissues of the diabetic patient described in my paper for the reason that a post-mortem examination was not permitted by his relatives. I am unable to say whether a blood count was made or not. I fully agree with Dr. Brown in his contention that the vast amount of work which is just now being done in the study of the therapeutic value of vaccines and in their use as agents for creating at least a temporary immunity by raising the opsonic index with reference to certain pathogenic bacteria is a phase of this subject which is of the utmost importance, and one which is giving—indeed, has already given—most encouraging results. As Dr. Rhein has said, however, I endeavored to concentrate my study and direct the attention of this audience to but one phase of this highly complex problem. With Dr. Rhein's remarks and with those of Dr. Brown I am naturally in hearty agreement.

I am at a loss to understand how it is that Dr. Patterson can draw from my paper the conclusions which he seems to have done. He apparently takes me to task for having given to those who are interested in the treatment of that group of gingival inflammations which we collectively speak of as pyorrhea alveolaris an excuse for neglecting their work by the effort which I have made to draw attention to one of the factors in its causation. That type of reasoning it seems to me is like contending that because the path of virtue and honesty may be shown to be difficult, an excuse is therefore given to humanity for immorality and dishonesty. It is true that I have not contributed largely to the literature of the surgical or local treatment of pyorrhea alveolaris. I have not deemed it necessary to do so. There is no sub-

ject within the domain of dental literature which has been more voluminously treated and more hopelessly treated. I have recently had occasion to read the page proofs of Dr. Guerini's "History of Dentistry" now issuing from the press, and the record in that publication is remarkably clear that diseases of the retentive structures of the teeth were recognized and known from the earliest ages of antiquity, and it is further shown that almost from its earliest recognition man has made abortive efforts to correct the disorder by local means. I have not felt it necessary, in view of all that has been done in connection with that aspect of the subject, to add to the general confusion by indicating some other means by which local surgical treatment of pyorrhea may be carried out. In the very beginning I take it for granted that everybody believes, just as Dr. Patterson says he believes, that local surgical treatment is absolutely necessary for the alleviation, and, if I may be permitted the use of the term, the cure, of pyorrhea alveolaris. I agree with all that he has said in favor of local treatment, but I find that, having granted all of that and admitted the possibility of the results which Dr. Patterson claims for his particular modes of treatment, he is nevertheless in agreement with my principal contention after all—for he says, "Whatever the systemic conditions, the proper surgical local treatment gives immediate and prompt relief; then let it be reinforced with the correction of the systemic condition in whatever way best suits the patient." I admit that local treatment gives relief promptly, or as Dr. Patterson puts it, "immediately," but I am convinced that such treatment is not of permanent value in preventing a recurrence of the disorder where malnutritional errors exist, and that these must be corrected in order to produce a result which may fairly and honestly be dignified by the name of "a cure." In making this statement I make the distinction between that class of gingival inflammations which are wholly and distinctly the result of filth conditions and due directly to the impingement of accumulations of tartar and infected food débris upon the gingival borders. The cases which I have in mind are not of that type, but are such as I have discussed in the paper which I have had the pleasure of presenting to you.

I hardly know how to characterize the critical remarks of Dr. Bryant. I do not wish to misjudge his attitude of mind, but I infer that he takes me to task for presenting a paper before the National Dental Association dealing with the subject of pyorrhea alveolaris from a standpoint involving terminology which he does not understand. That is to say, he seems to have called me to account for telling him something that he did not know.

The two principal misdemeanors for which I seem to have been indicted in the discussion are, first, that I have omitted to discuss the local surgical treatment for pyorrhea; and second, that in presenting the subject from another angle of view I have done so in terms that are not intelligible to some of my hearers. For the first, I have already explained that in view of the hoary antiquity of the subject of local surgical treatment for pyorrhea I did not think it necessary to add to the volume of material already written upon that aspect of the question. I have reason to believe that when Ecclesiastes refers to the coming on of that time when "the grinders shall cease because they are few," he referred to or had in mind the loss of the dental apparatus through the agency of senile pyorrhea, and if he had been less poetic and more technical he would have added some directions for the local surgical treatment of the disorder, and I suspect also that had the "sweet singer of Israel" been engaged in a discussion of the same topic and had been met by the criticism that he was presenting the subject in terms not generally understandable he would apply to that criticism the remark which he has recorded with reference to another matter in the one hundred and thirty-ninth Psalm—"Such knowledge is too wonderful and excellent for me; I cannot attain unto it."

A Side-light on Professional Interest.

By JAMES McMANUS, D.D.S.

I WAS very much surprised to receive from our president an invitation which, as a loyal member, I considered to be virtually a command, to read a paper at this meeting. I have never made pretentions to either scientific, literary, or inventive ability, but some of the older members know that I was a delegate member to the American Dental Association in 1864, and have kept up a paying membership in that and the National Dental Association, and have missed but few of the annual meetings since that year. My desire to obey the president was strong, my ability to prepare a paper that would interest questionable, until the thought came to me that possibly my long membership and my interest in dental associations—city, state, national, and international— ought to give me the privilege of speaking to you concerning the past, and of offering some suggestions as to the best possible course to be pursued in the future in order to broaden the social and professional life of the individual dentist, the college, and the associations throughout the land.

It is easy to find fault, and to criticize harshly; many have done so in the past, and now I am going to indulge in criticism to an extent that I hope will cause those who hear me, and those who may possibly read what I have to say, to reflect seriously and to make new resolutions to live and act in the open as dentists, doing the duty that many have for years deliberately shirked. And first I would throw a few side-lights on the past.

For many years I have known dentists who have held high rank in the state military service. To gain that rank they had to give up one or more evenings in the month to attending drills, frequently days to parading, and a week to the yearly encampment. They had to pay promptly the regular assessments, the cost of uniforms, and incidental extra expenses. With very few exceptions these soldier dentists had neither time to attend dental meetings nor disposition to contribute in any way toward the uplifting of the calling in the practice of which they earned the money that procured them food.

Another illustration, not quite so brilliant as the military but fascinating for many dentists, is membership in the various social clubs, lodges, and uniformed orders. There are expenses connected with all these organizations, especially if one desires to hold an official position, and the money to meet those expenses is earned in the laboratory or at the dental chair. I believe in social clubs, lodges, and uniformed orders; I believe that men should band together for mutual benefit, and that such organizations are powerful for good, their influence being felt and feared by politicians and governments. I have still all the old-time boyish admiration for military men and officers, and the various society regalias are always attractive and interesting, possibly from the fact that I have known so little about them or what they represent. But with the passing years I have learned to respect and honor the men who show to the world that they are proud of the calling they follow, and who are earnestly anxious to perfect themselves by study and association with their fellow workmen along the line of work to which they have devoted their life. There might easily have been a successful social dental benevolent organization long ago in this country, if a thousand dentists had banded together and had contributed as liberally to its support as have the military and society dentists to the organizations they are connected with.

I have watched with keen interest since 1864, and have never ceased to wonder why more of the dentists of the country could not see the advantages and benefits that society membership would give them. Societies will always rank first for extended educational work, and since society membership and work has made it possible for the calling of dentistry to be classed with the professions, the fact that such a large number of practicing dentists are not society members tells an educated and observant public just where they may place these practitioners among the craftsmen of the world.

The first dental society was organized in 1839 by dentists who had high ideals and who were earnest workers, but the growth of dental societies has been very slow, and their influence, both socially and professionally, is yet quite limited. All that could reasonably be desired might have been gained if those who joined societies in years past had kept up at least a paying membership. We cannot blot out the record of men who have dropped membership; it is decidedly unpleasant to recall that you have helped —some of the time innocently—members and societies to elevate to office men who on completion of their term coolly retired on their laurels, forsaking the friends and societies that gave them honors.

During the sessions of the American Dental Association held in Chicago in 1865, I well remember the reception given by Dr. N. S. Davis at his home to the members, his earnest kindly welcome, and his serious talk and forecast of what the association might and should do along educational and professional lines. The lectures given by Dr. Brainerd and the eye specialist, Dr. DeLaskey Miller, at that time surgeons of Chicago, were intensely interesting, and for the first time doctors and dentists fraternally grasped hands before the public. Those who attended the receptions given in the home of Prof. J. H. McQuillen of Philadelphia, from 1865 until his death, had the pleasure of meeting many of the medical and surgical celebrities of that city. Again, Dr. N. S. Davis of Chicago, then president of the Ninth International Medical Congress during the sessions held in Washington, D. C., in 1887, in his address of welcome to the members of the large Dental section, told of his continued and hopeful wishes for the success of dental educational associations. I remember the earnest work done by the committees, especially those on finance, in arranging for the success of the Dental section, the enthusiasm of those who were in attendance—numbering four hundred—and the generous contributions given by the members of the section toward defraying the large expenses of the congress.

The four hundred dentists who attended the medical congress in Washington, D. C., in 1887 were jubilant, and felt almost sure that dentistry had been recognized by medical men as a specialty of the healing art. Of that we are not so sure today. What we are sure of is this: The success of twenty-two dental schools awakened at that time in some of the medical teachers of the country an idea of what they might gain if dental departments were added to medical schools, and now lecture and other fees are paid by all the students of about fifty-six dental schools to over five hundred medical men whose names are printed in the announcements as professors and lecturers, and whose interest, with few exceptions, in dentistry is a financial rather than a professional one, and is limited to the hours engaged in preparing and delivering at most three lectures a week. I cannot recall of late years an occasion where medical men or college medical men have shown any special interest in dental affairs, and the fact that the large majority of the doctors of dental surgery who are heralded in college announcements as professors, lecturers, and demonstrators are not seen either at state or national meetings gives unmistakable evidence that they are not in unison with and will not meet or work with society men for dental advancement.

There are fifty-six dental schools in the United States, and each of these schools ought to have an uplifting influence over the dentists in their immediate neighborhood. Each of these schools through their announcements and advertisements ask the dentists of the country to send them students, and there is no doubt that earnest students can gain a technical knowledge in any of them, but in order to succeed in business, in public affairs, and in social life, the young graduate must give evidence of a broad and liberal training which three years of student life under conscientious teachers would imply. If the graduates of past years had been fully impressed with the stubborn facts that they had, and always would have while they practiced dentistry, much to learn, and that the local, state, and national associations were advanced postgraduate schools open to them at all times, which it was their duty to support as active members and in which they would be certain to hear the best teaching and see chair and table clinics, and where they should have, and could have, all the advantages of fellowship with the best teachers and leading scientific men and operators of the country, my paper would have no excuse for existence. During the past twenty years the dental schools have graduated many thousands, and just why the state societies, and especially this National Dental Association, has not had a large increase in membership is a question which I propose to open for consideration.

The pioneer Baltimore College started out with four teachers in 1839, to blaze an educational pathway that has since broadened to a magnificent boulevard that gives ample space and opportunity for dental colleges to parade over 1500

Membership in N. D. A. in Relation to the States Having Large Societies and Colleges.

STATES.	Number of Dentists.	Societies.	Colleges.	M.D. and M.D., D.D.S.	D.D.S.	Members of N. D. A.		Examiners Members of N. D. A.
NEW YORK	3930	28	3	33	70	'07	37	2
						'08	74	3
New York City	1324	..	..	..	..	..		..
Brooklyn	470	..	..	..	..			
Buffalo	224	..	..	..	..	..		..
PENNSYLVANIA	3260	23	5	54	55	'07	33	3
						'08	50	4
Philadelphia	1015	..	..	..	..	..		
Pittsburg	238	..	..	..	..	..		..
ILLINOIS	3081	39	4	32	115	'07	21	.1
						'08	49	2
Chicago	1441	..	..	..	..	..		..
OHIO	2236	12	4	88	49	'07	21	0
						'08	28	1
Cincinnati	247	..	..	..	..	..		..
Cleveland	306	..	..	..	..			
Columbus	120	..	..	..	..	..		
MASSACHUSETTS	1862	8	2	33	102	'07	12	0
						'08	47	4
Boston	727	..	..	..	..	..		..
MISSOURI	1469	7	4	44	128	'07	19	1
						'08	22	0
St. Louis	450	..	..	..	..	..		
Kansas City	205	..	..	..	..	..		..
MICHIGAN	1353	7	2	31	25	'07	7	..
Detroit	312	..	..	..	..	..		..
INDIANA	1179	10	1	9	16	'07	6	..
Indianapolis	175	..	..	..	..			
WISCONSIN	1169	9	2	13	51	'07	11	..
Milwaukee	276	..	..	..	..	..		..
KENTUCKY	748	2	1	13	11	'07	8	..
						'08	11	
Louisville	181	..	..	..	..	..		
GEORGIA	650	2	2	9	18	'07	27	0
						'08	39	1
Atlanta	110	..	..	..	..	..		..
TENNESSEE	605	5	3	19	24	'07	27	1
						'08	33	1
Nashville	82	..	..	..	..	..		..
Memphis	59	..	..	..	..	..		..
MARYLAND	498	2	3	311	123	'07	8	..
						'08	10	
Baltimore	358	..	..	..	..	..		..
WASHINGTON, D. C.	329	2	3	44	34	'07	14	2
						'08	31	0
VIRGINIA	472	9	2	13	51	'07	11	0
						'08	7	3
Richmond	54	..	.	..	..	..		..
TOTALS	22,841	165	41	419	872	'07	262	10
						'08	401	19

professors, lecturers, and demonstrators, and to flaunt their banners claiming special fitness and facilities for teaching students dentistry as a specialty of medicine. The number of dentists and the status of dentistry in states where dental colleges have prospered may be of interest.

The number of dentists in the states and cities and the number of societies given are taken from the last edition of Polk's Directory, and represent an under-estimate rather than an over-estimate of numbers. There are fifty-six colleges in the United States, whose professors and lecturers with the M.D., and M.D., D.D.S. degrees number over five hundred, and whose professors, lecturers, and demonstrators with the dental degree number over one thousand. In the fourteen states and Washington, D. C., as exhibited in the accompanying table (see opposite page) there are 22,841 dentists, 165 societies, 41 colleges, 419 men with the degrees of M.D. and M.D., D.D.S., and 872 men with the degree of D.D.S., but only 262 dentists* out of this large number are members of the National Dental Association.

As long ago as 1841, the dentists of the state of Alabama secured the passage of a dental law, and slowly the sister states followed her example. Connecticut's dental law was passed fifty-two years later. Each state seemed to be under the old influence of the doctrine of state rights when framing its law, and little thought or consideration was given to the possibility of any licensed practitioner ever finding it necessary to remove to another state. The hoped-for

interstate recognition is yet afar off, and there is little chance for a unification of state laws until it is demanded by the united and persistent efforts of the dental societies of the country. Each state so far has felt the power of political rather than professional influence in the appointment of state examiners. Men who work for or accept appointments as state examiners know that they have arbitrary power, and as President Hetrick said in his annual address in Boston to the Examiners: "We are an advisory body rather than legislative or educational." They should take an interest in the National Dental Association and become members thereof. They should know men from the different states, consult with them, act with them, show their interest in the calling which they officially represent. As the record now reads, of 230 state examiners in 1907 only 23 were members of the National Association.

While we might occasionally hope that more interest might be taken in dental societies by some of the medical teachers in dental colleges, we do know and we have a right to expect that there should be more active, earnest and helpful work done by a larger number of the doctors of dental surgery whose names are printed in the yearly college announcements as teachers and demonstrators of operative and mechanical dentistry. Their individual personal interest is on record, and should be supplemented by public professional interest in society work.

The pioneer dentists who started the educational movement and desire for professional recognition may not have foreseen the splitting up of what was then known as dentistry into pseudo-science specialties. The few who started out to

---

* In 1907 there were 262; in 1908, at the Boston meeting, 401.

ignore and render the old-time title "dentist" obsolete and to exploit the titles "stomatologist," "orist," "orthodontist," and "prosthetist" have now many followers, and between the professional man who ought to know how to do many mechanical things, but does not, and the artizans and mechanical workmen who know how to do them, a barrier or dividing wall seems inevitable. Professional dentistry is all right in theory, but the conditions under which artificial teeth and mechanical appliances are now turned out from dental kitchens suggest commercial rather than professional relations. Dentistry means first the saving of teeth, and the mission of the colleges is to graduate men competent to do well the ordinary operative and mechanical work—that is, the class of operations and mechanical work that so many of the old-time dentists did so well, the kind of work and service that the great majority of the human family need all over the world. Dental colleges are striving to do too much, they are striving to cover too large a field, and students are not held down as closely to the study of the principles of dentistry or given the thorough training they should have in performing the more common class of operations demanded of the dentist. Medical colleges graduate students not as specialists, but as men educated in the principles of medicine and surgery. They teach them how to study, but their diploma and license does give them a legal right without any experience to amputate limbs, remove tumors, operate for appendicitis, or treat serious and infectious diseases, if they have the courage to accept such cases. It is to the credit of the medical men that they buy books and are generally students, and that many of them take postgraduate courses. There

are no other graduates from whom so much is expected as from the dental graduates, and no other class attempts to cover so much in the college course. The new porcelain and gold inlay work, crown and bridge work, which when actually required and properly done are so satisfactory, represent a class of operations that dentists of long experience often find most difficult to make satisfactorily, and the correction of irregularities, while demanding the most careful study and judgment, is purely and wholly mechanical. Training in the fundamental principles and practice of dentistry and oral hygiene, the saving of teeth by operative treatment, and the making and adjustment of artificial teeth are what colleges are expected to teach during the entire course. These are the essentials for dental practice. If microscopy, histology, bacteriology, carving of block teeth, and orthodontia are essentials, then a four years' course is absolutely necessary, and under that ruling only students with means or those having backers may hope to enter dental colleges. It is fortunate that state laws do not require more than average ability from general practitioners, and state dental examiners are not likely to turn down applicants for license unless they are very deficient in theory and in average operative and mechanical skill. That out of 602 who applied for license in 1907 and 1908, 113 failed, gives opportunity to question whether the system of education was faulty, or whether the graduates were thoroughly incompetent to absorb instruction.

To the older dentist it has for years past been glaringly apparent how few among the many dentists are interested in either general or professional literature; and the one opportunity to get each year a valuable book, and their names for reference and indorsement as members on the roll of the National Dental Association, still fails to awaken in them a sense of duty or interest in their calling. A few years ago in conversation with a leading bookseller, I was surprised to learn that he sold few books of any kind, general or professional, to dentists, and that he did not consider dentists reading men. Again, later, in talking with a prominent dentist and teacher in one of the western cities, I learned that a bookseller told him the same thing, and then I recalled that at dental gatherings in years past I saw no dental or professional books on sale, which made good the statement of the booksellers. At the annual meeting of the Northeastern Dental Association held in Hartford last October, for the first time an agent of a publishing house appeared, and to the surprise of many took orders for a number of volumes. I have been told that after college examinations you can always find a goodly number of medical and dental books in second-hand stores, and that may in part account for so many failures in state examinations. As I recall the kindly advice often given to students by Professors McQuillen, Flagg, and that rare anatomist, surgeon, and philosopher, Garretson, to keep up their studies, to read and own books, to take advantage of the public libraries, to become members of a dental society, and to keep, if possible, in touch with medical men, I feel confident that if similar advice has been persistently given in years past to graduates, the majority of them have completely ignored it, failing to appreciate its value and importance. It has been a serious mistake to let so many graduates leave the colleges uncertain as to the relations which they might hope

to enjoy in the future with the men who had been their teachers during the three most impressible years of their life, and whom they had learned to respect and love. The "good-by" and added cheery words, "I want to see you often in the future, surely at society meetings, especially at the National, which I hope to attend often," would be a pleasant memory and a constant incentive to their becoming working society members.

One of the peculiar traits which may be rightly called a dental inheritance, which was so noticeable in the early days and which held back dental progress so effectually, was the deliberate cultivation of the secretive disposition. Other craftsmen are more united and sociable, and where they number fifty, or even less, in cities and towns they secure a home place for meetings and social gatherings. The quickest and surest way for dentists to get consideration in a community is to have a society home like other organizations. A room in a central office building, secured at a moderate rent, has been the home of the Hartford Dental Society for the past eight years. Most of its furnishings had already done duty in the homes of some of the members. Books, bookcases, and chairs were bought; rugs, a clock, pictures, a table for magazines and one for clinic purposes, a writing-desk, and cushions were all contributed, and give the room a comfortable and homelike appearance. Each member has a key, and the room is accessible at all hours of the day or night, Sundays included. We have our regular meetings there, and a pleasant feature is the Monday club night and registration of members and guests. It is an inexpensive club-room where all are on an equality, and sociability so far has reigned supreme. We are proud of our dental home, for we all realize fully how much we have been benefited in our calling, as well as how much we have enjoyed the comforts and pleasure of social companionship.

The large number of dentists that have been called together in New York, Philadelphia, Washington, Chicago, Minneapolis, St. Louis, Boston, and frequently in Asbury Park, under the auspices of the American and National Dental Associations and other gatherings, under the management of state and local associations, particularly in New Jersey, Chicago, and St. Paul, tell what efficient, earnest men have been able to do, and also what it would have been possible for them to do if they had put a little of their surplus energy into organizing a dental benevolent association. Many claim that American dentists, dentistry, and dental organizations lead the world. A glance at the record of what has been done in England will cause them to change their opinion. The British Dental Association for several years past has published a successful and profitable professional journal. It has maintained permanent home quarters for many years in London, open every day, except Sundays, for the use of members and friends, and in 1883 a Dental Benevolent Association was organized, in which only registered dentists are eligible to membership. In 1907 there were 4472 dentists registered, and 1200 of them were members of the association. The association has received some gifts, but owing to the depreciation of some of its bonds within the past few years, the amount invested is now only about $15,000. The annual dues are $5 a year, and the income about $3000. The disbursement to beneficiaries in 1907 was $2600. Only the members of the committee are supposed to know who receive benefits. When one recalls the brilliant and at one time very successful dentists who were cared for by the contributions of a few friends during the past twenty years in and about New York alone, and realizes the possibility that many in years to come may sadly need assistance, it is strange indeed that a movement for such an organization has been so long delayed.

The actors in this country have set a noble example, for they have had such an organization for years past, and in the large cities have given yearly benefit performances to increase its funds, and the leading actresses and actors vie with each other in their efforts to make it a grand artistic and financial success. If only one-tenth of the dentists in this country would unite and contribute once a year the fee received for one gold operation, a fund would be secured large enough to help to cheer and sustain many an unfortunate man and family in their time of trial, sorrow, and want. That two such associations should be firmly established in this country seems a duty. We know of the success of the one in England with a membership of 1200 drawn from a registry list of less than 5000. The New England and Middle states, with a registry list of 12,300, and the Western and Southern states, with a registry list of over 20,000, ought to have at least 1000 men in each section who would be glad to become members of such an organization. Such organizations would bring about the assurance that wherever there were fifty practicing dentists they had a dental home and were united in sentiment and purpose, and the public would quickly recognize that they had citizens, as well as dentists, whose wishes were to be considered and respected. In Boston the Academy of Dental Science and other local societies hold their monthly meetings in a hotel. In New York the Odontological, the Stomatological, and the First District societies hold their meetings in the Academy of Medicine, and in Chicago the largest local society in the world holds its meetings in rooms in the Public Library building. Surely in each of these cities the dentists are numerous enough, if they were united, to have suitable rooms for their exclusive use, and suggestions, petitions, or protests emanating from such home quarters would command instant attention and consideration, from not only citizens and civic authorities, but also from representatives and senators in Washington.

Today we look backward and briefly recall a few incidents in the history of the American Dental Association organized just fifty years ago. During all these years the ethical standard of professional gentlemen has never been lowered. Until this year, to become a member a dentist must have proper credentials from the officers of his state society, and the limit was one delegate to every five active members of the society represented. One very important fact stands out that should not be forgotten and should be carefully considered in passing judgment: Never since the organization of the American or National Dental Association has any state succeeded in any one year in having a full delegation report for membership, and but very few of those that did attend chose to become permanent members. During all these years, with the membership very far below the constitutional limit, the treasurer has never been overburdened with anxiety as to how he should invest surplus funds. Yet, limited financially as the association always has been, it has never yet failed to cheer-

fully help along all the scientific investigations, experiments, and practical work that the proper committees reported as being worthy of aid. Every judicious movement made for the uplifting of dentistry has been cheerfully and financially assisted, and when San Francisco was so fearfully afflicted, the association promptly and liberally sent assistance, while the members of the association became active agents in raising funds, dental materials, and other necessary articles, which were forwarded for prompt distribution among the unfortunates. Members from this association journeyed to London in 1881 to unite with the English and Continental dentists to make the Dental section in the Seventh International Medical Congress a great success. In 1887, the Ninth International Medical Congress held its sessions in Washington, D. C., and the Dental section there was under the auspices and management of members of this association. That Dental section attracted 400 dentists, including the foreign delegates, and was thought then to be a great success. The expenses of that section were large, but they were met by the liberal contributions of the members, who also contributed more than generously to the expenses of the general congress.

The Columbian Dental Congress was held in Chicago in 1893, under the auspices and management of members of the American and Southern Dental Associations, and all who were there will recall how prompt and full were the published daily reports of the papers and discussions, and what a large, varied, and beautiful display of dental instruments, appliances, etc., was exhibited by individuals and manufacturers, showing what had been done in other countries as well as in our own for the betterment of dental service. The success of the Columbian Congress raised dentistry to a higher level, and led dentists to take a broader view of men, of life, and of personal duty. In 1904, under the same auspices and management, the St. Louis Dental Congress was held, easily ranking first among dental gatherings. From all parts of the world educators, scientists, mechanics, and practicing dentists were brought together; many of these were specially delegated and wore the orders conferred on them for recognized merit, and from our own country the largest number of ethical dentists ever seen under one roof was assembled.

The literary, educational, scientific, and historical papers, the section work and the clinics, the interesting historical exhibits, and the display exhibited by the manufacturers of dental goods, gave to the congress an educational character and value far exceeding the most sanguine hopes of the promoters and managers. Together with the closing incidents and the brilliant scene of the banquet at the Jefferson, we recall the manly, intellectual-looking men, the brilliant women, the inspiring music, the eloquent introductions by our own B. Holly Smith, the characteristic emotional responses by the foreigners, the singing of the national airs of the different countries represented, the eloquent words of welcome from our own representative men to the visitors, now most valued friends. All this will remain with those who were present as pleasant memories while life lasts. The same auspices and management were largely in evidence at the successful Jamestown dental gathering, and have also been recognized and appreciated at the dental gatherings in Europe for several years past. "Lest we forget," I recall these incidents and

events, for they illumine the past, they tell unmistakably what has been done for the uplifting and betterment of the calling of dentistry throughout the world, by and radiating from the American, Southern, and National Dental Associations. Not a few of the 40,000 dentists of the country are saying what these associations ought to have done. The working members of these associations know well what might have been done with a larger membership. The younger men have a future, and it is to be hoped that they will make good, always keeping in mind that all that has been done, all the true progress that has been made in every department of dental science, literature, and art, has been given out to the world through the publications, discussions, and clinics given before or under the auspices and management of members of these associations during the past fifty years.

I have been proud of the old American, the Southern, and the National— for they are one, and I hope that our National body will rank in the future, as it has in the past, as the first and best organization in the world. If reorganizing with a new constitution and by-laws will increase its efficiency, usefulness, and influence, go ahead and reorganize! A new constitution and by-laws, if you can induce all the new and old members to read it through carefully twice, ought to do them good and arouse them to greater activity in getting and striving to hold the old and the new members through life.

Members—permanent, paying members, and more of them—is what has been wanted for years past to make this association influential and powerful. The medical men of the country do not all attend their National Association meetings, but a very large number do keep in touch with the secretary and treasurer, and their yearly subscriptions gain for the *Journal* of the association a large advertising patronage, powerful influence, and a full treasury. And this association might easily have been a good second to the medical, if a broader and more active personal interest had been taken in society work by authors of dental works, contributors to dental journals, state examiners, and the faculties, lecturers, and demonstrators of the numerous dental colleges of the country.

Medical men take a just pride in their calling, setting an example that many members of our profession might follow to their advantage.

Discussion.

Dr. J. Y. CRAWFORD, Nashville, Tenn. This has been, in my opinion, one of the best meetings that the National Association has ever held, and one of the contributions of most value is the paper by Dr. McManus. In addition to the value of that paper from a semi-historical standpoint, the underlying spirit of high fraternity seems to be most important, but in addition to the value of that contribution and its timeliness, we have an object lesson in connection with the paper that I regard of more important value—I refer to the distinguished essayist. If I were called upon to designate one of the most marked and distinguished dental surgeons in America from every standpoint, if I were forced to designate one man that I wanted to lead out and introduce as one of the very best type of dental surgeons, taken altogether from the standpoint of his accomplishments, of loyalty, of physical health, I believe I should select Dr. McManus of Hart-

ford, Conn. In addition to his constant work of forty-four years as a member of this association—I suppose he is the oldest member present—for forty-four years he has been a regular *bona fide* member of the National Dental Association of America, as the present organization is simply a continuation of the old American reinforced by the loyal support of the Southern Dental Association, which was a national organization as well, and it is our particular pride that we of the South took the initiative toward the amalgamation of the two associations, and as a result brought into this body a group of southern men, men in sympathy with the southern idea. I do not offer this as an offense, but to show that in the South we have been interested in the maintenance of the national phase of these questions. It has always seemed to me that Dr. McManus' life was made more beautiful and emphasized more markedly by the fact that he lived in Hartford, Conn., where anesthesia was contributed to the world by a member of our profession. He took an active part in commemorating that event, and when I went to the town of Hartford especially to see him and to pay tribute to Horace Wells—that is the only place where there is a monument in commemoration of that event—in the beautiful moonlight this gallant gentleman escorted me to the grounds occupied by the state capitol, and there in the moonlight I went on my knees and read the name of Horace Wells. Dr. McManus is more responsible for the erection of that monument than any dental surgeon in the world, and he has come here and has read us a paper imbued with fraternal spirit and presenting an historical phase of marked interest.

One feature that the essayist referred

to is the memorial to be founded in honor of the distinguished Miller, of which I heartily approve. The essayist also suggested the propriety of having an organization that would look after the welfare of the indigent dentists, and as well that of their families after they have passed away. We have a report or two every year from the Committee on Necrology, supplementing ordinarily the President's address, in which the sad demise of some of our members is recorded. I find that a very small number die annually, but we all have to die. On the left side of the thoracic cavity there is a great muscular organ known as the heart, which is constantly propelling through our organism the life-blood, but there must come a time when the pulsations of that organ will cease, and when we will be laid still in death. We have all to come to that finality, and one of these days the Committee on Necrology will refer to our demise. I think we should adopt the spirit of this paper, and when we have a report from the Committee on Necrology, each member of the National Dental Association should be willing to walk up and lay a coin of one hundred cents upon the table of the presiding officer, as a gold offering for our indigent members and for the families of those who have died. Dental surgery is a poor profession; we shall always be poor. The element of manual labor enters more into our life-work than into that of any other profession in the world, and that fact will necessarily keep us very largely poor. If we could send to the families of deceased indigent members a nice contribution each year, and if every member knew that when he shall journey to that bourn whence no traveler ever returns, his family, if in need, will receive a contribution from each member of the National Association, that would form a bond of union; we could bring the families of the defunct here, and have them conduct a memorial service, and at that service the treasurer of this organization could present them with a check toward which each member of the association has contributed; that would be better than sending stereotype memorial resolutions, flowers, or something of that kind; it would be a kind and at the same time effective measure that would result in making the young men of the country seek membership in the National Association, and instead of having a few hundred, we should have eight or ten thousand members. The spirit of this paper, if promulgated and acted upon by the members of the National Dental Association and the profession in America, would result in increasing our membership more than anything that we have done in the past. This kind of paper and the life-work of this distinguished member of the profession is a good pattern. I do not believe in imitating, but I believe that every young man of our profession should take the life and character of this distinguished gentleman as a pattern in order that his life may fully develop, and may add to the effectiveness and to the strength of the profession he has chosen.

Dr. C. S. BUTLER. Buffalo. N. Y. Dr. McManus paid me the very distinguished honor of sending me a copy of his paper some two weeks ago, with the request that, if I considered it of sufficient importance. I should discuss it in a few words. I regret that I have not been able to give to the paper as much thought as it deserves, because of necessary duties, and I feel embarrassed in attempting to discuss it. But my very great regard for the author, if nothing else, would prompt me to say a word at least in commendation of his paper. I have the feeling that we shall regard the paper which Dr. McManus has presented, as we have opportunity to read it more at our leisure, as one of the most valuable presented to this association. Truly enough, it deals largely with the association of the past, but it also projects itself into the future in that it indicates a line of work which would be well for the profession to follow.

It is very proper indeed that this paper should be presented at this meeting, it being the fiftieth anniversary of the organization of this society. You understand of course that this is the American Dental Association organized at Niagara Falls in 1859, and continued simply under another name, so that this is the fiftieth anniversary of organized dentistry in the United States as applied to a national association; and while many of us grow impatient sometimes and feel that we are not making the progress that we should, yet if we will but run back over these fifty years of history, I think we shall be astonished at the marvelous progress made by the association and the great work accomplished. Perhaps I can indicate in a moment or two a few of the things, which possibly may have been forgotten by some, which the association has undertaken and carried forward during these fifty years.

In the first place, the National Association has developed—or rather, its members are the men who have developed the scientific side of dentistry. Catalog in your minds the scientific men in dentistry in America, and you will find that every one of them, I think without a single exception, has been a member of our National Association. It is the members of this association who have devel-

oped our periodical literature, our dental journals. It can be said that there is no dental journal today of any importance that is not edited by a member of this association, and the same can be said without doubt with regard to our more permanent scientific and mechanical literature. This is also true with regard to our educational institutions. Who are the men of the past as well as of the present who have built up our colleges, who have buttressed the profession in every time of stress and strain? Members of our National Association. And it would seem, as we review these facts, that they must awaken a feeling of pride and gratitude for what our association has done for the development of the profession.

Reference was made in the paper to the *personnel* of the teaching faculties of our colleges, and it was regretted by the essayist that we must to such a large degree depend upon medical men for the education and instruction of our students. Probably this could not have been prevented in many of our institutions, yet I hope to see the time when we shall have at least one dental school in this country in which every member of the faculty will be a practicing dentist. I was made cognizant of a fact this morning which I have every reason to believe to be true, considering the source from which it came; that is, that it is impossible to trace thirty per cent. of the graduates of our schools beyond three years succeeding the date of their graduation. Now, if this be a fact, it seems to me that there is a responsibility of great moment to the profession resting upon the faculties of our colleges. What becomes of the thirty per cent. that disappears within three years of the date of their graduation? I do not attempt to say, but it seems to me that if our college men could realize what this great loss means, they would by some method keep a more constant and definite watch over their graduates. While in college the students are surrounded by men engaged in the same kind of work, and have also the encouragement of the faculty to keep them in line; but the moment they get out into the world an inherent weakness exerts itself, and they go down in the struggle for existence. I have long felt that there was one element lacking in the education and preparation of our students for professional work which should be strengthened. I mean the development of a higher moral sense. As a profession, and this I believe has been the leading thought of the paper, the one thing which we most vitally need is a higher appreciation of the professional value of integrity. "Moral integrity as a professional asset" should be so instilled into the mind of the student as to be the governing principle of his after-life. That is the purpose that should be constantly in the minds of our college teachers. They have very largely the molding of not only the present but of the future of our profession, and while we commend them for the great work they have accomplished in the development of our educational institutions and systems, still we must go forward, not only along the lines indicated by the essayist, but in the development of a higher and fuller appreciation of the value of the moral integrity of the men who are to practice in our profession.

This paper is valuable to us in that it holds up the best there is in our profession, and indicates that we are not only progressing in the right direction, but are progressing more rapidly than we oftentimes ourselves appreciate.

Dr. J. P. Gray, Nashville, Tenn. I wish to correct a mistake that I think Dr. Butler made in reference to students dropping out of sight. He evidently made a mistake when he said that thirty per cent. of them are lost sight of within three years after their graduation. I believe that seventy-five per cent. of the dentists stick to their profession—fully that many, if not more. I know that this has been the case with schools with which I have been connected, and you will probably find it to be true with others. At present we find more dentists that continue in practice after graduation than ever before in the history of our profession, and they are doing better work.

I want to thank Dr. McManus for speaking with reference to the teachers, bearing more particularly upon the moral condition of the students. I believe that this side is being more carefully considered every year by the teachers. They are realizing more and more the very great responsibility resting upon them in this respect, and the profession is now beginning to appreciate the good work that is being done by the schools. It is only a few years since everybody in the associations was censuring the schools, but today they are speaking kindly of the work that is being done, and I believe that the time is ripe, as the essayist says, for great progress to be made. The association can do much in this direction by sending a better class of men to us and encouraging men of ability to enter the profession, and giving them to understand that when they have finished their school work they are not perfect dentists, but have been given simply a foundation to stand upon, and that is the best we can do. They must not think continually of the money side of their work, of making money and of reaping riches from it. Dr. McManus will approve of the suggestion that the foundation must be laid in the schools, and that the superstructure must be built by the students afterward and by the encouragement of this body.

Dr. EDWARD C. MILLS, Columbus, Ohio. We have a dental library at Columbus which, in addition to being one of the most complete, has the distinction of being the pioneer of the many public libraries now scattered throughout the country. As secretary of our Library Association, I received an autograph copy of a pamphlet by Dr. James McManus, "Early Record of Dentists in Connecticut."

After perusing that pamphlet, I was impressed with the unselfish interest and vast amount of labor necessary to gather together all the data and information relative to those pioneers in our profession, and to place it in that permanent form for the use of some dental historian at some future date.

Besides hearing his valuable paper, it is an equally great pleasure for me to look upon an old Roman of the dental profession like Dr. McManus, who in spite of his years of toil for the interests of dentistry, still remains the embodiment of great physical strength and endurance. His recreation during a long professional career has been along such lines of work that his name will go down to posterity as the Nestor of dentistry in New England.

Among the many subjects referred to in his paper, one of great interest to us in Ohio is the matter of the Miller memorial. We are entirely in sympathy with this international movement. The great success attendant, and the conditions that have made possible the many triumphs of surgical art during the past

few decades is due in a large measure to two men from the ranks of our profession. These great benefactors to suffering humanity have transformed the operating room from a chamber of horrors into a place where one can lie down to pleasant dreams.

Memorials to Horace Wells and W. T. G. Morton were established some fifty years after their discoveries in anesthesia, at a time when anesthetics had come into such general use that the laity assumed them coeval with the practice of medicine, and the memorials did not do just honor to the discoverers. For these reasons, in order to do full honor to the memory of Dr. Miller, it seems important that immediate action be taken. The profession in Ohio will always feel a sense of pride in the fact that Dr. Miller was one of Ohio's sons, and his name will be added to the galaxy of names which our state has given to dentistry.

I do not hesitate to bring this matter to the attention of this association, especially since this meeting is held in the hospitable South, for which I feel a close affinity. It is with no small degree of pride that I state that in my veins flows the same blood as flowed in the veins of Daniel D. Emmitt, author of Dixie.

This association, I believe, is the representative body of our profession in America. Its deliberations are echoed and re-echoed through our subordinate or local societies from ocean to ocean. Speaking of our profession as an organism, this association is the heart; from its pulse-beat, and from the blood that flows through it, the entire profession receives its stimulation and life. It makes for the oneness and perfect unity of the entire body.

Our willing response to its appeals

welds into one harmonious unit the entire body of the profession, just as our patriotism and allegiance to a common flag tends to perfect our civic relations. The strongest link forged to bind forever the interests of the North and South was left to the indirect agency of Spain during the recent war. Spain being shorn of her rich and magnificent colonial possessions, which had been her pride in the days of her ascendancy, still held Cuba and a few patches of territory scattered about the world.

Her oppressive and unjust rule in Cuba precipitated the clash with the United States, and in spite of the prediction that a foreign war would cause a rupture between the North and South the sons of the veterans who wore the blue and of those who wore the gray marched together under General Joseph Wheeler to victory. There is no North, there is no South, except for geographical distinction.

You will remember the story of the three Americans at a dinner in Paris, toasting to their country. The first American said the United States is bounded on the north by the Dominion of Canada, on the south by the Gulf of Mexico, on the east by the Atlantic Ocean, and on the west by the Pacific Ocean. The second American, feeling that the first had rather a limited conception of the greatness of his country said that our country is bounded on the north by the north pole, on the south by the south pole, on the east by the rising sun, and on the west by the setting sun. The third American arose and was gratified to know that the last speaker had a more glorious conception of the magnitude of our country than the first, but to him the horizon seemed even yet too narrowly drawn. "Our great coun-

try," said he, "is bounded on the north by the aurora borealis, on the south by the precession of the equinoxes, on the east by primeval chaos, and on the west by the day of judgment."

Our great profession, as it has evolved from the mysticism of the past, is ever expanding in scientific knowledge, and its possibilities are unfolding proportionately to the demands made upon it by each succeeding generation.

In our onward march, some day we shall approach that western boundary where all science, and art, and religion shall have arrived at a state of perfect development; then we shall find that Willoughby Dayton Miller has contributed materially to the perfection of our noble science. Let us give him an international memorial; after that, gentlemen, let us give him a monument in America.

Dr. B. HOLLY SMITH, Baltimore, Md. I feel privileged to say a few words in regard to the able and entertaining paper read by our dear friend, Dr. McManus. I prize as the most delightful heritage of my professional career the recollection of incidents, experiences, and associations with the older members of the profession of dentistry—many of them have gone to their reward—men who were intimately associated with the distinguished essayist, and the sentimental references to incidents in the life of our association deeply touched and appealed to me.

At our meeting in Boston there appeared before the Executive Council some gentlemen who were not so familiar with the history of the organization of this association, and who talked ruthlessly and almost rudely about the reorganization of the National Dental Association, as if the association had failed of its mission, as though the life-work of these men of honorable repute, the sacrifices they have made for the perpetuation of this association, were for nothing. A proposition was made for such a reorganization of the National Association as would exclude all possible continuance of our delightful affiliation with the Southern Branch of the National. I saw some time ago that there had been a meeting of modistes, women who meet in council for the propagation of correct forms of dress, and it was suggested that it would be desirable for the ladies to resort to some surgical operation for the removal of the ear, because it was in the way of the high collar now coming into fashion, and they proposed to have the ear removed so that the collar might be extended above the usual location of the ear. It seems to me quite as reasonable— for our present body is the union of the American Dental Association and the Southern Dental Association, with all of the delightful reminiscences of the history of these two bodies—that we should propose to cut off our association with the Southern Branch.

Reminiscences of the history of this association bring me to a very tender consideration, one that the members of this association would perhaps not mind my mentioning. Among us, at almost every meeting, we have had for years a man whom we all love and who because of sickness has been prevented from attending our meeting this year—I refer to our beloved friend, Dr. Frank Holland—and I move that the secretary of this association be authorized to send to Dr. Holland the greetings of this association, with the information that we love him and that we miss him.

Dr. Smith's motion was carried unanimously.

Dr. EMORY A. BRYANT, Washington, D. C. Following my friend, Dr. Smith,

I wish to say a few words in regard to the movement to reorganize this association. When I came from the great West into the eastern part of our country I came for one purpose, and that was to try in my humble way, through my inventions and methods, to do something to aid in the progress of my profession. It was my one ambition, from my college days on to the present time, to do something in my professional work which should receive the recognition of my profession, to gain their esteem and to make a name for myself that would hold an honored place in the history of dentistry. Though I started practice in a mining camp in the Rocky Mountains under the worst conditions that could confront a young man beginning professional life, it did not dampen my ambition, and thinking I had invented something of interest, I traveled East to show my invention, and one of the first men to take me by the hand and encourage me in the work was Dr. McManus of Hartford.

Like others of the West, I concluded that the environment and the opportunities for professional advancement were better here, and I established myself in Washington, identified myself with the local society, and became a member of this organization as its delegate, with the idea that it furnished the associates and the opportunities to bring out the best in man for the benefit of all.

I gave clinics, read papers, and added to my inventions, bending every energy to accomplish the ends I had in view, when unfortunately political topics became involved and I found myself, much against my inclinations, compelled to shift my energies from legitimate professional progress into the whirlpool of dental society politics and organization jealousies, with their attending demoralization of the scientific and practical progress of our professional work, as well as of its workers.

Perhaps I might say, without being wrong, that for the past five or six years I have been engaged in a controversy that may not at the time have appealed to some of the members to be a matter of progress for the profession, but I wish to assure you that one idea has prompted my actions from the start to the finish, and that was, equal rights for all, special privileges for none. The effort to obtain what I have struggled for, as far as this organization is concerned, started at St. Louis some five years ago and ended at this meeting—that was, that every member of this association should receive equal consideration, the protection of its constitution as well as its penalties, and when matters of general or special interest were brought before this association which involved its membership as well as the dental profession throughout the country, that each member should receive the same consideration as any other member, and receive the same courtesies. While my professional life has also been involved, the principles enunciated have been the predominating feature of the fight I have made. We have practically gone around the circle, and while doing so have encountered those things that appear from time to time in every organization, creating little troubles that, as a stone thrown into still water produces little rings that spread out and grow into seeming billows, cause dissatisfaction with the advancment being made, produce ill temper, prejudiced actions, and apparently demoralization; but notwithstanding all this, we have made decided advances in the material work of our organization. Some of us wanted a re-

organization based upon the plan of the American Medical Association, to enlarge the influence, better conditions, and create better progress, just in the same spirit that the gentleman who preceded me reorganized the old American Dental Association and Southern into the present National organization. There has been no movement within my knowledge that has in any way tried to disparage the Southern Branch of the National Dental Association, or in any way to reduce its influence throughout the country. I have been charged with being in sympathy with such a move, but if you will read my letter in the *Items of Interest* of the last issue you will find my position fully stated, as well as my views upon adopting the proposed plan of the American Medical Association.

I am not impressed with the idea that the terms of a constitution are more essential than its observance after adoption, or that the success of the organization may be jeoparded by their close observance at all times. I say to those who are in control of our organization that if they will be considerate in their treatment of the younger members and not mix in local society squabbles, they will have no such antagonism as has permeated this organization for the past five years. I do not want to occupy too much of your time with my personal views, but before closing I wish to say a few personal things: I have always wished to work in harmony with this association, and when I have not done so it was because I was forced not to by circumstances over which I had no control. I have in the past said things that have been harsh, but the Lord knows I have had harsh things said against me and without justification. I have been forced to do things that I have been sorry for, and I have done things unthinkingly that I would have apologized for if given the opportunity to do so. Among other things, I have been fighting a fight for my professional life, and I have used every legitimate means and method of warfare at my command to gain my fight, for which I have no apologies to offer; and while I have been engaged in this battle I have to the best of my ability promoted everything that made for progress and the recognition of every member upon an equality. Now, I have done some missionary work through the issuance of a little journal that I published for four months—the *National Dental Critic*—to call the attention of the dental profession and the members of this association to its methods of proceeding along lines that to my mind were not proper. I did not do this with the intention of stirring up strife, but simply to call the attention of the association to matters which they could remedy themselves, and that have been remedied. At St. Louis an amendment to the constitution was offered, which was adopted at Buffalo by a small majority vote, excluding members of local associations from becoming members of this association. When the error of this was demonstrated, this amendment was amended to take in all the members of state societies. This has not fulfilled expectations, and now, with the adoption of the report of the Committee on By-laws, we will have gotten back to where we started—into troubled waters.

Now, let us get together and work to make this body a representative organization, put every shoulder to the wheel, forget our personal troubles, and work as a unit for the betterment of all. Let us proceed by the best methods, straightforwardly, honestly, and progressively,

that every man can freely lend his aid and encouragement to every action we may take. As I said before, I may have done things that were wrong; I may have taken actions that were severe, but I wish to say before sitting down that if I have ever hurt the feelings of any member of this association, I most humbly apologize for it. I wish to say that I want to work in harmony, and I hope that we can go onward without any more of these controversies that in the first place never should have been brought before this association.

Dr. TRUMAN W. BROPHY, Chicago, Ill. Just forty-two years and five hours ago I entered upon the study of dentistry in the city of Chicago, and I have witnessed with a great deal of interest the advancement of the profession since that time. It was my privilege to know many of the men whose names have been presented here today, and to gather from them inspiration that has assisted me in my work. I do not intend to enter into a discussion of the achievements of these men any more than to say that their lives have been to us a great heritage; they have furnished us with material, have enriched the literature of the profession, have enriched our lives by what they have achieved, and we are doubly grateful to them for what has been left us. The dental profession would be indeed very poor had it not been enriched by the lives of the great men that have gone before. Then I was only a boy, less than nineteen years of age, and today I find myself among those regarded as the aged members of the profession. At that time there were no colleges in the South and only one in the West, the one at Cincinnati. Today there are fifty institutions of dental learning in the United States. Then this association, which may be regarded as a continuance of the old American Dental Association, had only a few members. Today it is enlarged, but I believe that the usefulness of this body would be greater were the membership increased still more. In the city of Chicago we have a local society in which there are about eleven hundred members, and I see no reason why our National Dental Association should not have at least four or five thousand members, and I believe it should be increased to not less than five thousand members in a country where we have thirty-five thousand dentists engaged in practice. We have a disadvantage, however, in the fact that our country is so broad and so long that men cannot attend national meetings as readily as they can the local associations.

In conclusion, I want to pay tribute to my friend Dr. McManus, who has done so much to bring the dental profession prominently before the scientific world. There are probably young men here who do not know what I am about to state. Dr. McManus is the only man in this world who began and successfully carried through the movement toward having erected a monument to the memory of one of the greatest benefactors of the human family. It was Dr. McManus who took steps and pursued them so diligently that in the city of Hartford there stands in bronze a monument to Dr. Horace Wells, the discoverer of anesthesia, and I believe that I am right when I say that it is the only monument erected to a dentist in the world. But he has not finished his work, we are all glad to know, and as the years go on we may expect from him and from his distinguished son a rounding out to the full of the historical literature of our profession which we will all read, as years go by, with satisfaction and with profit.

Dr. McManus (closing the discussion). I hope that I can really give a slight idea of what my feelings are after listening to the many complimentary remarks that were made about me.

I wrote this paper at the request of our honored president. I did not want to do it, because I have done my share in the past, as some may realize from the remarks made by others, and I felt it was time that I should sit in the background and not offer any more papers before this association, but I could not refuse the request of our esteemed president. I did not know what to write about until I had the inspiration that I might be able to offer something of interest by throwing a side-light on the question of professional interest. I wrote the paper, and therein I have given my views, and I want to say that in this, as well as in every paper which I have presented before the association, I wanted to stay as near the truth as I possibly could, and for that reason I wish to make a correction in regard to one thing that I stated. My reason for making this correction is that I have received information this morning—and it was worth coming to this meeting to get that information alone—regarding the number of dentists in this country. I have said that there were forty thousand, but we have not so many in this country. It was a surprise to me to hear this, and it was also a surprise to hear regarding the number of dentists who in three years after graduation seem to drop out of professional life. That may partly account for the membership in the associations of the country being not larger.

I want to say that my object in writing this paper was to call attention to certain facts. In my past career I have tried to uphold as far as possible the action of the colleges, and I have never to my knowledge criticized them uncharitably, and never want to; but the time seemed to have come when it was proper to state some facts before this association, and I am happy to say that the character of the association this year and the number in attendance is a great surprise to me, and a very pleasant one. But, as I say, I wanted to state some facts regarding the work of the colleges, which I have felt of late years have not quite lived up to their opportunities. I do not care to criticize unless I have the facts, and I am now going to make some statements in regard to the colleges situated near where I live, in order to show you the lack of professional interest on the part of those connected with the colleges. Massachusetts has, according to Polk's Directory, 1862 dentists in the state, and 727 in the city of Boston, and I believe both of these statements to be very nearly accurate; these two colleges, one of which is a university that stands very high in regard to its demand for preliminary instruction and to the general character of its teaching corps, Harvard College, and Tufts College, have together considerably more than one hundred men connected with the teaching and demonstrating faculties, and yet in the entire state of Massachusetts in 1907 there were only twelve members of this association. Last year at the meeting held in Boston special efforts were made, and at that meeting forty-seven members of this association were present. That is the record of last year; out of 727 local dentists and 1862 practitioners in the state, forty-seven were members of the association. Does that show that the members of the profession and the professors and members of the teaching faculties are much interested? Any excuse they may make for not attending the meetings is of no avail when we look around here and see Dr. Black, Dr. Smith, Dr. Carr, Dr. Kirk, Dr. Patterson, and others who have come from long distances, as they have done in the years past, in order to attend these meetings. The men connected with the institutions of the country have not done their duty. However, I said in my paper, and I wish to emphasize it here today, that judging from the interest that was taken in the meeting last year, from the character of the meeting this year, and from the number in attendance. everything looks bright and prosperous for the future.

I have sat here and listened to the kind words spoken about me, and had it not been for the fact that Dr. Crawford in his remarks occasionally put his hand on my shoulder, I should have wondered who it was that he was complimenting so highly. I assure you, gentlemen, that I most highly appreciate what you have said, and I cannot express to you how much I value the kind treatment I have received from the members of this association from all over the country.

Management of the Teeth and Mouth from the Age of Six to Adolescence.

By L. G. NOEL, M.D., D.D.S.

BEING aware of the impossibility of properly covering so much ground in the time usually allotted to an essayist on an occasion like this, and realizing that I am addressing an audience that is not only well posted in the text-book and journalistic literature of this subject, but well acquainted with its manifold phases and difficulties through actual experience in practice, and knowing furthermore that this familiarity with the practical details of each division of this subject will necessarily render you very critical, I feel somewhat timid about presenting my own methods of practice; but I shall be content to be the subject of adverse criticism—yes, even ridicule—if in the discussion of this effort new light may come to some of us, and better methods of practice may follow.

I would refer you to a short paper in the January issue of the *Dental Brief* on "The Management of the Deciduous Teeth," which should be read in connection with this, and which brings us to the period of the eruption of the first permanent molars. This is a critical period, and the dentist will watch with interest the eruption of these first permanent molars, which, from their great importance as props to the jaws and as factors in determining the position of the other teeth, have been termed the *principal* molars.

The period of eruption of the first permanent molars is subject to some variation, but is usually about the sixth year or a little later than the sixth year— often as late as six and a half. This is the period given by that careful observer, Dr. Black,* who notes cases of wide variance, and mentions one case in which the four first permanent molars were in occlusion at four years of age. The teaching of Dr. Black's latest text-book in regard to the normal position and special function of these molars† is so valuable that I must call your attention to it, but time will not permit me to invade the field of orthodontia. I can only stress the great importance of correct occlusion of these molars, and cite the above-mentioned article, in which it has been so forcibly set forth.

The growth of the roots of the permanent teeth has been carefully studied by Dr. Black, by Dr. C. N. Peirce, and others,‡ and the work they have done on

* "Operative Dentistry," vol. i, pp. 259, 260.
† *Ibid.*, p. 263.
‡ *Ibid.*, pp. 258, 259. Also Burchard's "Dental Pathology and Therapeutics," p. 164.

this subject is a safe guide to the practitioner as to the possibilities of pulp-removal and root-filling in young subjects. The illustrations they have made to demonstrate root-growth should be indelibly fixed upon the memory; furthermore, they should be enlarged and hung up in every dental office for reference.

If children are placed under the care of a competent dentist (one who shall have charge of them without change or interference) it will generally be his fault if carious cavities become deep enough to cause the death of a pulp; for if he does his duty toward the child, he will insist upon seeing it often enough to fill all defective fissures and carious spots in the enamel sufficiently early to prevent pulp-irritation. His whole treatment and instruction should be directed to the maintenance of oral cleanliness and the prevention of decay. If this is accomplished—as I have seen in many cases—the dentist should not be called upon to essay the impossible either in root-filling or contour restoration, except in cases of accident or fracture, for all necessary operations will be simple and easy of accomplishment.

The stomatologist on whom is placed this sacred trust, the continuous care of the teeth of growing children, must be a man of experience and ripe judgment, not a faddist and experimenter.

CAVITIES IN FIRST PERMANENT MOLARS.

If the deciduous teeth have been properly cared for and oral cleanliness has been maintained, no caries should attack the mesial surfaces of the first permanent molars, but owing to structural defects we shall usually find the disease attacking the fissures of their occlusal surfaces, and sometimes the buccal pits of the lower molars.

Occlusal and buccal cavities. These cavities should be carefully excavated, and as a rule should be filled with the best obtainable cement. I am now experimenting cautiously with the silicate cements, and am at present favorably impressed with them in shallow non-sensitive cavities on the occlusal and buccal surfaces of these first molars. Many worthless zinc phosphate cements are now being sold as the *best,* some of which stain the teeth like amalgam if worked with steel instruments.

The experienced operator will know his material, and if there be much sensitivity of the dentin he will probably decide to fill these occlusal and buccal cavities of the first permanent molars with zinc oxyphosphate. The rubber dam should be adjusted, sensitive dentin coated with a suitable varnish, and the oxyphosphate allowed to set fully before removing the dam. The therapeutic effect of cements in these cases is to cause tubular calcification, an effect much to be desired before introducing gold fillings.

Mesial cavities. When the mesial surfaces of the first permanent molars require filling before the bicuspids have advanced sufficiently to obstruct access, it is the custom of many eminent practitioners to fill with gold when the child is manageable, urging this time as an opportunity to be eagerly seized before it is gone forever. Some eminent writers have not only urged filling with gold at this tender age, but have also recommended extension for prevention.

I should not expect to have one of my young patients return to me for another operation after such treatment, but this is not the chief reason for its being disapproved of.

The terminal nerve filaments are more sensitive at the dento-enamel junction than in any other portion of the dentin, and in placing a gold filling there at that tender age we run great risk of setting up pulp-irritation. The risk is greatly increased when the surface is extended. These spots of decay should be prepared if possible as simple cavities, *i.e.* without extension to the occlusal surface, and filled with either gutta-percha or cement, the usual care being taken to adjust the dam and to varnish the cavity if it is hypersensitive. For gutta-percha work a varnish of resin dissolved in chloroform will be found most useful, rendering the surface adhesive. For cement, cavitine or gum mastic may be used.

If, after six months or one year, a cement filling on one of these surfaces shows wasting, a gold filling may be substituted provided the patient is manageable and the access is good.

CAVITIES IN INCISORS.

Lingual cavities. The lingual pits in the upper lateral incisors may be defective, and require filling shortly after eruption. Here the excavation should be most carefully conducted, for there is much danger of exposing the pulp or of irritating it by a too near approach. A good cement is the safest material, and should be worked with the same caution as mentioned above.

Labial cavities. If proper care as to diet and oral cleanliness has been taken, we should not find caries on the labial or approximal surfaces of the incisors before the eruption of the canines, but alas, how often do we find that our warn-

ings have been disregarded! or it may be that the little patient comes to us for the first time for the treatment of cavities on these surfaces.

When the labial surfaces are carious, a carefully selected silicate cement will prove the most esthetic material, and— if our confidence be not misplaced—the most lasting. It must be remembered that these silicate cements are highly irritating to the pulp, and therefore the cavity should be varnished with cavitine, or some other good stainless varnish.

Approximal cavities. The dentist is sometimes greatly shocked when after a short interval his patient, over whom he thinks he is keeping watch and ward, returns with dangerously large cavities in the approximal surfaces of the incisors. Sometimes it is difficult to discover the cause or causes for this sudden destruction of tooth structure, but it will usually be traced to errors of diet and habits. It is generally traceable to over-indulgence in sweets, too much sugar in the food, too much syrup at table, and indulgence in candies between meals. Such habits encourage bacterial growths in the mouth, and favor the progress of caries; but inquiry will often disclose other and greater violations of hygienic laws, such as too much forcing at school, insufficient outdoor exercise, insufficient supply of oxygen in sleeping apartments, irregularity of meals, and indulgence in rich lunches between meals.

All these errors tend to vitiate the oral fluids, to favor bacterial growths, and to lower the vital resistance of the individual. It is the imperative duty of the dentist to seek out and correct these hygienic errors, for upon this will depend his future success in his practice with that family, and besides, to a great extent, their health and happiness.

These approximal cavities should be reached by forcing the teeth apart with rubber, tapes, cardboard, or wooden wedges, and the excavation should if possible be conducted so as to leave the enamel margins unbroken to protect the fillings from friction.

The cavities should be filled with gutta-percha, if they be hidden well from view, or with cement. If with the latter material, a colorless varnish like cavitine should be applied to the surfaces of the cavities before introducing the cement.

I have high hopes of the silicate cements, but they are new, and until they have been further tested should be used with great caution. My own experience leads me to consider them dangerously irritating to pulps, and knowing this, I am cautious to protect them with a varnish or a layer of zinc phosphate. Gutta-percha has a good record through many years of service, and when protected by the knuckling together of the teeth I have known it to stand for twelve or fifteen years.

Insist upon *frequent examinations.* The dentist should have an understanding with parents that the children shall be brought in for examination not less than four times per annum. These periods are best marked by the changing seasons. These opportunities for removing stains and bacterial plaques are to be seized with eagerness by the dentist, and he must not fail to correct faulty habits that in his judgment menace the welfare of the teeth and general health.

During this time, from the ninth to the twelfth year, the deciduous molars and canines are giving place to the bicuspids and canines, and the jaws are lengthening backward to give place to the permanent molars, while at the same time there is a general development of all the bones of the face.

At about the age of twelve we expect the second permanent molars to appear—contemporaries, as it were, of the canines.

FISSURE CAVITIES IN THE BICUSPIDS.

The bicuspids frequently present faulty occlusal fissures that early show signs of decay. These fissures should be carefully excavated as soon as decay is apparent, and should be filled with the best cement that can be obtained.

Here, again, I have high hopes of the silicate cements, and some cases which I have treated with this material show no perceptible wasting after a test of twelve months. Good oxyphosphate cements would probably show as well, and I do not consider this a decisive test.

At this age, many of our patients are sufficiently manageable for the introduction of gold or tin, but until the growth of the roots is complete, I prefer to combat caries with cements. The residence and circumstances of my patient might cause me to change materials. For those patients whose residence will permit the frequent examinations mentioned above, I prefer the cements.

THE MOST IMPORTANT AGE FOR CORRECTING IRREGULARITIES.

At about the age of twelve the canines and the second molars put in their appearance, and the dentist who has conducted the young patient thus far will be much concerned about alignment and occlusion.

Many cases will present irregularities of arrangement, calling for mechanical devices for correcting these defects, and mature judgment should first be sought, then prompt action taken to remedy such defects.

As before remarked, I do not propose to enter the field of orthodontia, but I must insist upon the importance of correct alignment and occlusion of the teeth, with the need of expanding some arches in order to obtain this, and urge the general practitioner to seek the aid of the specialist in difficult cases, to the end of health, usefulness, and beauty. This is perhaps the most important age for correcting defects of arrangement, and the opportunity should be considered most precious.

OCCLUSAL CAVITIES IN SECOND PERMANENT MOLARS.

The second permanent molars frequently present defects in their occlusal fissures, and in the buccal pits of the lower ones, that should be treated early with cement. The same reasons set forth in speaking of the bicuspids will apply here.

My desire to prevent deep and destructive caries is so strong that I frequently fill notably defective fissures with cement before these teeth are in occlusion, watching and re-filling more perfectly when it becomes possible to apply the dam.

The period from the twelfth to the fourteenth year requires extraordinary vigilance on the part of the dentist, for it is usually a period of rapid growth, of animal-like carelessness on the part of children, of abundant ropy saliva full of mucin—in short, a period presenting every condition that favors fermentation in the oral cavity.

PREVENTION OF DECAY.

Cement fillings are apt to be of short duration under these conditions, requiring frequent renewals. It is the duty of the dentist to make these things clear to parents, and insist upon regular attendance upon the dentist, aided by redoubled home care.

By these means we may be able to avert the disaster of approximal decay, but the dentist should be ever on the alert for evidences of the beginnings of enamel softening on the approximal points of contact. If detected early, it may be arrested by a thorough polishing with wood points or with fine strips applied so as not to flatten the points of contact, only removing the etched portions of enamel without cutting to the dentin or destroying the natural rotundity. This can only be accomplished with wood polishers and strips. Disks in the dental engine are sure to flatten the surfaces, inviting a recurrence of the trouble.

Incipient decay upon the enamel of the lower teeth, and in all situations out of sight, should, after such polishing as above described, be treated with silver nitrate. In treating approximal surfaces the dam should be applied and a saturated solution of silver nitrate applied with sufficient exposure to light to secure a deposition of silver upon the surface.

The age of puberty is, as a rule, early enough to commence gold operations—a rule admitting of some few exceptions—and these should be performed only upon such teeth as have about completed the growth of their roots. Strict adherence to this idea will, at first, almost limit gold fillings to the first permanent molars, for there will be few cases where we shall find it wise to use gold in the incisors.

Wasting cement fillings in the first molars may now be replaced with gold, and new cavities of moderate depth in these teeth may be treated in like manner.

Passing on to the age of fifteen and sixteen, we have to deal with years of similar susceptibility to dental caries, and our vigilance should never relax.

In spite of all our efforts, cavities will sometimes be found on the approximal surfaces of the incisors and canines, and on the approximal surfaces of the bicuspids. These cavities between the incisors and canines should be treated in the manner above described, filling them with gutta-percha or cements. Approximal cavities upon the bicuspids will usually have to be reached by cutting from the occlusal surfaces, and the preparation of such cavities should not be undertaken without first obtaining sufficient separation to get a good view of the surfaces involved. The softened area should be fully embraced in the cavities, which should be extended buccally, lingually, and gingivally until the area of safety is reached. If the teeth are hypersensitive they should be filled with cements guarded at the gingival margin with gutta-percha. These should be permitted to remain—under constant surveillance—until a wasting demands their removal, when they must be permanently filled with gold.

The treatment of hypersensitive cavities with cements, and with combinations of cements (zinc oxyphosphates) and gutta-percha, is worth all that it costs the patient in the beneficent effect produced upon the dentin and pulps of the teeth thus treated. Hyperemia of the pulp is thus allayed and tubular calcification of dentin is thus brought about, before the teeth are subjected to the shocks of thermal and electrical irritation induced by metallic fillings.

Eagerness to introduce a so-called permanent filling has caused the loss of many a tooth. Cavities on the distal surfaces of the second bicuspids and mesial surfaces of the molars will sometimes be met with as early as fifteen or sixteen, and later. These should have the same treatment as that outlined above.

If the teeth are hypersensitive, and the oral conditions are such as to seemingly favor rapid and destructive caries, they should be first treated with combination fillings, either of cement and gutta-percha or cement and amalgam. In lower teeth and when the filling is out of view, the latter is preferable.

Caries at from sixteen to eighteen years. Approximal decay is often met with in the molar teeth as early as sixteen to eighteen years of age. When the structure is markedly faulty, and caries is riotous in the mouth, the wise dentist who values his own reputation and his patient's teeth will follow about the same line of treatment as set forth above, with the exception that amalgam will probably be used as the permanent filling.

Buccal cavities in the molar teeth may be filled with gutta-percha until it is deemed wise to risk a permanent filling of amalgam or gold. Cavities on the contact surfaces of the second and third molars are usually best filled with amalgam, and occlusal cavities when they occur will generally be treated with the same material.

In speaking of cements and amalgams, I have been unable to refer to those which I have found reliable, time and space forbidding. Suffice it to say that many of the materials offered by dealers are worthless, and the dentist must *know* that he is using the best that can be obtained.

From eighteenth to twenty-first years.

From the eighteenth to the twenty-first year the dentist may replace with gold all cement fillings that are wasting or otherwise defective, provided conditions are such in his judgment as to warrant such procedure. Simple approximal cavities in the incisor teeth should be approached from the lingual aspect by first obtaining a free separation, then a slight beveling or planing away of the fragile enamel from the lingual margin. The labial enamel should be so conserved as to conceal the gold from view.

When possible—and this is so with all simple cavities—these approximal cavities should be filled with non-cohesive gold.

This is the time for permanent fillings of gold wherever indicated; for extension for prevention within reasonable limits when required, and for so-called permanent operations wherever plastics are found wanting.

Discussion.

Dr. T. P. HINMAN, Atlanta, Ga. I read with a great deal of interest this paper, and believe it to be one of the most valuable that has been offered to the association at this time. I agree with a great many of Dr. Noel's remarks, but in some respects I must say that I take the opposite view.

The necessity for the care of the teeth, especially of the first permanent molars, is an opinion with which I thoroughly agree. This is an old question that has been long under consideration; quizmasters used to ask, What is the best time to extract these molars? The answer today is, Never. It is of the utmost importance in every way, from the standpoint of orthodontia, mastication, and sanitation, that the first molars should be preserved. In reference to how this should be done, someone said the other evening that the child should be under the care of the dentist from the sixth to the sixteenth year. My practice is, when possible, just as soon as the deciduous teeth begin to appear in the mouth to request that the child be brought to the office. I think the deciduous teeth should receive as much attention or more than the permanent ones, because during the time of their usefulness the formative period of the child is taking place, and unless the child has the proper organs of mastication we cannot expect health. But the question is, how to do this. The method I have used, and one which I understand is in vogue in the practice of other men, is to have what we term a call-list, which is simply a book in which are kept the names of all patients and children in alphabetical order. For instance, if a certain child is to be called in the month of May, and if that child's name begins with "H" it is put under "H," and the word "May" is put after it. At the proper time the assistant writes a card to the parent, calling attention to the fact that the child is due at the office at a certain time, and the day and hour is designated. In this way the patients are seen in some instances once in two months; all of them are seen four times a year, and in that way I have been able to bring children from about the second year up to the twelfth or fourteenth or sixteenth years with scarcely a cavity occurring in the mouth. If care is taken of them during this period, and oral hygiene insisted on, it is really astonishing how much can be obtained by this method. You cannot depend on the mother or the parents of the child to bring them to the office. It does not make any difference how strongly you impress this on their minds, they will simply forget it, but if you send them a positive engagement for a certain hour, you find that you will be able to give more care and attention to the deciduous and permanent teeth during this period than by any other method.

Something was said last night with reference to educating the public in reference to oral hygiene. To my mind there is only one way to do that. It is very beautiful to have this brought before us in the way it was, but to my mind the only practical way to do this is for the individual dentist to teach the individual patient oral hygiene; then it will be disseminated. Therefore, in the care of children's mouths and in the care of the teeth, I instruct the parents how to take care of the teeth, and if they realize the necessity of this as fully as they should, good results can be obtained in all instances.

The essayist had something to say on the subject of the silicate cements. Many hailed this as the panacea for all dental ills, and I began using it and thought from the results obtained at first that we had at our command a material that would take its place in our professional work, but unfortunately for me—possibly it may have been on account of my unsuccessful use of the cement—the percentage of failures in the use of silicate cement was so great as to make me absolutely abandon it. That is my individual experience, and the observations I have made in the mouths of patients coming from other cities, seeing the work of other operators who use silicate cements, absolutely confirm what I have just stated. One of the first things I noticed in regard to the silicate cements is the fact that they will discolor in proportion to the amount of

pigment that is in the cement. In other words, a perfectly white silicate cement does not discolor in the potassium sulfate solution, but just in proportion to the amount of pigment that enters into it does the silicate cement discolor in the potassium sulfate solution. Again, the question of the danger to the pulp arises: If the cavity is large and the silicate cement is brought into close proximity to the pulp, it will certainly devitalize the latter.

I do not believe in the use of cement *per se* as a filling material in approximal cavities in incisors. I may say that I have practically abandoned the use of cements alone as a preservative agent. I prefer inlays in most cases. I may be a crank on inlay work, but I prefer inlays. I have been asked how I treat approximal cavities in incisors at the age of ten years, and I simply say that I want to produce a permanent operation there, and that it has therefore been my practice for the last five years to make permanent porcelain inlays in these teeth, and the results I have obtained seem to justify this procedure.

The use of a cavity lining, especially under silicate cements and amalgams, I believe to be an admirable thing, but instead of using cements in small cavities in the coronal surfaces of molars it seems better practice and insures a more permanent operation to use amalgam. Gutta-percha also can be used in some instances, although I use it very little. In the lingual pits of incisors, gutta-percha is sometimes indicated in early life because of the fact that it is so easy to expose the pulps in these cavities. In some of these cavities, if we are not careful, we penetrate into the pulp before we know it. The filling of fissures in the coronal surfaces of the bicuspids I believe is best accomplished by the use of non-cohesive gold for a permanent operation. The operation is not so severe as to produce shock in the pulp. If there is a deep cavity the bottom should be lined with cement, and over this the gold should be used, in this way preventing reaction from thermal changes. This seems the best practice along this line.

I believe that frequent polishing of the teeth is necessary for their care from the sixth to the sixteenth year or to adolescence, also a careful regimen for their cleansing during this period. One thing for which I have to thank my friend Dr. Kells, has been of great benefit to me in caring for these teeth during this time, and that is the use of plain simple lime-water. By the thorough cleansing and polishing of the teeth when you see indications between the incisors of discoloration that will eventually become decay because of one of those little gelatinous plaques that Dr. Miller speaks of, by the careful separating of the teeth and thoroughly polishing with strips of linen covered with pumice, you can practically polish out a great many cavities; then use lime-water at least three times a day. You will find in many cases where you use the lime-water that you will obtain better results. I believe that in many cases where we see white decay the frequent use of lime-water will arrest this decay.

A MEMBER. How do you use it?

Dr. HINMAN. Brush the teeth and rinse the mouth with it.

A MEMBER. Swallowing a certain amount too?

Dr. HINMAN. A certain amount is absorbed, but I believe that from direct contact of the lime-water in the mouth the enamel absorbs a certain amount, and in proof of that I wish to tell you this incident, which goes to prove to a certain extent that the enamel absorbs lime-water. Dr. Head put two incisor teeth in orange juice and kept these in the incubator for forty-eight hours, after which time he found that the enamel had to a certain extent softened; but when the teeth were taken out of the orange juice and put into normal saliva which contained a certain amount of calcium salts, the enamel re-hardened. I do not say that this is true, but why not?

In the treatment of approximal cavities in bicuspids and molars, I do not believe in gutta-percha or cement at the cervical border, but prefer the practice of partially filling the cavity with cement and then restoring the proper contour with amalgam, thoroughly polishing, and in this way obtaining a perfect preservation of the tooth by the cement covered with amalgam.

Dr. G. S. TIGNOR, Atlanta, Ga. In commending this paper to the members of the association I shall not take issue with anything that has been outlined in the methods of practice, nor shall I take issue with anything that has been said in the discussion, but I wish to state that the methods as outlined in this paper are excellent, and that some of the methods Dr. Hinman spoke of in his discussion are no less so.

Dr. Osler was asked on one occasion what to his mind produced more permanent damage to the constitution, the use of alcohol in maturity or the neglect of teeth in childhood, and he answered unhesitatingly. "Aching teeth in childhood." That must be true, because there is nothing of consequence that can be accomplished by anyone who is suffering with toothache. It is impossible for the constitution to develop as it should in childhood when the patient is subject to toothache night after night, and if we secure the adoption of methods such as Dr. Hinman has outlined, of having youthful patients see us early and often, and systematically, we can prevent this trouble. I have never had toothache in my life, owing to the fact that I was born in a family of dentists, and my relatives who have practiced for us have always seen us early and often in order to prevent any trouble that might have arisen.

I have a few patients that have been in the hands of some Boston and Canada dentists all their lifetime, and these children have never experienced such a thing as toothache. It is simply a delight to practice for those who have enjoyed this care from our profession.

I wish to bring out the fact that if we are to make progress in the practice of dentistry, here is the field in which we can accomplish it. For fifty years we have made improvements in the replacement of lost dentures, filling teeth, and restoration by crowns and bridges; but we can prevent the greater portion of this trouble. The greatest difficulty is to induce the children to come to you. This can be accomplished by the adoption of a systematic method such as Dr. Hinman speaks of, and should we fail in this, we then can do no more than display our skill in artistic replacement by artificial dentures.

Dr. Noel (closing the discussion). I have only a few words to say in closing the discussion, and these few words should have been written as a preface to the paper. I apprehended that you would probably misunderstand my object in treating the subject in the manner adopted. My whole object was to emphasize the importance of caries of the teeth, and our ability to prevent it, for I believe that there is no disease that is so preventable as caries. My entire object was to emphasize the importance of seizing every opportunity for minimizing the cutting and destruction of tooth-structure. Some years ago, Dr. Flagg, endeavoring to impress this idea upon the profession, referred to the fact that wherever cement fillings are used in a cavity, there is only the waste of the filling material itself, and that we should realize that tooth-structure is valuable and precious, but that filling material is abundant and cheap. This is the idea that I wished to present to you: By treatment with cements, as I have practiced it for a number of years and as I have set forth in the paper, you save tooth-structure. By treating cavities in the manner described and temporarily bringing about tubular calcification, and especially during the childhood period, when it is difficult to do even that much, you can accomplish something for the patient without entirely demoralizing him, probably to such an extent that you could do nothing else for him. Minimize the operation of extension for prevention at that age with a view to putting in large gold fillings later on! In that way I believe we can accomplish something, instead of inserting inlays, when we must necessarily sacrifice large amounts of tooth-structure, which I certainly should never advocate in the treatment of young patients.

I wish to thank you for the kindly manner in which my paper was received and for the attention given to it.

Doctor of Dental Science.

By W. STORER HOW, D.D.S.

INDIVIDUAL self-certified medicators, surgicators, and denticators, as crude and rude practitioners, were evident in Egypt and India millenniums ago, but ages elapsed ere the authorized distinction of "Doctor" became a title of honor for the learned, irrespective of the function of communicating knowledge. "The word had long been used, even in the universities, as a general expression for teachers, ere it came to designate a degree or rank in the learned hierarchy to which only the united body of the teachers could advance or promote the candidate. Then formal promotions commenced at Bologna in the eighteenth century. In later times the title 'Doctor' has been applied almost everywhere to the three faculties of theology, law, and medicine."

The early practitioners of medicine and surgery were lower in rank than the members of the theological and legal professions, and when in modern times the new title of honor was becoming, those doctors unbecomingly refused to dentists recognition as fellow alleviators of the ills to which humanity is heir.

A brief relative consideration, however, will show the medical doctor to be principally a prescriber, who depends upon the patient's *vis viva* to do the healing.

The surgical doctor, while a positive personal agent in many operations, also must depend upon the patient's recuperative powers; his chief field of practice is comprised in destructive extirpations and dismemberments, after which the excised organs cannot be renewed, and the lost limbs the surgeon cannot replace, but leaves the rescued wreck to the inventive skill and ingenuity of the surgical substitutioner.

In the beginning of dentistry the initial operations were somewhat surgical; hence when the incontestably professional sanction of a dental college graduation was achieved, the American degree of Doctor of Dental Surgery was publicly conferred on commencement day, with the indicative abbreviation of D.D.S., in a diploma couched in the Anglo-American language.

Thenceforward, leaving physic to the other doctors, the domain of physics has been explored by the postgraduate with professional enthusiasm, studious learning, constructive skill, and an inventive ingenuity that has raised the dental doctor to the plane whereon he now stands as the pre-eminent professional prosthetist; for he replaces destroyed teeth-crowns and the singly or serially lost dental organs of one or both jaws, with artificial restoratives which are simulating substitutes in lifelike appearance, conformation, and their preparatory working operations as providing for bodily sustenance, speech, and song! He might therefore be termed Doctor of Dental Substitution.

There is yet further distinction in prospect, for the prophet surely foresees the future graduate dentist professionally in continuous serial supervision from the natal to the mature and terminal periods of human life; so that the conforming parents' progeny as patients, or in person, may practically possess, employ, and enjoy an efficient and a comely natural denture uninterruptedly—excepting, of course, loss or defacement by systemic or regional lesions, surgical operations, neglect, or local casualties.

Aberrant variations in dental developments may be orthodontially corrected, and incidental defects be rectified, without infraction of this conditional optimistic prophecy.

Therefore, taking into the account the combined and correlated prescriptive, surgical, operative, restorative, orthodontic, prosthetic, and stomatological professional functions, and generally learned qualifications of the constructive, inventive, accomplishing, and duly providentially endued D.D.S., he or she is justly entitled to be honored with the specific distinctive designation, Doctor of Dental Science.

At present there are fifty-five colleges and university dental departments in the United States conferring dental degrees under various titular designations. But the actual achievements and inventions —headed by original anesthesia—which have related and systematized real knowledge as an operative and applicable fundamental equipment for the positive professional control and doctoring of all dental diseases and disorders, requires and justifies the appellation Dental Science.

The book, journalistic, and contributory literature is voluminous, the American dental journals numbering twenty-one. One, the *Dental Cosmos*—"a monthly record of dental science"—is now in the second half-century of its honorable forecast and advocacy of dentistry as a *science*.

The National, Southern, state, and local dental associations aggregate eighty, one already termed "The American Society of Dental Science."

Who can imagine to what refinement of physical personal restoration, correction, prevention, substitution, and developing supervision the skilled scientific dental specialist may, by the grace of God, attain, and be found having on his hands the active organs of human life ingesta, and also of soul and spirit utterances, as a benefactor of his kind in its infancy, youth, maturity, and to old age, through ages to come! Why should not such special and successful scientist be deemed worthy of this honorably won collegiate degree, Doctor of Dental Science?

The studious, practical, self-experimental demonstrator of blessed anesthesia, Dental Doctor Horace Wells, 1844, caused the famous historian Lecky to write: "It is probable that the American inventor of the first anesthetic has done more for the real happiness of mankind than all the moral philosophers." He might well have included all of the physic, and physical philosophers, since Dr. Wells made tributary all future practitioners in every specialty of human healing and life-saving professional scientific service the world over;

the Doctor of Dental Science standing at the head as the saving stomatologist of a kindred and aching humanity!

He is professionally master of both the natural and artificial masticatory means for man's manually made maintenance, while also professionally providing for the proper pronouncing of the products of man's mental manufactory for those wonderful words of soul and spirit life which are the gracious gifts of God by His Son and Holy Spirit.

There appears in the Standard Dictionary, a "List of Degrees conferred by Colleges, Universities, etc." There are two hundred and twenty-five degrees, indicative initials, titles, and term courses: several titles are alternative; as D.M.—M.D., Doctor of Medicine; D.S.—Sc.D., Doctor of Science. The list contains sixteen degrees of Science, as shown in the following table:

have continued national; and now, Doctor of Dental Science may become so, superseding all the others, and retroactively be made exchangeable for them equitably.

CONCERNING "SCIENCE."

Broadly viewed, Science is: "Knowledge gained and verified by exact observations and correct thinking, especially as methodically formulated and arranged in a rational system." "Science is any department of knowledge in which the results of investigations have been worked out and systematized."

"Absolute science: Definite knowledge of things as they actually exist." "Abstract science: Theoretical knowledge—pure science." "Active science: Systematic knowledge put to actual use." (Stand. Dict.)

The modern, original, singular, hu-

Degrees of Science.

B.A.S.[1] ....Bachelor of Applied Science.			
B.A.S.[2] .... " " Agricultural Science.			
B.B.S. .... " " Business " 4 years.			
B.C.S.[1] .... " " Chemical "			
B.C.S.[2] .... " " Commercial "			
B.L.S. .... " " Library "			
B.N.S. .... " " Natural " 4 "			
B.Sc. .... " " Science.			
D.S.—D.Sc.—Sc.D. ....Doctor of Science. 4			
D.Sc.D. .... " " Science and Didactics.			
Dr.Nat.Sc. .... " " Nat. Science, European.			
Dr.Phy.Sc. .... " " Physical Science.			
D.V.S. .... " " Veterinary " 3			
M.S.[1] ....Master of Science.			
M.S.A.[2] ....Mistress of Science and Arts.			
M.L.S. ....Master of Library Science.			

The absence of Medical Science and of Surgical Science is noteworthy at this date, 1909.

Obviously the original American degree, Doctor of Dental Surgery, should

mane Dental Science, is systematic knowledge put to professional positive humane actual use by dental college graduates, "actually existent" and qualified to consider the condition of dental organs

Dental Degrees.

D.D.S.	Doctor of Dental Surgery.	3 years.
D.M.D.	" " " Medicine.	3 "
L.D.S.	Licentiate of Dental Surgery.	3 "
M.D.S.	Master " " "	3

in the mouths of patients, to competently determine what is needful, and to promptly personally perform the skilled scientific service.

In what other professional vocation is the operative and laboratory equipment so inclusive of aids, appliances, apparatus, instruments, contrivances, constructions, chemicals, correctives, medicaments, materials, anesthetics, substitutes, and curative adjuncts as are immediately at hand and requisite for the personal practice of up-to-date Dental Science. It is a far cry from the old surgical screaming sacrifice of hollow or sound teeth, to the new, soothing scientific service which renders salvable any tooth or root requisite for a useful and beautifying denture.

Prof. Elisha Townsend, D.D.S., dean of the Philadelphia College of Dental Surgery, in his eloquent commencement address to the graduates of 1854 (like his prophet namesake) foresaw and foretold the future of the new profession when he said: "Dentistry is usually spoken of as a branch of the great healing art, but in point of fact it has grown, not out of the stem, but up from the root of the tree of *remedial science*— Doctor of Dental Surgery is a comparatively new patent of nobility in the heraldry of *science*. Our profession has advanced from a sheer chaos to the form and order of a regular systematic art; so founded upon *principles,* and so justified by *experience,* as to entitle it to the character of *an integral science.*"

That distinguished doctor's jubilant forecast waited half a century for the jubilee of that graduate class to give occasion for a formal proposal that thenceforward the graduate D.D.S. should be honored with the title "Doctor of Dental Science."

The present comprehensive and practical program of the thirteenth annual meeting of the National Dental Association is adduced as evidence, cumulative with the scientific comprehensive curricula of the fifty-five dental collegiate American institutions, that the degree of Doctor of Dental Science should become the honorable and trustworthy title of every duly and legally qualified graduate.

Dean Townsend declared that the graduate should "Keep steadily before him the connection of *all the departments of physical and remedial science which our own involves,* and depends upon for its completeness and further progress."

Dr. Maurice H. Richardson of Boston, addressing the National Dental Association meeting in Boston, July 28, 1908, said in conclusion:

"We think that the dental profession, like all other professions, is most productive of good when it is most liberal in its education, and when the degree of D.D.S. should rest, in both theory and practice, upon a broad foundation, not only of medicine and surgery, but of the *arts and sciences.*"

"In behalf of President Eliot and Harvard University, and on the part of the Harvard Medical School, I extend to you our cordial greetings and good wishes."

With this courteous and highly authoritative advanced professional indorsement of the proposed degree, it awaits only collegiate and legislative realization. All hail, Doctor of Dental Science, D.D.Sc., *in futuro!* Then he may stand up for his calling as being in an eminent degree, also G.G.L.—Guardian of the Gateway of Life!

SECTION I:

Prosthetic Dentistry, Crown and Bridge Work, Orthodontia, Metallurgy, Chemistry, and Allied Subjects.

Chairman—H. E. KELSEY, Baltimore, Md.
Secretary—J. S. SPURGEON, Hillsboro, N. C.

SECOND DAY—Wednesday, March 31st.

IN the absence of the chairman, the first meeting of Section I was called to order by Dr. H. H. Johnson, Macon, Ga., at 10 o'clock A.M., Wednesday, March 31, 1909.

The first order of business was the reading of a paper by Dr. GEO. H. WILSON, Cleveland, Ohio, entitled, "The Principles of Retention of Artificial Dentures," as follows:

The Principles of Retention of Artificial Dentures.

By GEO. H. WILSON.

THE retention of artificial dentures is purely mechanical and is based upon the laws of physics. Indirectly, however, the personal equation is an important factor, in that the patient may not be able to control the laws of physics. These vexatious cases are often spoken of as awkward or clumsy, but such patients will eventually succeed in overcoming the difficulties provided they have sufficient perseverance.

The physical laws that play a more or less important rôle in the retention of artificial dentures are atmospheric pressure, adhesion by contact, leverage, tenso-friction, and adhesion or cementation. These forces are not equal in value, nor can any one principle be depended upon for retaining a denture. There will be a primary principle selected to bear the burden, and one or more secondary forces evoked or unwittingly included. These secondary forces may be either positive or negative. Thus atmospheric pressure may be selected as the primary retentive force, but adhesion by contact must be an associate retentive force whether it be so designed or not, and eventually will entirely take the place of atmospheric pressure in any given case. The principle of leverage is always associated, through antagonization, with whatever may be the primary method selected. This force especially may be considered as positive when the arrangement of the teeth is such that it tends to force the denture more securely to place, and as negative when the arrangement is such that antagonization tends to loosen the denture.

To consider this subject in its entirety would require too lengthy a paper, therefore we shall define these five physical laws as applicable to prosthesis, and consider some of their practical applications.

ATMOSPHERIC PRESSURE.

As is well known, atmospheric pressure is the weight of a column of air resting upon an object. The weight of a column of air at the sea level is 14.7 pounds to the square inch, and decreases in the ratio to the height above sea level. As this pressure is equal in every direction upon and within the human body it is not perceptible. Whenever a portion of this column of air is removed from a circumscribed portion of the body, its effect is immediately felt. No substance can be placed between the atmosphere and the surface, or a portion of the surface of the body, and remove the pressure of the atmosphere from the body, as the intervening substance, being contiguous, would be held against the surface of the

body by the full weight of the column of air resting upon it. Thus we may justly conclude that an artificial denture perfectly adjusted to the tissues of the mouth would be retained by the full weight of the column of air, or approximately fifteen pounds for each square inch of surface covered; also that a chamber cut in the maxillary surface of the plate would be a positive detriment, because it would be an air-chamber equalizing the column of air upon the external surface of the plate to the extent of the air-chamber. However, there is a fatal obstacle to this perfect retention of an artificial denture, for it is a physical impossibility to exclude the film of air between the soft tissues of the mouth and the hard base-plate except by substituting a fluid for the film of air. By this substitution of a fluid for the film of air the law of hydrostatics is introduced. The law of hydrostatics is, that a pressure placed upon a confined liquid is equal in every direction. Therefore a mechanically perfectly adapted artificial denture having a fluid contact cannot be so retained, because the intervening fluid equalizes, within and without, the atmospheric pressure.

Atmospheric pressure *may be utilized* to retain an artificial denture, but through the medium only of a vacuum chamber. Since an absolute vacuum is an impossibility, the amount of retention by atmospheric pressure is contingent upon the square surface of the chamber and the vacuity obtained. To produce any degree of vacuity it is necessary to have the plate surrounding the vacuum cavity perfectly adapted to the soft tissues. The extent of exhaustion of the air from the chamber is governed by the power of the muscles of the tongue and the ability of the patient to apply them. The exhaustion is produced by forceful swallowing.

Retention by atmospheric pressure can only be temporary, and maintained only so long as there is a partial vacuum. The effect of the vacuum chamber upon the tissues of the mouth is the same as cupping in medical practice. As soon· as the atmospheric pressure is reduced upon a circumscribed portion of the body, it acts as an excitant, causing an increased blood pressure in the part, with a temporary swelling, and if continued a proliferation of tissue cells, producing a permanent growth until the chamber is filled. When the chamber is filled by tissue and the fluids of the mouth, atmospheric pressure can no longer exist; the denture is then retained only by adhesion by contact. While the term "suction plate" is not so euphonious as "atmospheric pressure plate," it more nearly expresses the truth without attempting an explanation of how the suction is secured.

As the amount of retention of a vacuum chamber stands in direct ratio to its square surface, so its relative permanence and its injurious effects stand in direct ratio to its depth.

ADHESION BY CONTACT.

This retentive force is too often confused with atmospheric pressure, whereas it is an entirely different principle. Atmospheric pressure retention is contingent upon a chamber which is more or less evacuated of air, while adhesion by contact is conditioned by uniform pressure and absolute contact. To comprehend this principle of retention, the molecular forces of attraction and repulsion must be appreciated. These two molecular forces, to a greater or less extent, exist within and between all bodies. In solid matter attraction predominates over repulsion, whereas in liquids the two forces are equal, and in gaseous matter repulsion predominates over attraction. Attraction is always stronger between like atoms than between unlike atoms. (This last fact is beautifully illustrated in the low-fusing alloys composed of tin, lead, bismuth, and cadmium. These metals range in fusing point from 442° F. to 617° F., yet when they are properly combined they may fuse at 135° F., thus demonstrating that the molecules of these metals create a marked repulsion for each other, and that it takes but a low degree of heat to render attraction and repulsion equal, that is, to fuse to a liquid state.) When like atoms are brought into atomic relation to each other, they are said to be held together by cohesion; when the interatomic space is exceeded, they can only be held together by adhesion, either by mass attraction or an intervening adhesive substance. Thus it is apparent that the expression "uniform pressure" and "absolute contact" are misnomers, because absolute contact is an impossibility; but when these terms are used, they signify the closest mechanical contact of the mass, and do not refer to the atom relationships. When masses of matter are brought into mechanical contact and are caused to adhere by a film of non-adhesive fluid, it might be thought that the adhesion is due to the strength of the fluid, but this is not the case, because the thinner the film the greater the adhesion. That this adhesion is not due to atmospheric pressure can be demonstrated by suspending two masses of matter adhering by contact in the chamber of an air-pump and exhausting the air, when the adhesion will remain the same as under normal atmospheric conditions. Therefore, through an understanding of these axioms regarding attraction and repulsion, we can appreciate how artificial dentures are retained by the so-called adhesion by contact.

LEVERAGE.

In mechanics the lever is a rigid bar working upon a pivot. The pivot is called the fulcrum, and the bar is considered as two portions called arms—the one called the power arm and the other the work arm. There are three groups of these factors, fulcrum, power, and work arms, called classes. In the first class the fulcrum is between the power and the work, whereas in the second class the work is between the fulcrum and the power; in the third class the power is between the fulcrum and the work. In prosthetic dentistry the lever of the first class only need be considered, and it is of great importance. This principle of physics is involved in every case of prosthetic restoration, either in its positive or negative sense, and too often in both. In complete artificial dentures the alveolar ridge constitutes the fulcrum, and the retention of the base-plate by either atmospheric pressure or adhesion by contact constitutes the power; the portion of the base-plate upon which these retentive forces exert their influence constitutes the power arm. The teeth form the work arm, and antagonization is the work. In partial artificial dentures the remaining natural teeth and roots may be the fulcrum or even fulcrums.

The law governing the direction of energy should be taken into consideration. The law is: Energy moves in a straight line and at right angles to the surface from which the force emanates. Thus in the lines of energy there may be great resistance, while laterally there would be but slight resistance. (This is well illustrated by two plates of glass held together by adhesion by contact, which will offer much resistance to an effort to pull them directly apart, but only slight resistance to lateral pressure.)

The anatomical relation of the mandible to the maxilla is a peculiar one, and offers many problems in physics. As resorption of the alveoli progresses, these adverse conditions become exaggerated. Therefore it follows that artificial substitutes should be inserted soon, that is, within a few weeks—two to six—after the removal of the natural teeth. As the resorption of the alveolar processes progresses, the summit of the alveolar ridge of the upper jaw recedes upward and inward, whereas the summit of the alveolar ridge of the mandible recedes downward and outward. Hence, if the artificial teeth are set in the position occupied by the natural teeth, the problems in leverage become very serious. It is apparent that if the upper teeth could be arranged with their buccal surfaces just inside the summit of the alveolar ridge, it would be impossible to dislodge the base-plate by direct occlusion, no matter how hard or circumscribed the bolus of food; but as it is not practical to so arrange the teeth, it is desirable, from a mechanical point of view, to approach this condition as nearly as the individual case will permit. If, after the alveoli have thoroughly receded, the upper artificial teeth are mounted upon the base-plate in their normal distance from the rhaphe, the work arm of the lever is relatively much lengthened. Therefore to overcome this untoward leverage, the teeth are drawn in toward the summit of the ridge. There is a limit to the inward drawing of the lingual surface of the teeth, for undue encroaching upon the domain of the tongue will ensue. That this work arm may be still further shortened, the artificial teeth bucco-lingually are made narrower than normal. As the shortening of the radius shortens the circumference of a circle, it becomes necessary to select artificial bicuspids and molars a little narrower mesio-distally than the natural teeth which they replace. This is but one of the reasons for the reduced size of the grinding teeth. The other reason for reducing the size of these teeth has to do with their power, and should not be discussed together with the principles of retention. We have already stated that motion—force—moves at right angles to the surface from which the motion emanates, therefore the shaping of the facets of the occlusal surface of the bicuspids and molars is an important factor in the problems of leverage.

TENSO-FRICTION.

This term is used to cover all those cases where retention is obtained by contact, but the surface of contact is too insignificant to constitute a factor. It includes all forms of clasps, removable plate-bridge attachments, spiral springs, and spring plates. It implies that the retention is obtained by friction through tension. The simplest form of tenso-friction is the spring clasp, in which the narrow strip of metal grips a tooth by friction through the tension in the metal. Further than defining this term, we will not discuss it, as it is in itself a subject for a lengthy paper.

ADHESION OR CEMENTATION.

This term is used to denote that an adhesive substance, as cement, is used as the means of retention. All kinds of fixed bridge work and the so-called "alveolar dentistry" are in this class. This phase of retention will not be further discussed in this paper.

PRACTICAL APPLICATIONS.

It is often said that the difficulties of retention of artificial dentures are in direct ratio to the number of teeth supplied. Broadly speaking this is true. In the remainder of this paper we shall confine ourselves to edentulous jaws and to the first two methods of retention—namely, atmospheric pressure and adhesion by contact. Leverage has to do with the arranging of the teeth upon the baseplate, and antagonization therefore will not be discussed. Thus we have reduced our subject to the consideration of the retention of base-plates upon edentulous jaws.

There are four factors to be considered in the retention of base-plates: Size—that is, the amount of surface covered; soft tissue; fluids of the mouth; and, of the least importance, the shape of the portion covered.

Size. In any given case the amount of retention by adhesion by contact is, like atmospheric pressure, according to the area of the surface. Hence, other things being equal, the larger the denture the better the retention.

Soft tissue. No one factor has so much to do with retention of artificial dentures as the soft tissues. These may be divided into three classes—muscles and their attachments, submucous tissue, and the mucous membrane. As an axiom it may be stated that a base-plate cannot rest upon a muscle which impinges upon or draws over the periphery of the plate, as the contractile power of the muscle is greater than the retentive force of ad-

6

hesion by contact. The muscle attachments should always be observed in examining the mouth prior to taking the impression; then, in taking the impression, the muscles should be marked in the impression, so that the base-plate may secure a close adaptation about the muscle attachments and yet not be dislodged thereby. As adhesion by contact is in the ratio to the surface covered, it is apparent that the base-plate should extend as far in every direction as the attachment of the muscles will permit, but not so far that the muscles when placed upon their greatest tension will impinge upon the periphery sufficiently to dislodge it. This may give a very irregular outline, but the proper outlining of the periphery of the base-plate is one of the important operations in adapting artificial dentures. Beginning in the median line, the labial flange of the upper base-plate should be well cut away for the labial frenum, then gradually ascend to the canine eminence, where for cosmetic effects it must be as high as possible. After forming the outline of the canine eminence, the border of the flange abruptly drops to accommodate the buccal frenum or levator anguli oris. The remainder of the border to the tuberosity must be kept as high as the attachment of the buccinator muscle will permit. In passing around the tuberosity, if there be one, the edge of the base-plate must not impinge too much upon the soft tissues. After trimming the base-plate to what seems to be the proper outline, it should be tested by moistening the maxillary surface, placing in the mouth, and instructing the patient how to exhaust the air from between the base-plate and soft tissues upon which it rests. The patient should then be requested to vigorously work the mus-

cles of the lip and cheeks, and see if in any way the base-plate can be dislodged. If so, the patient should again attach the base-plate, the operator grasping the lip and cheeks, one portion at a time, between the thumb and finger, and firmly extend the tissues outward and downward until the point or points that are not properly relieved are discovered.

The lower base-plate is of horseshoe or crescent shape, and necessarily covers much less surface than the upper one; but if the impression is properly taken and the periphery properly adjusted for the muscle attachments, the base-plate can be seated, and sometimes considerable adhesion obtained. Some writers would lead one to believe that all lower artificial dentures should have a deep lingual flange, while other writers would have the lingual flange almost entirely removed. Both are correct, because some cases require the one treatment and other cases the other method. In those cases in which the crest of the alveolar process of the mandible is pronounced, and the attachment of the mylo-hyoideus muscle is low upon the lingual wall, the lingual flange of the base-plate can and should be carried well down, for adhesion by contact is according to the area of the surface, and the larger the base-plate the greater the resistance to the force of mastication; but if there is excessive resorption of the process, and the attachment of the mylo-hyoideus is at or very near the crest of the slight ridge remaining, or if there is a sharp edge representing the union of the lingual plate of the mandible and the remains of the alveolar process, there should be almost no lingual flange to the base-plate. If in taking the impression the mylo-hyoideus is compressed and depressed, the apparent space for a lingual flange will prove very delusive and troublesome; also, if the base-plate is carried over the sharp lingual edge often found upon the mandible, much irritation will be produced. In these cases the only means of success is to cut away the lingual flange, if one has been formed. In constructing the superstructure upon this properly fitted short lingual flanged base-plate, an extra retention flange of one-sixteenth to three-sixteenths of an inch in width may be extended horizontally into the mouth, when the glands and folds of mucous membranes resting upon this enlarged base-plate will often be of much aid in retention. The buccal flange should be kept as broad as the muscle attachments will permit. The same tests applied to the upper base-plates should be used with the lower.

Submucous tissue. In this class is included all the soft tissue of whatever histological formation—except the muscle tissue just considered—lying beneath the mucous membrane upon which the base-plate rests. When a moderate amount of soft tissue is evenly disposed beneath the mucous membrane, the very best condition possible as far as this tissue is concerned is presented. In some mouths the rhaphe of the maxillæ will be found over-developed, and covered with a thin, tensely drawn mucous membrane, while upon either side there may be an area extending well toward the base of the alveolar process with more or less submucous tissue, and a portion of the alveolar ridge composed of soft flabby tissue only. If a patient representing such a mouth has not long since acquired the knack of wearing artificial dentures, the chances of his success are very unfavorable. The treatment for such a case would be to relieve the pressure upon the whole length of the rhaphe; let the soft

tissue in the vault alone and increase the pressure upon the soft portion of the alveolar ridge. A vacuum chamber in such a case, placed over a portion of the tense membrane in the highest portion of the vault would be a source of irritation and useless.

Mucous membrane. This membrane must bear the burden of supporting all complete artificial dentures, therefore an appreciation of its capabilities is an important factor to the prosthetist. In examining the mouth prior to taking the impression the condition of health of this tissue over which the base-plate is to be placed should be noted, and if necessary, the required attention should be given. There are two qualities of this membrane to be considered—tone and tension.

Tone. This membrane is much influenced by the health of the individual, and may be quite an index of the condition of the general system. The patient will learn that when the general system is vigorous and rested, the denture will have its maximum retention, but when the system is debilitated or relaxed from temporary exhaustion—tired—the retention of the denture will be poor and troublesome. When patients complain that their dentures are not "sticking up" as well as they did, it is well to investigate the tone of the system and explain this principle. When the mucous membrane loses tone for any reason, the retention of the denture will be correspondingly affected. When dissolution is about to take place, it may be noticed that artificial dentures cannot be retained at all. Because of this quality of tone, other conditions being equal, the younger the patient the better the retention. Aged patients in a debilitated state of health and unacquainted with the use of artificial dentures should not be encouraged in having their mouths fitted to new dentures, for the tax upon their vitality may be too great, and hasten their death.

Tension. When a surface upon which a denture is to be worn is covered with healthy mucous membrane, evenly underlaid with a medium amount of submucous tissue, and the tone is good, as far as the tissues are concerned, the very best conditions exist for retaining an artificial denture.

When the soft tissues covering the roof of the mouth are thin and tense, the case is much more difficult. In the former case the tissues will quickly conform to the hard base-plate, and if there has been a reasonably skilful construction of the appliance, the retention will be satisfactory. In the latter case, with the most skilful construction it will often require an hour or two before the mucous membrane conforms to the unyielding material of the base-plate. It is this class of cases that tempts the dentist to use velum rubber lining to the periphery of the plate, or to resort to the patent soft rubber retainers. As this condition of the mouth is the only logical one in which these retainers are permissible, little harm is done if they are never used where not indicated. In these cases of tense mucous tissue no sharp edges or localized increased pressure by any means whatever can be tolerated. Carving of the cast is contra-indicated.

When the mucous membrane is excessively underlaid with soft tissue over the roof of the mouth, and deeply fissured, the case can justly be classed as unfavorable for retention. The cast of such a case may be carved with impunity. The object sought in carving is to cause the periphery of the plate to embed itself more firmly, or to raise a bead just inside the periphery. This temporarily creates a large vacuum chamber, but as soon as the raised portion becomes embedded into the soft tissues, adhesion by contact is secured. In some cases the bead acts as a barrier to the ingress of an excessive amount of fluid.

Many cases presenting will have areas of thin tense tissue and other areas of excessively soft tissue. The treatment for this class of cases has already been stated, that is, relieving of the pressure upon the tense tissue in the proximity of the rhaphe, to the extent of its entire length. This can usually be accomplished by the addition of one or two layers of No. 60 tin foil. The soft areas over any portion of the vault should not be changed, but an excessively soft tissue upon the alveolar ridge should be compressed. Rarely should any hard portion of the alveolar ridge be relieved, then only when very circumscribed.

Fluids of the mouth. The normal thin watery fluid of the mouth is most favorable for retention by adhesion by contact. This fluid makes the contact, but does not hold the base-plate so far away as to interfere with the adhesion by contact. When the fluids are vitiated, thick, and ropy, they may have sticky properties, but not enough to compensate for the interference with adhesion by contact. Temporarily these vitiated secretions can be removed from the mouth by thoroughly washing with an alkaline solution, then inserting the denture well moistened with cold water.

Shape. The shape of the vault of the mouth is a minor factor. The size, tissues, and fluids are the factors that govern adhesion, with one exception. A high-pitched compressed vault is unfavorable in shape, because the resistance to stress is lateral instead of being at right angles.

Summary. The essentials of retention of complete artificial dentures may be summarized as: Properly diagnosing the conditions, a suitable impression, carefully preparing the cast, accurately adjusting the base-plate, carefully mounting the case with the face-bow and bite-gages upon the New Century articulator, proper antagonization, and infinite patience and perseverance while educating the patient in their use.

Discussion.

Dr. S. L. RICH, Nashville, Tenn. I cannot but feel that a great honor has been conferred upon me in that I, one of the younger members of the profession, was called upon to open the discussion on this most excellent paper written by a man whose attainments in the field of prosthetic dentistry have placed him in the front rank of his profession. While I feel deeply the honor conferred upon me, I realize that a difficult task has been assigned to me, because Dr. Wilson's papers are so complete that they leave very little for other men to say. I heartily agree with every suggestion offered in his paper, and the best that I can do is to try to emphasize some of the points which he has made.

In the first place, we know that we cannot depend entirely upon atmospheric pressure for retaining artificial dentures. That was for a long time the current idea in the profession, but we now know that adhesion plays a most important part, especially in the retention of full upper dentures. The essayist also tells us that the force of adhesion depends directly upon the area of surface contact between the denture and the tissues of the mouth, and for this reason we should secure as much contact as possible by ex-

tending the denture in every direction as far as is practical. In some cases where the ridge is not high we should even extend the lower denture inward along the floor of the mouth and underneath the tongue, in order to increase the surface contact and so receive more retention from adhesion. However, in extending our dentures we must not impinge upon the muscular attachments, because the force exerted by the muscles is greater than the force of adhesion, and consequently the denture would be displaced rather than held in place as a result of the extension.

I do not wish to commit myself to the statement that atmospheric pressure plays no part in the retention of artificial dentures, for I believe that in the upper jaw it plays an important part, especially until the patient has learned to use the teeth properly.

I agree with the essayist's view concerning the early insertion of artificial dentures to overcome the disadvantage of leverage; that is, however, only one of the many important advantages to be gained by the early insertion of artificial dentures.

Dr. F. W. STIFF, Richmond, Va. I have little to say on this subject, for the same reason as Dr. Rich gave. The profession is to be congratulated upon having among its members a Wilson, a man who is willing to devote his time and labor to scientific research in this unpopular but necessary domain of our profession—prosthetic dentistry. We who teach in the schools know how difficult it is to induce students to take an interest in this work, and we are continually urging them to give more time and attention to prosthetic dentistry.

When a paper is read before a society each member of the audience is weighing the arguments and the evidence adduced, and comparing them with his own preconceived notions on the subject. I must confess, as did Dr. Rich, that the views of Dr. Wilson are so nearly similar to my own that I have little to say about the paper except in commendation of it. I have long ago discarded the use of vacuum chambers in artificial dentures, believing that they are not necessary, but that the plate is retained by adhesion of contact and more largely by atmospheric pressure than I think Dr. Wilson claims. I do not think that his experiment is entirely conclusive. In regard to the test which he made of suspending in a vacuum two substances attached by adhesion, I should like to ask the question whether or not he made a comparison between the power necessary to separate these two substances in the vacuum and the power necessary to separate them in the air? If you will try that, you will find that it will take less power to separate them in the air than in the vacuum. Adhesion or contact in my opinion plays a very important, in fact the most important part, in the retention of dentures, but throughout the wearing of a denture, temporary or permanent, atmospheric pressure forms an auxiliary to the retention.

The personal equation which the essayist mentioned in the opening portion of his paper has a great deal to do with the retention of plates. I had a patient who wore a partial plate with four incisors ; the plate was broken entirely across lingually of the incisors into two pieces, yet the patient for several years wore that plate in two pieces. I think that without the assistance of nature, and persistence, particularly of our lady patients, we should have a larger percentage of failures than we really have on account of faulty adaptation.

Dr. A. J. COTTRELL, Knoxville, Tenn. I am very sorry that my friend called attention to me, because I believe that brevity is not only the soul of wit, but that, in the discussions at least, it contributes largely to the success of a dental meeting.

First I want to thank Dr. Wilson on behalf of myself and the profession for the careful study which he has devoted to this subject, and I say to you gentlemen who want practical subjects expressed in a practical way that Dr. Wilson has brought to you in this paper the milk of the cocoanut. It will be well worth your time to secure this paper after it has been published, and to study it carefully. I am glad to see that in these days, when mechanical dentistry has become so unpopular, a few men are still left who know how to construct artificial dentures, and who are still willing to perpetuate knowledge along these lines. The young men practicing today go wild on the subject of bridge work, porcelain, orthodontia, etc., and absolutely forget all about prosthetic dentistry, but as long as people live and as long as people lose teeth, somebody must be able to construct well-adapted dentures, and those of us who possess that faculty may consider themselves fortunate indeed.

I shall pass over the question of adhesion by contact and atmospheric pressure because they are accepted facts, and will refer just briefly to the one factor of leverage that the essayist mentions, and which the average practitioner overlooks in the construction of a denture. This is the rock upon which many pieces of bridge work and many prosthetic appliances have been wrecked. I have seen teeth that were protruding a quarter of an inch from the ridge; the farther they protrude the more adverse the influence of leverage. In proportion as the teeth are set toward the inner side of the ridge, the principle of leverage becomes an aid, because then the denture is forced deeper into place. The alveolar ridge acts as a fulcrum, and the opposing jaw is the force on the lever. If the teeth are set on the outside, a fulcrum is established which displaces the denture, while if they are inclined to the inner side as much as possible a fulcrum is established that will drive the denture into place. This is a point that we should look after very carefully, and that is very often overlooked. Of course, for cosmetic reasons there is a limit to the advantageous use of this influence, but it should be utilized to the greatest extent possible.

Another point that the essayist has accentuated is the desirability of extending the plate over the surfaces as far as the attachment of the muscles will permit. This necessarily gives the retentive benefits afforded by the undercuts at the canine fossa and the maxillary tuberosities. These factors contribute greatly to the retention of the upper denture, and yet they are often entirely overlooked. You have all seen dentures in which the prosthetist has failed to take advantage of a well-developed maxillary tuberosity.

The character of the soft tissues was also mentioned and analyzed. There was a time when we constructed all dentures alike, but we now understand that if we would be successful we must consider the character of the soft tissues in each individual case and proceed accordingly.

Let me close as I began, by advising everyone who intends to construct artificial dentures to secure this paper and study it closely, because it will be well worth while.

Dr. J. P. GRAY, Nashville, Tenn. I wish to congratulate the association on this excellent paper, because we have so few men who understand prosthetic dentistry. I am not surprised that many people go to the shops to obtain artificial dentures, because there are so many men who do not make plates very much better than the shops do. Many practitioners go into their laboratories when they are tired, postponing that work until the very last, and often until night, and then try to make a piece of prosthetic work. I dare say that when Dr. Wilson begins a piece of this work, he does it at a set time, and when he is in the best condition for that work.

There are three principles which must be considered in the making of a set of teeth for an edentulous mouth: First, we must remember that the articulation must be proper; next, that we must restore the features to their normal conditions; and third, vocalization must be considered. To all of these points little attention is given. Some make plates too thick and destroy vocalization in all of its forms of speech, others forget all about the muscles of the face; yet no good set of teeth can be made unless all three of these requirements are fulfilled.

The essayist entered into the question of thorough retention of the teeth. One little knack may be of help to the younger men especially; that is, in a lower plate run a string around the outer rim, commencing back at the angle of the jaw and passing around the entire edge of the plate. Invest that in the wax, and in this way you will secure a V-shaped space into which the muscles will drop, and which aids in holding the plate. In the course of a week the muscles will be lying in that space in such a way as to produce almost a complete suction. This is especially useful if.the lower ridge is almost entirely gone, and if the plate is to be left as flat as possible.

As to Dr. Wilson's ideas on the articulation of the teeth, no one will of course attempt to disagree with him. I always bow to him when he speaks of prosthetic dentistry, because I regard him as one of the greatest prosthetic dentists in this country.

Dr. J. Y. CRAWFORD, Nashville, Tenn. In addition to its value this paper seems especially appropriate just now, since mechanical dentistry or the consideration of artificial dentures has never been more important in the world's history perhaps than now. It has been said that we shall always have edentulous mouths. That is true, but the important point to which I wish to call your attention, in addition to indorsing the paper, is that the proper appreciation of this subject is one of the best tests of the dental profession and its capacity for meeting the wants of the general public. If I, a humble teacher of dental surgery, were called upon to designate what clinical proposition would best test the practitioner's powers in regard to clinical diagnosis, I should probably say: Take a typical patient who has passed the meridian of life and has perhaps been unfortunate from the dental standpoint, and determine whether his natural teeth should be preserved or whether it is time to substitute an artificial denture. This to my mind is one of the strongest arguments that can be raised in support of the idea of keeping dental surgery together. Any man ought to be a better practitioner of operative dentistry if he understands mechanical dentistry, and any man ought to be able

to do better mechanical dentistry if he is competent in operative dentistry. If a man devotes his life to the preservation only of the natural teeth, he will go too far in that extreme, and if he devotes his entire life to the practice of mechanical dentistry, he goes to the other extreme. One man will sacrifice teeth that he should save and the other will attempt to save teeth that he should sacrifice.

In order to derive the proper benefit to humanity from both branches of dental surgery, we ought to hold consultations more frequently than we do, when the time comes that we have to determine whether a patient should have an artificial denture, and we should call upon men like Dr. Wilson. If that idea is inculcated in the minds of the younger men, a higher professional status in dental surgery will develop. In this respect the other professions should be a lesson to us. Take the profession of law for instance. If today a great question of law arises in which human labor is involved, we immediately procure a lawyer, who will procure assistants to help him. If it be a condition of surgery in which human life is involved, not only one surgeon, but two or three will be called into consultation. But in dental surgery, where the matter of practical consultation would be of more advantage than in any other profession, how many consultations does a practitioner in this country have in a year? There surely is a decided lack of such consultations. In the practical application of mechanical dentistry to the wants of the people and in its professional aspect, there is nothing more valuable to patient and profession alike than a rational, properly conducted consultation. This would increase the reputability of dental surgery and give it more influence. People would say that if the dentist is so much interested there must be something in it, and dental surgery will rise in public estimation.

Dr. E. M. KETTIG, Louisville, Ky. The subject of the retention of artificial dentures is one of very great interest to those of us who like prosthetic dentistry. I am sorry to say that there are few of us who really do love that branch of dentistry, probably because prosthetics is attended with so many difficulties, disappointments, and despairs that the men who take up that work become discouraged. A very large percentage of the men who start out in the field of dentistry fall in love with operative dentistry, but very few become prosthetic dentists, on account of the vast number of difficulties to be overcome.

Probably one of the greatest troubles we have, and one easily overlooked in the retention of upper dentures, is the fact that we usually try to secure an impression of the mouth with the tissues in a state of repose, whereas we should bear in mind that when the plate is about to be used in mastication, when stress is about to be brought to bear upon it, a different condition arises than when the mouth is in a state of repose; therefore in taking an impression of the mouth we should try to use about as much pressure as is exerted upon the plate during eating. That is often overlooked.

Most dentists use plaster for taking impressions, yet in many mouths, in my experience, plaster is probably one of the poorest materials we have. So many conditions arise from the varying degree of hardness of the roof of the mouth, and for these we should make provision. If we can get a plate that will fit in the roof of the mouth and resist stress equal to the amount of force used in mastica-

tion, we have solved that problem to a large extent. If plaster will not solve that problem, we should use something else—modeling compound. My method is to take a modeling compound impression of the mouth, then cut out a thin layer of the compound so as to form a matrix that will fit almost perfectly the entire area of which I wish to get an impression; then I take an impression compound of a lower melting-point, and spread a thin layer of it inside of that matrix that I have first prepared. The outer layer of compound is cool, and the inner layer must be applied somewhat hurriedly, so as to keep it warm, before the bottom layer becomes soft. Then the whole is put in place, gradually and with precision, and a great deal of pressure is used in bringing it against the roof of the mouth. In that way full advantage is gained from the compressibility of the tissues, without displacing them. A plate made from a model prepared from such an impression will be retained in the mouth during mastication. In lower dentures I believe the outer buccal portions of the lower rim of the plate should not be so prominent, but the posterior lingual portions of the plate should extend under the lower portions of the tongue, still allowing the tongue enough room to perform its function.

Dr. WILSON (closing the discussion). I wish first to thank the association for the kind consideration of this subject.

I wish to call attention to the fact that we do not always make the proper distinction between atmospheric pressure and adhesion. In order to have atmospheric pressure, we must have a vacuum cavity and the air partially exhausted from it. As soon as the cavity is filled by any means, atmospheric pressure ceases. After an artificial denture has been worn for a time, the fluids make contact with the maxillary surface, and as atmospheric pressure ceases the retentive force must be something else. As there is always moisture between the soft tissues and the plate, atmospheric pressure must cease to operate because of the law of hydrostatics.

The strong statement was made in the discussion that plaster is the worst material that can be used for taking impressions. I would say just the reverse. I consider it the best material that can be used. The difference is this: One man can probably obtain better results from one material and another from another. It is simply the man behind the material.

I believe that plaster is the best when properly used, because in it the action of the soft tissues can be more readily indicated. A compound impression lined with plaster is often improperly called a modeling compound impression. You would not speak of an impression as being a block tin impression simply because the block tin tray held the compound. It is the part that comes to lie next to the tissue that should give the name to the impression.

The next order of business was a paper by Dr. H. H. JOHNSON, Macon, Ga., entitled "Observations on Crown and Bridge Work," as follows:

Observations on Crown and Bridge Work.

By H. HERBERT JOHNSON.

IN an unguarded moment I allowed myself to become obligated to write this paper. Since promising to do so the slight inclination felt at the time, which was mistaken for inspiration, has about departed, and I find myself in the deplorable condition of being unable to creditably proceed and too far obligated to gracefully decline.

With much regret thus to have to impose on this section, I shall take advantage of the only remaining avenue of retreat and make the effort very brief.

Upon making a deliberate survey of the subject, it is quickly discernible that little can be said that is either new or that would make even an interesting résumé. It would be tedious and tiresome to my hearers to introduce any detailed points of the technique such as is pursued in the making of bridge work

that might come within my knowledge, as all practitioners of even slight pretensions are now familiar with the general ideas of construction. About the only thing apparent, therefore, and indeed all that I shall attempt, will be to introduce some old but as yet unsettled questions for discussion, in the hope of thus shedding more light for our future guidance.

As the comfort, the durability, and the strength of crown and bridge work depend upon the success of the method employed in making the abutments, pillars, and attachments, it has been decided to deal principally with that portion of the subject. Experience of many years has taught us valuable lessons concerning the amount of anchorage required to retain for a reasonable time pieces of work of varying extensiveness.

When bridge work was first introduced, common sense seemed to indicate that as few remaining abutment teeth or roots were to be relied upon to perform the work of those lost as well as their own, a bridge would require a very strong and rigid attachment, and that nothing short of gold telescoping crowns and strongly banded roots would be sufficient for such support. With these ideas firmly fixed in our minds, in some instances great injury was wrought in cases of misfits, of teeth with short crowns, and roots broken down to or beneath the gum margin. In the firm belief that a broad surface of band was necessary for support, the bands were often cruelly driven far beneath the gum, resulting in inflammation, finally recession, and in many cases premature loss of the teeth or roots supporting the structure. Those of us who have been in practice a sufficient length of time to observe results are quite familiar with this class of cases. During that early period, also, the lack of good reliable cements had something to do with fixing these banding ideas in the minds of the practitioners, as it was thought that when bands were driven well beneath the gum margin, this covering would form a protection which would prevent the disintegration of the cement.

Viewing the progress of cases of many years' standing, these valuable truths are revealed to us. In almost all cases where bands of extraordinary width were fastened about teeth, even when this was done as skilfully as would be reasonable to expect, the result was a gradual recession, until these bands now do not reach to the gum, and in most cases have disclosed misfits that are a surprise to the makers. Time has also shown that where bands and crowns have been carefully and neatly fitted, the cement has not disintegrated any faster after the margin of the band or crown has been deprived of its supposed gum protection than it did while thus covered. This, together with the observations gained in porcelain inlay work and other cemented fillings, would seem to prove that cemented bands and other attachments, when neatly fitted, last as well when not driven beneath the gum margin, and that the gum covering affords no special protection to the cement. It is further observed, as has been remarked, that all bands and telescoping crowns driven beneath the gum or extended farther over the tooth result in a misfit which increases the farther the band passes above the neck of the tooth. Then, as there will always be a dissolution of the cement for a certain space beneath such ill-fitted bands, it is plainly evident that the piece only receives support as far as there is any cement attachment, and that the extended margin of the band from which the cement has been dissolved gives no further support at all, and only proves an irritant which finally weakens the strength of the living attachment to the jaw itself. As the permanence of the work must rely at last upon the stability of the abutment teeth or roots in their living healthful attachment to the jaw, it is more than evident that nothing could be of greater importance than to look carefully to the preservation of this much-desired condition.

If this, then, is recognized as a proved fact, and further, if it is agreed that bands and other devices forced beneath the gum do create permanent harm, is it not high time that these irritating devices be forever discarded, and that we cast about for some better methods for the support of bridges?

The application of the more recent methods which so greatly simplify the making of half-caps, hoods, and molded fillings, will in a great many instances prove to be of advantage as a substitute for bands and ferrule crowns. It is gratifying to observe the firm support that can be obtained in even extensive pieces with long spans of bridge work by the exclusive use of molded fillings and small hoods, when these hoods and fillings are further strengthened by iridio-platinum pins of small size extending some depth into sound dentin. Then, too, with this kind of attachment every portion of the margin will be visible, and accessible in case of future disintegration from any slight defect.

These points of weakness, if any occur, can readily be repaired by the insertion of a small filling at the margin where decay or disintegration has appeared. Bridge work that has been inserted with telescoping and banded crowns has been subjected to much criticism on account of unhygienic conditions, and in many instances this criticism has been just, and none too severe. Another forceful argument that may be raised in favor of the simpler forms of attachment is that in all probability it will be less necessary to destroy the pulps in abutment teeth or to render them liable to die afterward from excessive cutting away of enamel and dentin.

It has been forcefully argued in the past that no tooth should receive a crown unless its pulp has been first devitalized. We are already familiar with the points in this argument—that the tooth cannot be properly prepared, that the removal of so much enamel and the contact of so much metal with the sensitive dentin will afterward cause the pulp to die, etc. I have always opposed this idea and have advocated at all times the preservation of pulps whenever possible, and I am

constrained to believe that it is entirely unnecessary to indulge in any wholesale destruction of pulps on account of crowning. There are many good reasons in favor of preserving pulps when teeth are to be covered with gold crowns, especially if these crowned teeth are to act as supports of much-needed bridges. The argument that a molar cannot be properly prepared for the fitting of a gold crown without devitalizing is not well founded. There are only a very few cases where this is positively true. Likewise my experience does not show that pulps die more often under gold crowns than they do in filled teeth, and certainly no one would argue that every pulp should be devitalized before filling a tooth. A sound tooth properly ground for the reception of a gold crown should exhibit no more sensitiveness to thermal changes after the crown has been cemented in place for a week, than if it had never been crowned. It is more than probable that those frequent cases of pulps dying under gold crowns are often brought about through some deep-seated cavity which had encroached upon the pulp, and was not taken into consideration. Of course in such cases the crown should not justly be held responsible. It must be remembered, also, that the cements may not be entirely free from contamination. With a cement of good quality mixed on a clean slab no trouble should arise.

A living pulp in a crowned tooth often gives a warning that results in saving a valuable bridge abutment for many more years of usefulness. It is well known that decay does frequently occur about the margins of gold crowns, usually after the piece of work has been worn for a number of years. If this should happen to a tooth containing a living pulp the warning is given by increased sensitiveness, and the necessary correction can be made in time to save the tooth. But suppose, on the other hand, that this should occur in a devitalized tooth. The patient is not warned, he neglects to undergo the necessary examination, decay progresses rapidly, many times more rapidly than in open cavities, and in a very short time the entire crown portion of the tooth is eaten away, and the first warning given is the sudden collapse of the end of the bridge under the stress of mastication. This may be

extensive areas, such as would be used in abutments for bridges, it is generally advisable to strengthen such attachments by the insertion of at least two pins or posts of iridio-platinum wire. When these fillings are to be cast from a wax mold, the operation of manipulating the wax will be greatly facilitated if the wire forming the pins is bent in the form of a staple, so that it may embed itself more firmly in the wax, thereby lessening the danger of displacement of the pins during the handling of the wax model

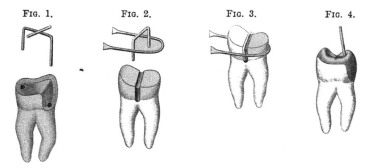

FIG. 1.   FIG. 2.   FIG. 3.   FIG. 4.

a much-needed bridge, probably the only resource for mastication, but there is no help for it, it must come out. Many of these cases have come under my observation, but never yet have I seen an abutment tooth entirely lost before warning was given in the case of a tooth containing a living pulp. This itself would be a strong enough argument to warn us to proceed carefully in promiscuous devitalizing. When we consider the other ill-effects from devitalized teeth, the argument should be even more than convincing.

In closing, just one or two practical suggestions will be offered that have proved to be helpful in practice. In making large cast gold fillings covering

for investment (Fig. 1). If the surface covered by the wax mold is broad, a cross wire may be attached, which will greatly assist in preventing the warping of the wax while finishing and shaping the wax mold on the tooth, as illustrated also in Fig. 1. If a hood abutment after the Alexander method is to be cast, it will be found to be almost an impossibility to perfectly adapt the wax without resorting to some such method as that suggested in Figs. 2 and 3. By the application of this crib of No. 20 iridio-platinum wire, the operation of making the mold is very much simplified. After shaping the tooth and cutting the usual groove, the staple is adjusted to fit rather loosely. A piece of the wire is next bent in the form of a letter U and passed around the tooth, the flattened ends projecting buccally, and forming, with the staple to which it is soldered on one side, what we might call the crib. Mold a sheet of wax over the prepared tooth, press the crib to place, embedding the wires into the wax, building up to the desired contour with extra wax melted and spatulated on. When invested for casting, the projecting ends of the U wire, which may be flattened to add security, will be embedded in the investment, and hold the crib in place in the mold after the wax has been melted or burned out. After casting, these ends can be cut off and saved.

Those who have had difficulty in such castings will find these methods simple and very helpful.

When molded fillings are to be used as abutments for bridges, it is often found difficult to keep these fillings in proper place while pouring the model from the impression or in the investment while soldering. Fig. 4 illustrates a method by which this can be accurately done. Place the fillings in the cavities and take the necessary bite for occluding the bridge. Then remove the fillings and attach a small piece of wire, projecting at right angles and soldered with a minute quantity of solder. Replace the fillings in the cavities and take the impression. These wires will be embedded in the impression material and come away with it. They may be left in place until the bridge is formed, to act as a·stay in the investment, when they can be removed and the bridge can be polished.

These little knacks have helped me over some great difficulties, and I offer them with the hope that they may be of some assistance to others.

Discussion.

Dr. H. T. STEWART, Memphis, Tenn. In the copy of the paper which he sent to me Dr. Johnson started out by assuming that he did not know anything about bridge work, and that he was inflicting himself on this section by offering a paper. I have always believed that a man who has a good thing should stand up for what it is worth. We all know that Dr. Johnson is an excellent dentist and a fine crown and bridge workman.

Dr. Johnson spoke of using the band under the gum. I think we all agree that if we could avoid the use of the band under the gum we would only be too glad to do so, but bridge work has not yet reached that stage where it is possible to do so. It is true that in the cases of the ordinary bands met with, the gums of the patients about the roots of the teeth would be better off without the band, but at the same time we must use it in many cases, and if it is made properly there is practically no irritation under that band. In my Riggs' disease work I have had to be especially careful on that one point, and I have long ago stopped making collars to go on the root. I first prepare the root in a conical shape, which is a great deal more easily said than done. The conical shape should be extended well under the gum, if necessary, with a bud-shaped bur. The floor and collar are both swaged in one piece out of pure gold, as thin as will bear the blowpipe. I generally use about No. 35 or 36 gage, taking the impression first with modeling compound, after having made a band that fairly accurately fits the root. This band can be made of any sort of material that you please, preferably copper or German silver, and after filling it with compound it is put on the end of your finger and pressed to place. After obtaining your impression, make a cement die and swage the floor and collar all at once. It makes no difference how careful you are in this, you cannot get an absolutely accurate fit. The most particular part of the work is the burnishing of the pure gold floor and collar to the surface of the root and under the gum. That should be done with exceeding care; the ordinary burnishers are not suited for that purpose. I use burnishers after the style of Dr. Reeves', designed for burnishing platinum into cavities for porcelain inlays. The gold must be burnished to the surface of the root as closely as in burnishing a piece of gold or platinum for an inlay. If the burnishing is done thoroughly the accuracy of the fit is certain. Another important step is the shaping of the root into a cone. We wish to restore the root to its original shape. The floor and collar are then laid on a second piece of gold and soldered to that piece, which is cut out a little larger than the other, invested, and flowed full of solder clear up to the edge of the band, thus restoring the original shape of the root, and bringing it clear out flush with the root where it has been cut off with the bur. In that way I find that the irritation is reduced to a minimum, and if the operation is carefully done, there is little or no irritation to the gum.

I heartily agree with Dr. Johnson in his statement that wholesale destroying of pulps should not be resorted to in crowning teeth. We have a great deal to learn in this respect, and Dr. Johnson's ideas, together with those of Dr. Alexander on preserving the pulps in such cases, are very acceptable. We have a great field before us in that line. While it is necessary in many cases to destroy a pulp, yet we should preserve it whenever we can, for many different reasons, not the least of which is that we cannot always thoroughly clean the root-canals, especially those in molars, up to the apex and then thoroughly fill them, in spite of the best of intentions. If we could take out teeth, especially molars, that we have filled to the best of our ability, some two or three years afterward, and could examine them thoroughly, we should be astonished at the imperfect conditions which the roots of these teeth would present.

The average lifetime, especially of molars that have been treated and the roots of which have been filled by the average practitioner, is far shorter than we are willing to admit. If in abutments for a bridge the pulps can be saved, it is usually far better to do so, unless these teeth are badly affected with Riggs' disease; in the latter case I do not hesitate under any circumstances to devitalize the pulp; it should be done in nine out of ten cases. In the first place, I think the teeth are better off. I have for years argued that when teeth that are badly affected with Riggs' disease are cut off, it is somewhat like cutting off the branches of a tree; the vitality is confined to the remaining portion of the teeth, and in that manner we obtain the best results. Moreover, if teeth, especially molars, are cut off, we can operate better around the teeth and can obtain much better results than if we try to operate on a tooth with a vital pulp.

Speaking of these bands reminds me of a paper on partial plates that was read by Dr. House before the Indiana Society, in the discussion of which Dr. J. D. Patterson of Kansas City made the statement that in his experience "the best partial plate was worse than the poorest bridge." He also stated that bands should never be used on the teeth, and that no tooth should ever be crowned without having first been devitalized. Such views are not only extreme but foolish. I can conceive of nothing worse than a poor bridge. As Dr. Johnson said, we often see ill-fitting bands and shell crowns extending beneath the gum with great shoulders under which large quantities of cement are held; I can conceive of nothing worse than that. Dr. Patterson also said that the band should never be used, and gave as one reason for his assertion that we could not secure the proper interdental space. I wish to emphasize, however, that you *can* secure the proper interdental space by constructing the bands in the way described; oftentimes we can obtain a much wider interdental space than exists naturally, especially if two adjoining teeth are to be crowned. The interdental space in such cases can be made so that the body of a small toothpick can be passed between the two teeth. So this is not a good argument against the band. While the band, as Dr. Johnson says, is wrong in principle, we have to do the best we can, as so far there is nothing that could entirely take its place.

Dr. T. P. HINMAN, Atlanta, Ga. In discussing this paper I wish to remark first, that the paper that has been presented to the association seems somewhat different from the one that has been sent to me for discussion; therefore some of my remarks will probably involve points that were not revealed in the reading of the paper.

In the main I thoroughly agree with Dr. Johnson in what he says with reference to bridge-work attachments, etc. There is one feature that he spoke of in reference to the failure of bridge work that seemed to impress itself more on my mind than anything else, and as he does not bring this point out clearly, I think it would not be out of the way to mention it at this time. The failure of the majority of bridges, the loosening of the abutments of which he speaks, is in my opinion not so much due to the fitting of the bands below the gums as to bad occlusion. If you have a molar attachment which is, say, one one-hundredth of an inch too high, the entire pressure of the jaw during the process of mastication is brought to bear upon this attachment, and in the molar region this pressure approaches one hundred and twenty-five pounds. You can therefore readily see how this continual impact will cause the loosening of the attachment, a diseased condition of the gum, and the failure of the bridge. Uneven distribution of the stress of mastication, in other words allowing the greatest amount of pressure to occur at one point, will certainly create inflammation and cause failure of the bridge.

I am thoroughly in accord with the essayist in the belief that it is not wise in a majority of instances to destroy the pulp for the purpose of making an all-gold crown, although there are certain teeth of a bell shape where it is necessary to destroy the pulps if an accurate fit of the gold crown at the gum margin is to be secured. The pressing of the gold band far beneath the gum certainly is, as we all know, bad practice, causing recession of the gum and subsequent decay. It is often the case, however, if a tooth is vital and recession and decay take place, that the tooth readily responds to sensations of heat and cold, warning the operator of the approach of destruction.

As for the half-banded crown, the so-called modified Richmond crown, I do not believe in that form of appliance. If for the purpose of strength we have to band a root, I believe the continuous band to be the better. As for hoods, inlays, etc., for bridge attachments, I have used these for quite a while. In the making of the hood, which I believe I designed, and in the making of inlays for the purpose of bridge attachments, instead of making a staple on the crown as the essayist suggests, my method is to put in two pins at the gingival border, which I believe makes a simpler and just as strong an attachment. In my observation the majority of operators make a mistake in attempting to cast the abutments out of 22-karat gold. Indeed, to attempt to cast inlays for attachments out of a low-karat gold means practically certain failure. The cast is not clear and clean on account of the oxidation, and consequently the attachment is not as strong as desired. A small proportion of platinum added to the pure gold will produce a much stronger attachment that will not oxidize, and will afford a more perfect fit.

In reference to cements, we very often hear the question as to what is the best cement for cementing crowns. There are so many good cements on the market that it is difficult to indicate which is the best, although I have my preference. Failure in their use is due to the fact that the operator is not familiar with the material which he is using; one cement in one operator's hands will give good results, whereas in another's hands it will not give good results, owing to the operator's unfamiliarity with that particular cement. Therefore, in a great many cases, especially of students who ask which is the best cement to use, my answer has been that they should select some good cement, become thoroughly acquainted with its peculiarities and learn how to work it properly, and then they will not be troubled with the cement washing out from under crowns.

Dr. JOHNSON (closing the discussion). I do not care to now add anything to it, and as the hour has arrived for the convening of the general session, we will simply consider the subject as closed.

Section I then adjourned until Thursday evening at 8 o'clock.

THURSDAY—Evening Session.

THE second meeting of Section I was called to order on Thursday evening, April 1st, at 8.30 o'clock.

The first order of business was the reading of a paper by Dr. J. CLARENCE GRIEVES, Baltimore, Md., entitled, "The Behavior of Certain Metals in the Mouth," as follows:

The Behavior of Certain Metals in the Mouth.

By CLARENCE J. GRIEVES.

"IT is much to be desired that the dentist should have a more definite knowledge of the behavior of metals and their alloys in the mouth; that he should make his metallurgy something not apart from, but a part of his daily practice."

With this idea foremost, these slides and this paper are modestly offered. If a lack of sequence in the facts presented and a greater lack of knowledge as to the primary and final causes of these phenomena affecting all metals exposed in and continually wetted by a salivary and decomposing food environment as complex as it is changeable mark this effort, no apologies are made, for the slides which were obtained from many fields examined show conditions not as we wish they might be, but as they really are— conditions observable by any busy dentist in the detail of everyday practice. Several important changes in the point of view are or should be the result of recent dental research, and not only our methods but our materials must be carefully reviewed and modified. Clinical data, physical laboratory tests of teeth and materials, and chemical analyses of saliva have shown that it is not so much a question of tooth structure, important though that may be, as of the environment of that tooth structure and of the associated operation. Prophylaxis, the product of sound pathological reasoning combined with common sense, looking not to one but to all mouth phases and lesions, has made evident and imperative

perfect cleanliness for both dental and general health.

If it can be established that a vitiated saliva, or even a normal saliva and its mucous contents, or the decomposition of food in the common retention centers, or a combination of all of these, affect the metals in use in operative and prosthetic dentistry in such a way as to bring about their corrosion, forming other retention centers to the minute but ultimate destruction of smooth surfaces, prophylaxis exacts of us that we correct the environment if possible, close all retention centers against the lodgment of filth, or substitute some material impervious to such action. The systemic danger from the continued ingestion of the by-products of metallic disintegration will be in direct ratio to the time of exposure and the amount of that disintegration. While noting the fact that an ingested metal is not as dangerous as its salts, yet it becomes a question of absorption of the metal by the mucosa and the solubility of the salts if formed.

It would be a waste of time to name the metals employed in the mouth. If used alone a few are apparently invulnerable; many in the salivary environment degenerate rapidly; alloying, which helps the situation in producing desirable physical characteristics, increases vulnerability to such a degree as to call for definite laws for the guidance of the manufacturer. *These laws must be furnished by the dentist, who uses, is responsible for, and should dictate the type of product.*

In proof of the foregoing the following may be cited and summarized from a recent paper:*

is significant when seen in the light of the table of Berzelius, gold and copper standing as highly electro-negative as op-

FIG. 1.

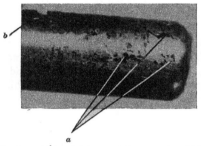

FIG. 2.

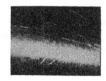

Section of buccal tube worn two months; 18-k. platinous gold, 5 per cent. zinc. *a*, Craters by electrolysis. *b*, Disk notch.

Section of 14-k. arch containing no zinc worn same period in same mouth, showing no disintegration.

(Figs. 1 and 2 were purposely made under the same light and lens.)

The alloy German or nickel silver was found by six assays of as many varieties manufactured to consist of copper 6.1, zinc 2.1, nickel 1.7, and iron 0.2. Exhaustive physical tests by the Bureau of Standards show this metal to be fit for all purposes in orthodontia, but it disintegrates in the saliva and hence is chemically unfit. Plain German silver examined with low powers after exposure of a few weeks in the mouth, in child saliva, presented craters in the centers retaining food; on longer exposure these craters extended all over the appliances—an arch bar for instance—even to the parts kept clean by the lips and tongue; corrosion was more pronounced and fixed than in removable appliances, and distinctly more violent and rapid, even to perforation of the metal, when gold plating, which was always defective, occurred.

That the added layer of gold should greatly increase corrosion, even granting some damage to the alloying in plating,

* "Base Metal *vs.* Noble Metal Appliances in Orthodontia," proceedings American Society of Orthodontists, *Items of Interest*, May 1909.

posed to nickel, zinc, and iron, which are electro-positive.

It was found that the craters were cut in the food-retention centers just as the

FIG. 3.

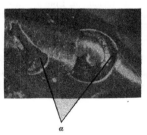

Deep disintegration of German silver wire "dutchmen" soldered in 18-k. bridge. *a* occurred on sheltered palatal surface and were flush when set in the mouth about eighteen months ago.

tooth was cut, but there the analogy ceased, for to conclude that this is an acid process *per se* is to admit either that the acid starting craters extends and is retained all over the appliance, even at the constantly cleansed spots, or a general mouth acidity as high as the retention center—a position entirely untenable, for all children wearing appliances do not have hyperacid mouths, while the corrosion of German silver is remarkably constant in all mouths.

Electrolysis is, then, the principal agent working toward the destruction of this alloy, with the acids of food decomposition first charging the battery, and with the saliva containing such, as a general electrolyte. This may be further established by the following facts:

First. An alloy containing approximately gold 18, platinum 2, the remaining four parts of the 24 karats being made up of equal parts of silver, copper, and zinc, after short wear under like conditions presents corrosion almost as pronounced as with plain German silver. (Fig. 1.)

Second. "Dutchmen" of German silver wire used to fill in bridge dummies surrounded by gold solder and exposed in finishing, present deep degeneration spots on otherwise smooth surfaces when placed in the mouth away from the abrasion of occlusion. (Fig. 3.) German silver crown posts when soldered in gold crowns and exposed to saliva degenerate quickly.

Third. Brass (copper 2, zinc 1, approximately) buccal tubes attached to plain German silver molar anchorage bands corrode much less than the bands, owing, possibly, to the fact that while

FIG. 4.

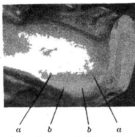

Palatal view of molar bridge dummy (18-k. gold solder) worn seven months. *b,* Lower part of saddle covered by gum hypertrophy free from erosion. *a,* Line of craters in the retention center just above the false gum margin.

FIG. 5.

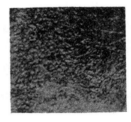

Greater detail of crater shown at *a,* Fig. 4.

brass has copper 2, electro-negative, to zinc 1, electro-positive, German silver has copper 6.1, electro-negative, to nickel 1.7, zinc 2.1, iron 0.2, all electro-positive.

Fourth. Brass wire ligatures crossing platinous gold arch bars disintegrate much more rapidly than when in contact with plain German silver arches in the same mouth.

Last, but by no means least, the study of a large number of 18-karat gold solder surfaces known to have been smooth when placed in the mouth by the writer, develops the interesting fact that whenever a food-retention center was created, as in saddle dummies, where gum hypertrophy has produced a false margin, corrosion exists to a marked degree. (Figs. 4 and 5.)

"Eighteen-karat" gold solders are really 16-karat gold, and nearly, if not all, contain approximately gold 16, copper 5, zinc 3.

It has thus been proved that German silver, with 15 per cent. zinc, 18-karat gold solder with 12 per cent. zinc, and all below such, and platinous gold alloy with 5 per cent. zinc, all corrode, with the human saliva as electrolyte, while gold plates of a much lower proportion of gold, such as coin gold

become pitted; that it is bad dental and general hygiene to have such pitted surfaces in the mouth; that the degeneration waste metal is ingested continuously, producing possibly systemic detriment, and finally, that because metallic poisoning has not been generally noted, this does not in the least affirm that it has not occurred.

The foregoing is particularly important when applied to bridge work or dentures which are fixed or worn in the

FIG. 6.

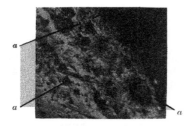

Degeneration of cast metal base surface in use five years. a, Deep pits cut in casting "faults."

FIG. 7.

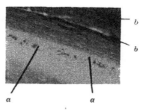

Deep section cut through rim of cast metal base worn three years, carrying vulcanite attachment. a, Deep defects in casting extending to surface. b, Vulcanite. c, Open joint between vulcanite and base.

(gold 90, copper 10) and the lower dental plates alloyed with metals all of the same electro-negative class as gold, with copper, silver, and platinum, do not degenerate under the same conditions. (Compare Fig. 2 with Figs. 1, 4, and 5.)

Zinc to the average extent of 5 per cent. is thus the disturbing element, and the following law may be safely deduced:

Metals violently electro-positive and negative to each other should not be used in alloy or apposition in the human mouth, with the saliva as an electrolyte; as, for instance, gold and zinc, copper and zinc, etc.

Corollary to this law stand the facts that it is absurd to spend time polishing surfaces which we are assured will shortly

mouth for an indefinite time, the metals occurring in mass; and while there may be greater food retention about fixed bridges, the argument that a minutely corroded metal denture may be removed and cleansed is misleading, since boiling is the only means for perfectly cleansing such corroded surfaces, which reek filth immediately when they are put to use, the craters becoming deeper with consequent loss of metal.

Most vulnerable among the metallic bases used in artificial dentures are the low-fusing "cast metal bases," with or without aluminum; they are classified by weight into those which are jarred or forced into the mold and those which displace the contained air by sheer weight. Of the latter, Wood's, Watt's, and Weston's metals are proprietary, but

FIG. 8.

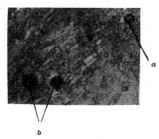

Palatal surface of cast aluminum plate worn eight months. *a*, Air bubble. *b*, Disintegrations beginning about blow-holes.

it can be assumed that they approximate in formula Kingsley's (tin 16, bismuth 1), Reese's (tin 20, silver 2, gold 1), or Bean's (tin 95, silver 5), fusing at about 700° F. Several such metal dentures were examined, more lowers than uppers, and presented after short periods of wear on all retention surfaces deep craters, many being filthy in the extreme. (Figs. 6 and 7.) It has long been common laboratory knowledge that after exposure for any time in the mouth these alloys cannot be fused and utilized, owing to the great amount of dross and their increased fusing-point, showing pronounced loss of certain elements.

The behavior of the cast metal bases with aluminum requiring pressure in casting, of which Carroll's formula is typical (aluminum 98 per cent., platinum, gold, and copper making up the remaining 2 per cent., fusing at about 1300° F.) is of particular interest because of the growing popularity of pressure casting with such metals.

Whatever casting machine is used, the results differ little in the mouth from those obtained in the older and more

crude apparatus of Carroll, as the slides will show, and we must distinguish between defects in casting, the metal ap-

FIG. 9.

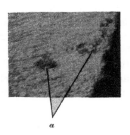

Section of cast aluminum base. *a*, Deep defects in casting.

parently chilling in the mold (Fig. 9), blow-holes from air retained or carried into the mold with the metal (Fig. 8),

FIG. 10.

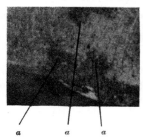

Disintegrations occurring at the gingival line of a swaged aluminum crown. *a*, Deep erosions.

and disintegrations in the mouth, which usually "start" one of these defects near the surface. (Fig. 8.) The rolling of aluminum into plates or the drawing of it into crowns seems to present but little better surfaces, as a section taken from a swaged aluminum crown worn for some time will prove; note how it has suffered at the dangerous gingival line. (Fig. 10.)

The least that can be said is that cast base metals should be most carefully inspected before being used, as nothing

FIG. 11.

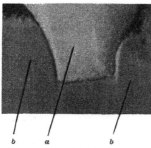

Buccal view of vulcanite plate worn ten years. Same enlargement as Nos. 6, 7, 8, and 9. *a*, Porcelain tooth. *b*, Pink vulcanite.

can be more filthy when they are porous; an illustration of a well-vulcanized rubber denture worn ten years is submitted in contrast. (Fig. 11.)

FIG. 12.

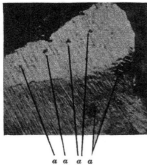

Deep section through 24-k. cast gold inlay cut at three angles. *a*, Defects.

It may be worth while to present a section of a pressure-cast gold inlay showing open spaces. These defects occur centrally as well as at the margin in both 24-karat and 22-karat gold (Fig. 12); they are obviously too irregular in outline to be borax pits (Fig. 13), and the method or machine appears to make little difference. The writer is informed that the porosity of gold cast under pressure has been known to the manufacturing jeweler for a long period, and that this is his chief reason for discarding the process.

It would be going too far to claim that any damage is done to the operation by such defects, unless there are numerous and deeply reaching caval edges; there is, however, a danger well worth mention in gold casting methods applied to the platinum pins of porcelain teeth, quite apart from that of "checking" the facing, and to platinum posts cast in copés for crowns.

If the wax of the "disappearing model" be high in carbon, if the carbon be not thoroughly burned off, or if the posts be rough in order to retain them,

FIG. 13.

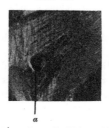

Surface section through 22-k. gold solder of matrix and solder inlay. *a*, Borax pit.

the high heat of pressure casting, the impact of molten metal in a closed chamber formed by the investment, or all of these factors together, serve to drive the carbon into the platinum, making a combination which is quite brittle, which fractures crystalline under slight strain, and is completely changed in its physical characteristics; a heavy root-post is thus totally unfitted to meet the stress for which it was planned.

This was noted by Cunningham years ago in the too generous use of the "brush" blowpipe flame on the pins of teeth, and is a fact familiar to the makers of porcelain furnaces.

We approach the question of the behavior of amalgam in the mouth with much hesitation. The field is broad, the

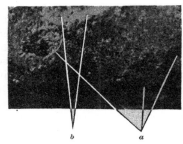

b   *a*

Well-finished cervical seat of amalgam into which, after set, was anchored gold foil filling. *a*, Craters adjacent to gold in amalgam. *b*, Beginning of gold filling.

causes are obscure, and we are but in the beginning; criticism of amalgam is not new, and clinically is prejudiced one way or the other. One fact only is assured, namely, that much needed physical research on this line has been accomplished out of the mouth, and there is room for even greater research chemically as to the behavior of this material after exposure to mouth environment.

Tin, the principal ingredient of amalgam alloys, when associated with gold cervically as foil under the influence of the saliva loses much of its physical character and becomes hard and brittle. Binary amalgam alloys (tin and silver) placed cervically as the base for gold foil

operations are changed along the same lines and to a greater degree. Tin, then, is the active factor, but who will say whether the force acting as to so modify metals is chemical or physical?—for these phenomena do not occur outside of the mouth.

The quaternary alloys, containing besides the usual proportion of tin and silver a small portion of copper, gold, or zinc, or any two of the latter, do not

FIG. 15.

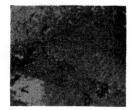

Craters on well-finished amalgam filling surfaces unassociated with gold.

harden as do the binary alloys in apposition to gold in the mouth; those containing zinc 2 parts show, when placed as a cervical seat for gold foil fillings, corrosion just about the gingival margin. These spots have been found on well-finished fillings from the hands of careful operators, and have been produced experimentally in the mouth by the writer. (Fig. 14.)

It may be noted that as far as these observations go, ternary alloys (respectively silver, tin, and a portion each of copper, gold, or platinum), while covered with sulfids, do not show degeneration as do the cleaner-looking quaternary alloys having a small percentage of zinc, with gold or platinum (the writer does not take the latter any too seriously). This is of particular interest, first, because mercury, silver, copper, and tin, the metals common, in the order named, to amalgam alloys, occupy a central position in the series of electro-positive and negative substances, being almost equal in potential, while gold and platinum are as far away and opposed electro-negatively from this naturally combined central group as is zinc electro-positively; second, these four metals combined have

dark salts, presumably sulfids, just at this line are the rule even on well-fitted gold caps and well-adapted gold fillings; below the line the gold is bright and as well finished as when placed; vulnerable alloys show a line of pits of disintegration at this point. In gold-plated German silver anchorage bands the row of craters is deeper at the line, with a few

FIG. 16.

FIG. 17.

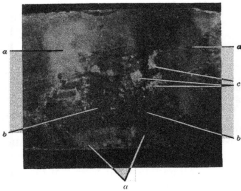

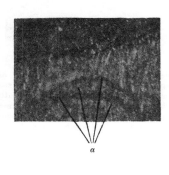

Approximal portion of gold-plated German silver molar anchorage band exposed three weeks in the mouth, showing damage at the gingival line. *a*, Gold-plating above the line. *b*, Line of craters of disintegration at the line. *d*, Perfect gold-plating below the line. *c*, Deposits of white salts.

16-k. gold solder surfaces with lines of corrosion at *a*, just under gingival margin.

long been known as producing the best practical results.

It is most difficult to condense amalgam without defects throughout the filling; pits of corrosion have been noted on amalgam fillings quite independently of contact with gold; these occur on surfaces which have been carefully polished, and do not resemble in the least operative faults due to lack of manipulation. (Fig. 15.)

The gingival line, and what occurs to metals above and below it, is of great interest in this connection. Deposits of

craters above it and with a loss of gold plating, which is absolutely intact below the margin and free from corrosion. (Fig. 16.)

Reference has already been made to 18-karat gold solder (Figs. 4, 5, and 17) and amalgam, and to the line of corrosion found on a swaged aluminum crown in this connection (Fig. 10), and in every instance, with the exception of the 18-karat solder, which maintained its finish below the margin, these alloys are dark with sulfids. The metals apparently suffer not unlike the teeth from a combination of the saliva and decomposition of food, and are protected by the

FIG. 18.

FIG. 18.

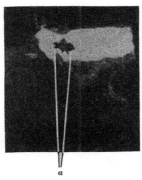

a

Section of the "knuckling contact" of amalgam adjacent to which later was set a gold crown. *a*, Lower third of deep crater. The bright crystalline state of the metal exposed in such craters is very different from the dull sulfidization found in operative defects.

gingival secretions. It would seem that this fact should have some bearing on the yet unsettled question of the begin-

FIG. 19.

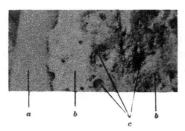

a   *b*   *b*

c

Surface of carefully finished oxyphosphate filling exposed four months in mouth subject to erosion. *a*, Enamel. *b*, Cement filling. *c*, Pits of disintegration.

nings of caries of the enamel, for all the metals vulnerable in the mouth are attacked at this line.

Carefully contoured and finished amalgam fillings (quaternary alloys) built by the matrix, approximally to which later on gold crowns were set, exhibit deep disintegration at the "knuckling," or point of contact with the gold surfaces. These crypts are typical, differing in no respect from the earlier illustrations of crypts in gold-plated German silver or platinous gold (zinc 2 per cent.), and are totally unlike operative defects. (Fig. 18.)

If it be not too elementary, the damage produced in gold crowns by the mercury in amalgam fillings, no matter how well these crowns are constructed, when placed adjacent to such fillings, may be mentioned. The gold degenerates in these cases as it does outside of the mouth, but in a less degree, possibly owing to the protection afforded by the colloid substances of the saliva coating the surface of the crown.

All operators will agree that there are certain mouths in which, no matter what amalgam alloy is used, there is a marked wasting of amalgam surfaces quite independently of the stress of occlusion or abrasion from dentifrices. Good gold foil fillings and the 22-karat plate of shell crowns highly burnished, in a short period after having been newly placed assume in such mouths a brassy, almost greenish hue, lose luster, and take on a dull "pumice finish." Chemical erosion with deep "cervical notching" is frequent. Fig. 19 shows the behavior of oxyphosphate in such a mouth. Abrasion from dentifrices as a cause is excluded, simply because careful inquiry proves that such have not been used. These are the mouths characterized by hyperacidity, usually in persons of middle life, in which sulfid staining is rare.

The case about to be reported, one of

a few examined, is of this type, complicated by the conscientious use of fourteen

of erosion fifteen years ago by one of the
best operators in this country. Hidden

FIG. 20.

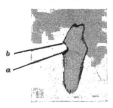

Diagram of lower central incisor showing
what was left of amalgam at *a*, and new
erosion at *b*.

FIG. 21.

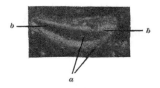

Remains of amalgam filling at *a*, Fig. 20. *a*,
Pits in amalgam. *b*, Deep notch cut in filling flush with tooth at *b*, Fig. 20.

FIG. 22.

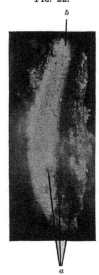

Enlargement of filling shown in Fig. 21. *a*,
Deep craters which appear all over eroded
amalgam surfaces. Note the marks of
brush, which are deeply continuous from *b*
to *a*.

FIG. 23.

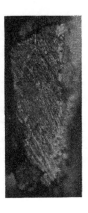

Section of tooth side of filling shown in Fig.
22, rubbed down on cuttle paper. Compare
the scratches here with those produced by
powder in Fig. 22, and note the absence of
pits and the well-condensed amalgam.

(These pictures were purposely made under the same light and lens.)

years of a popular dentifrice full of soap
and diatoms. Twelve good amalgam fillings were placed in the cervical notches

by high commissure and close lips, they
have fully justified the judgment of the
operator in selecting such a material, for

not a particle of recurrent caries resulted, but all these teeth were notched anew, including adjacent tooth structure.

The illustration presents what was left of one of these operations diagrammatically and actually, removed from the cervix of a lower central incisor (Fig. 20), the notching being in evidence. Fig. 21,

case, it is evident that tooth-brush abrasion alone and unaided could not cut cervically the typical notches which we call erosion.

The oral conditions are very similar in the second case to be reported—that of Mrs. X., age fifty-five, the mother of two sons, respectively twenty-four and

FIG. 24.

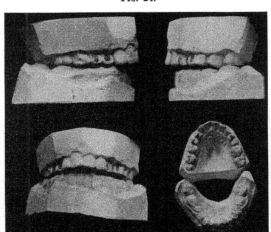

Casts taken two years ago. Sectioned gold fillings marked in black in bicuspids and canines. Left upper second bicuspid destroyed and crowned at this period. Note the good condition of the second molars, upper and lower.

with detail, shows the cut of the abrasive dentifrice, and what is of greater import, deep pits (Fig. 22) which are not to be seen in an illustration taken from a section of the tooth side of the same filling, the amalgam being condensed above the average (Fig. 23) ; so some solvent is at work in this mouth, reducing both tooth and filling, other than simple abrasive brushing. Further, if this solvent action of the mouth environment plus the known and continued use of an abrasive for fourteen years produces in amalgam only such damages as is presented in this

twenty-eight years of age, who are already showing mouth symptoms similar to those about to be described.

For over forty years the patient has been under the constant care of Dr. E. P. Keech, one of Baltimore's most eminent and conservative dental practitioners, who kindly permits the use of the casts and vouches for the data furnished herewith.

The element of mechanical abrasion either from occlusion or dentifrices is absolutely eliminated from consideration in this case. First, because at no time in twenty years has it been possible to bring the missing teeth in actual contact; second, but one dentifrice, the abrasive portion of which is precipitated chalk, has been used. (Fig. 24.)

The wasting process began early in life, simultaneously on the anterior upper and lower teeth labially, later buccally, and was met by the best of gold foil operations, as the writer can attest, having seen those extant in the mouth; these fillings lost substance and wasted just as did the caval and adjacent tooth substance retaining the filling until the small part remaining was lost owing to lack of retention. The lower incisors and canines and the contained fillings were the first to be destroyed, progressively from labial to lingual, cut level with and even under the gingiva; the wasting upper incisors were restored by four porcelain crowns, after which the process continued, sectioning both canines, exposing and destroying the approximal gold fillings previously covered by labial enamel, and cutting the buccal walls of the bicuspids to that half of the width of the crown, exposing and destroying, as the detail will show, the compound gold fillings that had been placed occlusally years before. We wish particularly to emphasize the progressive, equal, and regular destruction of both pure gold and tooth structure in this mouth, without mechanical cause, and to call attention to the fact that while all of the lower incisor, canine, and bicuspid groups are gone, even below the gingiva, and the upper incisors would likewise have disappeared had the four incisor porcelain crowns not stopped the process, *none of the molar group which are all "in situ" have been attacked except at the anterior buccal angles of the upper first molars.*

That mechanical abrasion has had

nothing to do with this case is further established by the fact that for at least twenty years these four molars have been the only teeth occluding, yet they present comparatively slight facets morsally, as noted in the illustrations.

The health of the patient during this period has been good; the salivary analysis could not be made, it being impossible to secure a specimen.

A definite anatomical relationship is shown in all erosion cases between a great loss of dental tissue—and in this case of gold as well, beginning labially and buccally and extending to all parts in direct contact with the fresh secretions conveyed by the ducts of the parotid and the submaxillary and sublingual glands, and particularly of the labial and buccal mucous glands —and the tooth-surfaces exposed to these secretions. This relationship is further emphasized by the fact that the buccal or molar mucous glands are described as being fewer in number than the labial glands, and diminishing as we follow the buccinator muscle to its distal insertion.

The continued immunity of the molars in this mouth, in which all other teeth have been destroyed, is most impressive, particularly if seen in the light of the foregoing statements and of the anatomy of the parts, which proves it to be more than a mere coincidence.

The writer resists the temptation to theorize as to these carefully observed phenomena, the causes for which he is totally at a loss to explain. Theories are fascinating, but not convincing. As a profession, we need a thorough chemical or electro-chemical investigation of the behavior of the metals in the mouth, as complete and final as the bacteriological work of Miller or the physical tests of teeth and amalgam by Black. Then shall we indeed suit our materials as we try to suit our methods—not only to the teeth but to the environment.

Discussion.

Dr. B. Holly Smith, Baltimore, Md. I should very much prefer to discuss the essayist than to discuss his paper. I was struck with the rather familiar way in which he called for the higher power and seemed to obtain it. I confess to no such familiarity with this higher power.

I am deeply interested in the subject of the disintegration of metals in the mouth, and I should deem it a rare privilege to have read the paper in the presence of Dr. Black, who knows perhaps more than any other man in this room about the behavior of metals in the compositions which we have presented to us as filling materials—he can help us, no doubt, to solve some of the complex problems involved. A little experience in the laboratory—where I had left a bottle of sulfuric acid unstopped, exposing some German silver to its fumes, which entirely changed the character of the metal, rendering it brittle—impressed me with the possibility of deteriorating influences of the oral environments on metals; not that we could have the fumes of sulfuric acid in any such concentrated form, but we know the influence of hydrochloric acid, which may be erupted from the stomach, affecting the metal used in the mouth. These observations give us a warning as to the advisability of using some of the base and low-fusing metals in appliances or fillings.

I confess to you that I am not capable of discussing this paper. I am not a metallurgist nor a chemist, and there

are many subjects that I should prefer to discuss, such as, for instance, Dr. Noel's paper. But Dr. Grieves' paper shows us that he and the others who are interested in this subject are trying to enable us to do better service for our patients than heretofore. It has not been uncommon practice in using porcelain teeth to set posts of German silver in zinc oxyphosphate, without a knowledge of the fact that the phosphoric acid would in a very little while destroy the posts. Unquestionably these defects, microscopic though they be, present a serious menace to the health of our patients. The salts produced by the disintegration of the metals enter into the alimentary tract and possibly have a deleterious influence upon the nutritive organs of the human body. I congratulate this association that this subject has been given serious consideration by one whom I know to be careful in what he says and conscientious in what he does.

I should like to hear Dr. Black discuss this paper, although I do not wish to put him ahead of our friend Dr. Head.

Dr. Joseph Head, Philadelphia, Pa. When our friend Dr. Smith speaks we all sit up and listen, and when he says what is true we all believe it, and even when he says what is not true we all wish it were so and half believe it. When he spoke concerning the grave danger of cementing German silver posts with zinc oxyphosphate, I confess that while I listened while he gave us most excellent reasons why the posts should deteriorate in a short while, I almost forgot that I had been setting these posts in zinc oxyphosphate for many years, and that many of them are now in position in the mouth. Still, I shall be cautious in doing it in the future. I have been reminded of the incident of the man who, when the locomotive first came into use, said that its real value would be greatly crippled, because he had worked it out with the utmost scientific accuracy that if a man traveled through the air at a speed greater than fifteen miles an hour, he would lose his breath and perish. It is similar with a great deal of our scientific work. We can give most excellent theories for anything under heaven, but every scientific experiment should be verified by accurate observation in the mouth, because the mouth observation is the final ultimate scientific test. We lead up to mouth experimentation as best we can by our laboratory work, difficult though it be, but we should always remember that in our laboratory work we are preparing for the great final arbitration of what we really find in the mouth, and I think that should be the keynote of all scientific work.

I can only most heartily commend this very excellent paper of Dr. Grieves on the deterioration by electrolysis. A great deal of his work will lead to far greater development in the future, and I hope that he will carry it on as he has begun it. I most heartily appreciate that he has not tried to explain the equation that we have in the mouth, where there are about ninety-eight unknown to any two known quantities. Often when the complicated processes of metabolism are explained by simple organic chemistry, we find that while the explanation is simple in the extreme, there is only one chance in a million, perhaps, of its being right. The great feature of Dr. Grieves' paper is that he has preferred to give the scientific data in a clear, concise, simple way, explaining what he could reasonably explain, and leaving the rest for the future to unravel. I have the greatest admiration and praise for

the author, and hope that his paper may help to stimulate more scientific work of a similar character.

The case cited in the essayist's paper which interested me most was that of a mouth in which he found that there was something which attacked the pure gold as well as the tooth-structure. Of course we all know that some of the base metals are very harmful if they are swallowed, but I should think that the patient in whose mouth gold fillings dissolved would at least not need the gold cure. It is strange that anything at all should be left in such a mouth, but I cannot help feeling that a great deal of that deterioration and wearing away of the gold may have been due to friction, even of precipitated chalk. Until the contrary is proved I should be strongly inclined to believe that the gold disappeared more from the friction of the tooth-brush. The tests Miller and a number of others have made in this direction show that while the tooth-brush applied with pure water has very little action, precipitated chalk will have a very decided effect. We all know from our laboratory work that precipitated, not the ordinary chalk, if applied on the brush wheel will rapidly wear away pure gold. There may be an acid in the mouth that attacks pure gold, but if that is the case, its presence is one of the most incomprehensible problems that have yet been presented to us. I also noticed that the front teeth were greatly affected and the molars not at all. Why should this electrolysis leave out the molars? In my opinion it is much more likely that these conditions arise as a result of the decalcifying action of foodstuff seconded by tooth-brush friction, its effect on the front teeth standing in direct ratio to the decalcifying action of the foodstuff on the teeth. I should feel very much inclined to ask such patients if they are in the habit of sucking lemons or oranges or other acid fruits, for it is well known that the fruit acids will soften the enamel so that very slight friction of the tooth-brush will wear it away with astonishing rapidity.

I cannot believe that Dr. Grieves' investigations entitle us to assume that there is in the mouth an acid strong enough to attack pure gold. I do not think that it is proved that electrolysis wears away the enamel and the tooth-structure. It must be at least the presence of decalcifying foodstuffs, perhaps together with the presence of decalcifying saliva, tooth-brush friction, and precipitated chalk, which produces just such a condition as the essayist has so scientifically and most excellently presented to us tonight.

Dr. G. V. BLACK, Chicago, Ill. It is with some hesitation that I respond when asked to talk about a subject in which we have so many conflicting data. We know very little about alloys. There are some phases about the metals, the most sensitive of all the elements, that we seem not to be able to understand. When I work with metals it seems to me that they are living entities; when they are pure they do certain things over and over again with an exactness that cannot be expected of any other elements, but when we turn them loose and let them run riot, mixing them with each other and with other elements, we never know what to expect. I have long been impressed with this, and hesitate to talk of the metals unless I can single them out, or pair certain ones together.

Pure gold cannot be dissolved in the mouth. Dr. Miller announced that his gold fillings were worn away by erosion just the same as the tooth material, by the tooth-brush and abrasive powder, as he supposed. I had been trying to stop erosion by gold fillings; the erosion would go on beside the fillings and leave the margins of the fillings standing there perfectly shaped without a trace of erosion. That went on for years, and I had never observed anything else. But some time ago I met a dentist whose teeth were badly eroded, and who had gold crowns put on because his teeth were so exceedingly sensitive. On one of these teeth the crown had been cut through; another crown had been put on and that was cut through, and a third crown had been put on, and that was also cut through. The patient maintained that no abrasive tooth-powder whatever was used in brushing his teeth. I would compare this with another observation: A gentleman of my acquaintance has a class of patients practically all of whom have erosion. I questioned one of his patients about the use of the tooth-brush, and he replied that he brushed his teeth three times every day, and brushed them well. Another dentist was examining that patient's mouth at that time, and saw the operator make a cross-mark with a chisel on the buccal surface of a molar that was thickly covered with filth. He called my attention to this, and four days afterward that cross-mark was still showing in that mouth.

Dr. HEAD. Was there erosion on that molar?

Dr. BLACK. No, sir.

Dr. HEAD. So that shows that friction did not act on that molar.

Dr. BLACK. That may be. We have so-called erosion by friction, undoubtedly due to abrasive tooth-powders. But we also have erosion though the patient does not brush his teeth. This can surely not be due to friction. There are a good many questions about erosion that I am in doubt about, but some of the horizontal lines that run across the teeth are in my opinion due to the tooth-brush and abrasive powders. I looked over Dr. Miller's work in his laboratory during his experiments on the artificial production of erosion, and I must say that if he had shown me these as cases of erosion that had occurred in the mouth, I would not have thought of questioning the correctness of his statement. But they are not of the character of many of the erosions which I have seen in the mouth. The characteristic cup-shaped erosions which we see in the mouth were produced artificially by fluids in motion, but we never observe such rapid motion in the mouth.

We have heard tonight a good deal about electrolysis, much of which is not electrolysis at all. If we take ordinary crystal gold such as Watts', place it on a tray, stick a pin through it and let it stand, the pin will fall off. It will be corroded at the surface of the gold, and will do so over and over again, though varying considerably in time in different trials. That is explained by the fact that the gold attracts acid gases and forms acid salts in its pores, and just where the pin comes to the air it will be corroded and fall off. This may be observed over and over again. We can analyze that which the gold has attracted from the atmosphere, if it is not too complex; sometimes it is so complex that it puzzles the best investigator. I do not know whether the gold fillings that were presented here tonight have been cut away by any acid in the mouth. You find this condition, however, quite commonly, and it is well to remember that we are very easily deceived in this respect, although the patient may have no intention of making false statements.

There is a great deal of misconception about amalgams. I have not been able to speak plainly enough to be well understood, and some phases have come up that have been overlooked in my early investigations and need to be corrected. I cannot understand why very many alloy makers insist on using two or three modifying metals in alloys while they should use but one, using metals that are incompatible with each other. Why should we mix our solders with zinc? Why should men want to place amalgam in a cavity and put gold over it? Why mix gold and tin? These metals are incompatible and will not work well together, and will destroy each other. If you take a block of silver of an inch square, rest it upon a block of tin of an inch square and put twenty-five pounds of pressure on it, you will find that the tin goes through the silver in a short time, and changes the character of the block. This shows that tin and silver have a very strong affinity for each other. But why mix gold with amalgam alloys? Gold will not harden in mercury. And you cannot make an amalgam of gold and platinum, so why put in these substances that will only cause trouble?

When studying amalgam alloys I asked the alloy makers to send me their alloys in ingots for examination. I laid these ingots on a piece of metal with a piece of tin beside them, and heated them up in such a way that the alloy and the tin received equal heat. I watched them until the tin had just begun to melt, then I took up the alloy with the tongs and knocked it on the table, and obtained globules of tin as big as a buckshot that had never been alloyed at all. Not half the alloys on the market at that time were true alloys; they were simply mixtures. There is a difference between an

8

alloy and a mixture. In alloy-making an alloy is one thing, and a mixture is another thing entirely. You may take a conglomeration or mixture of tin, gold, platinum, and what not, throw them into a crucible, and from this form an amalgam, and you will get such results as depicted; but if you take a silver and tin amalgam made from an alloy dependable results can be had, and you can always know when you have an alloy, if you are accurate enough in the weighing, because the alloy of silver and tin will always result in a condensation which will give you a higher specific gravity. This has been denied recently by some German investigators, but they have made the denial purely upon theoretical grounds, and I demand that they prove it by actual alloying and weighing.

Dr. E. A. BRYANT, Washington, D. C. I wish to say that in two cases I have met the very conditions which Dr. Grieves has brought before us in the last case cited. Not only was the pure gold disintegrated under these conditions, but an entire mouthful of crowns was simply wiped out, as Dr. Grieves has shown in his case. It seems to me that we have there the same conditions that are met with in depositing metal electrically. Dr. Head and Dr. Black have said that pure gold could not possibly be so dissolved, but I have seen several of these cases, and one of them is now living and in the hands of one of the leading dentists in Washington.

Dr. HEAD. I wish to add a remark on the deterioration of German silver in zinc oxyphosphate, about which my esteemed friend Dr. Black spoke. I can readily imagine that German silver would be deteriorated by the fluid oxyphosphate, and I have never questioned that, but when that mixture becomes set, it is inert and does not affect the German silver.

Dr. SMITH. When you set the pin in the oxyphosphate, it is in a fluid state.

Dr. HEAD. Only for a short time, and there is not enough acid left in the zinc oxyphosphate, and not enough time for the fluid to work upon the German silver so as to in any way affect it. As a matter of fact we have again and again taken the pins out immediately after setting them, or within six months, if we could get them out, and have found them to adhere firmly. If there had been any deterioration of the metal on the surface, the pin would have become loose. While Dr. Black may have seen these various phenomena, I have seen green teeth that did not have any German-silver pins in them; it may be that he has seen pink or sky-blue teeth, still he or I would not attribute that to German silver.

Dr. L. E. CUSTER, Dayton, Ohio. I have worked with German silver, platinoid, and metals of the higher melting-point, also with pure nickel. You may take a piece of German silver, which today is as fine as any metal you may wish to use in practice, and lay it away for six months, then bend it, and find that it has become brittle. This is because it is an alloy. Nickel as we ordinarily find it has a melting-point in the neighborhood of 2700° F. If pure nickel is used for regulating appliances instead of German silver all these difficulties which have been spoken of tonight will be overcome. It is not quite as rigid and strong as German silver; it possesses, however, some of the properties of the platinum pin in the Logan crown. Hammering or bending imparts to it a temper. Pure nickel is hard to obtain, and cannot be secured in this country, as far as I know, except from a firm in New York city. From this firm I have been able to obtain absolutely pure nickel, which I use instead of German silver, and if you will use it in your regulating appliances, you will overcome all the trouble referred to.

Dr. H. C. FERRIS, Brooklyn, N. Y. We are indeed to be congratulated upon this essay. This paper could be discussed for two or three days, and then we would have only commenced, as it contains so many discussable statements. I am going to briefly touch the subject from the physiological standpoint. The essayist makes mention of the physiological conditions resulting from the amount of solvent in the German silver being present in the mouth, and the deleterious effects upon the constitutional conditions. We all know that German silver dissolves in the mouth, and we also find that saliva containing the product of this solvent action has a germicidal effect upon the bacteriological product in the saliva. I have made some investigations along this line, Dr. Dexter, a pathologist of Brooklyn, carrying out these experiments for me. He put a band that had been worn in the mouth for two or three weeks into a gelatin culture, and found a negative result after incubation. He took the band again, scraped off the surface, put the scrapings in a gelatin culture and the band in another gelatin culture, introduced both into the incubator at the same time, and found that the scrapings had developed bacteria, the band none. This can be proved more easily by taking a specimen of saliva from a patient who is wearing German silver bands; you may allow that saliva to stand open for three or four days, and will perceive no odor from that specimen, or comparatively little. If, however, normal saliva from a normal mouth is left standing, in a night and a day it will drive you

out of the room. Again, saliva from a patient wearing a regulating appliance may be taken, filtered, dialyzed, mounted on a slide and examined under the microscope, and crystals of copper will be found in it. That proves that in such mouths copper is present, which has a bactericidal action on the saliva.

Dr. GRIEVES (closing the discussion). I am more than honored by Dr. Black's presence and his courtesy in discussing my paper.

I shall not take much time in closing, but would try to clear up a misunderstanding on the part of my friend Dr. Head. I had no idea that electrolysis had anything to do with the dissolving of the gold—I did not know what it was, and I think the paper which we are now going to hear from Dr. Ferris may throw further light on this question.

I have worked along this line and have presented this paper, feeling that dentists did not know the environments in which they were working, that they have been putting all kinds of things in mouths and did not know what was going on as the result of this. My thought is that dentists should make tests of the saliva, in the same way as the medical men make tests of the urine. They can do this in most cases, but occasionally they run across a hard case that they will have to send to some laboratory. Just as the medical men are making tests and are finding acetones and different acids in the urine, so we can test the saliva. Dr. Ferris, as chairman of the Committee on Scientific Research, is the man to tell us about such tests, and I am glad that his paper follows mine.

The next order of business was the Report of the Committee on Scientific Research, by Dr. H. C. FERRIS, Brooklyn, N. Y., chairman, as follows:

Report of Committee on Scientific Research.

By H. C. FERRIS.

YOUR committee has organized, and has taken up the study of "Salivary Analysis," as being the most important subject before the profession at the present time.

To intelligently study the pathological conditions of the oral cavity, we deem it necessary first to determine the normal. To accomplish this aim it is necessary to have more accurate information, together with a more simple and definite technique in the examination of saliva for its physical and chemical properties, in order that one investigator may work in the same field with another. That this may be accomplished a systematic examination of thousands of cases is necessary.

It is the opinion of your committee that the work done to date, from a pathological standpoint, cannot be of scientific value, as the normal constituents of the salivary secretion are unknown. Several chemical analyses have been made by physiological chemists, but comparatively little time has been spent upon this secretion, the importance of which as a factor in diagnosis has but recently become recognized.

In review of the methods used in salivary analysis, your committee are of the opinion that errors in technique are numerous. We have outlined a plan for the systematic study of the subject, in order to secure results that may be uniform and that a definite end may be attained. It will require painstaking work on the part of a number of investigators examining thousands of cases to produce results that can be considered of scientific value.

It is unnecessary to take up your time by relating in detail the extent of the experiments performed by your committee to attain the present method. Suffice it to say that we have detected errors in the method of determining the specific gravity. There has been no instrument devised for obtaining the specific gravity of the saliva. Findings have been reported lighter or below the specific gravity of water; if this be true, an error in technique remains to be proved.

To accomplish this object we have devised a salivary hydrometer whereby the specific gravity may be ascertained from 0.990 to 1.030, and requiring but a small quantity of the given specimen. The instrument is composed of a glass tube fitted with two compartments, one sealed and the lower one corked. The lower section holds $3\frac{1}{2}$ ccm. of water, the corked one is weighted with mercury so that when floated in distilled water at a temperature of 70° F. the scale in the stem will stand at 1000. Substituting the specimen for the water, one may read the scale, plus or minus. With this instrument one is able to determine the specific gravity of small quantities of saliva which are lighter or heavier than water. Care must be taken to fill the receptacle so that the bottom of the meniscus registers on the line, as the instrument is extremely delicate.

We also found errors in the method of

taking the acid and alkaline reactions with litmus paper, and in the ordinary method of titration with phenol-phthaleïn taken with sodium hydrate, owing to the presence of carbon dioxid.

In order to eliminate this property, a definite quantity of hydrochloric acid was added to the specimen, which was then brought to a boiling-point, so that the acid estimation would be more accurate by the elimination of the CO_2. This technique is explained in chart No. 1. (See end of report.) For determining extreme alkalinity, 1 per cent. solution of methyl orange may be used as an indicator, titrated with 1/40 normal hydrochloric acid solution.

We suggested to Dr. H. Carlton Smith, professor of chemistry at Harvard Medical College, that he devise for us a more definite scale for the quantitative analysis for sulfocyanates, so that the estimation of these properties of saliva be uniform and the findings be intelligible to the scientific world. The instrument which he devised is here illustrated. It affords a fair estimation by color reaction.

The instrument is constructed with a 4 mm. cell cemented in the center of a disk of glass 2 mm. in diameter. The cell is filled with aqua destillata and six definite amounts of potassium sulfocyanate added, with two drops of ferric chlorid (5 per cent.) as a reagent. Another disk of glass is placed on top of the cell, so as to eliminate all air-bubbles. The color reaction was then painted in oil on the under surface of the upper disk, leaving the center free. By substituting saliva for the aqua and adding your reagent, you compare the color obtained with those found on the disk, which will give you an approximate estimation of the quantity of potassium sulfocyanate in your specimen. The instru-

ment is practical in high percentages, although it is of limited value in dilute solutions, owing to the limited number of colors on the gage.

Your committee are greatly indebted to Dr. Smith for his assistance.

Your chairman, assisted by Dr. Schradieck of Brooklyn, has devised another scale for this reaction, which is composed of two glass tubes of the same caliber, with white glass backs and with a blue line running through the center.

Tube A is scaled to receive 1 ccm. of the specimen to be examined. Tube B is scaled in multiples of 1 ccm. divided into tenths.

The method of estimation is as follows: In tube A put 1 ccm. of the specimen to be examined. In tube B put 1 ccm. of a standard solution of 1:2000 sulfocyanate of ammonia, then add two drops from the same pipette of a 5 per cent. solution of ferric chlorid as a reagent. The color struck in tube A will be lighter than that struck in tube B. By adding sterile water to tube B to the second volume you will have reduced this quantity one-half, or 1:4000, and so on. This reduction continues until you match the shade of reaction in tube A. You will then be able to read from the bottom of the meniscus, in thousandths and ten-thousandths, the quantitative value of sulfocyanate in the specimen. With this instrument one is able to determine quantities up to 1:20,000, but if you dilute your standard solution of sulfocyanate of ammonia one-half, or 1:4000, and proceed as before, you can estimate a quantity of 1:40,000, the instrument being as sensitive as one drop of your color reagent in 1 ccm. of aqua.

The same scale may be used to determine the quantity of ammonia or organic matter, using Nessler's reagent instead of ferric chlorid.

Your committee has adopted this scale for the estimation of these chemicals, until it is proved defective.

The present estimation of ammonia with Nessler's reagent is incorrect, as Nessler's reagent strikes a color with any vegetable or animal matter in solution, epithelial cells, etc.; we have therefore substituted the term "ammonia or organic matter." In this connection your committee are cognizant of the fact that Nessler's reagent varies materially as made by different manufacturers, therefore it is advisable to procure it from the same chemical supply house.

In order to further this object we have devised a set of examination sheets with directions for the technique, making these as simple as possible, so that any careful practitioner may pursue this work. No. I—Method of Technique; No. II—Salivary Record for each patient examined. These records may be procured from the committee.

To further facilitate this method on your part, we have arranged with Eimer & Amend of New York city to construct a salivary analysis set, which will contain a special 5 ccm. burette and stand, 11 tubes each fitted with a rubber-stoppered pipette, a 10 ccm. graduate, a 10 ccm. graduate, corked, with a double scale; a salivary hydrometer, a colorimetric scale for ammonia and sulfocyanate; a glass mixing-rod; a set of beakers; 1 oz. of each of the twelve reagents, and a white porcelain minim examination slab. These may be procured at an expense of $17, or fitted in a wooden case with removable sections, $20.

Your committee wish to call for volunteers to work with us. We should be glad to have the gentlemen interested in this work report their findings in ten cases of normal mouths which show normal reaction in urinary excretion (two examinations to be made, three days apart), and as many cases as possible of pyorrhea alveolaris and interstitial gingivitis, the examinations to be made every three days during treatment. If such reports be furnished to your committee by January 1910, a tabulation of results will be made. We also solicit all the criticism that can be backed by scientific proof, both chemical and physiological, upon this technique, which we consider as being far from perfect, yet as marking an initial step in the scientific consideration of this subject.

In order to emphasize the value of investigation of this character and the interesting results following, we wish to report a case of orthodontia examined under an inferior technique to that which we are presenting, together with a urinary analysis, examinations having been made twice a week for nine months. You will note the changes in time of delivery of the specimen, the specific gravity, the acid index, sulfocyanates, and ammonia or organic matter—all those properties which are recognized as pathological being eliminated with the exception of a trace of albumin, at the end of this report [exhibiting]. The final result you will here see illustrated in the patient.

Such reports as these are being duplicated every day throughout the country, and from our clinical experience we know what must take place. But if we desire to be considered scientific men, it behooves us to prove our work in a scientific manner.

We trust we may be able to interest you gentlemen in this field, so that we may be enabled to determine the normal, and establish a system of diagnosis that will be practical.

[I.]

Directions for Making Analysis of Saliva.

(Prepared by the Scientific Research Committee of the National Dental Association.)

History of chronic disease:

Description of teeth and mucous membrane:

Character of decay:

(1) *Time of day:* (2) *Time to deliver 20 ccm.:*

Amount:

Consistence: [Sticky, thick, or thin:]

Odor: [Fetid, ammoniacal, resembling garlic, or other peculiar odor:]

Specific gravity: [May be taken with a salivary hydrometer (Eimer & Amend):]

Precipitate: [Whether large or small quantity:]

Test for acid index: Should be ascertained as soon as delivered. Use 1-40 normal sodium hydrate solution in 5 ccm. burette. The degree of acidity is obtained by taking 5 ccm. saliva and adding 2 drops of phenol-phthalein solution, neutral, then drop by drop NaOH (1-40 normal solution sodium hydrate) until a rose color is produced. Having noted on paper the number of ccm. of the NaOH in the burette before and after the rose color is obtained, the number of ccm. displaced multiplied by 20 and divided by 4 (in order to find the number of ccm. NaOH necessary to reduce 100 ccm. saliva) equals the degree of acidity—normal being alkaline.

To attain a more accurate result, add 1 ccm. of 1-10 normal HCl solution and boil to drive off the CO_2; titrate as before and subtract the acid index of HCl from result.

Test for alkalinity: Proceed as above, substituting 1:40 normal HCl for sodium hydrate and methyl orange for phenol-phthalein, and titrate.

Sulfocyanate: Use the colorimetric scale (Eimer & Amend), 1 ccm. of specimen in tube A, 1 ccm. of 1:2000 sulfocyanid ammonia in tube B; add 2 drops of 5 per cent. ferric chlorid to each tube, add aqua destillata until color in B matches that of specimen. Read scale in thousandths and ten-thousandths. Care must be taken to have the bottom of the meniscus on the line.

Ammonia or organic matter: Use colorimetric scale, 1 ccm. of specimen in tube A, 1 ccm. of 1:2000 ammonium chlorid in tube B; then add 2 drops of Nessler's reagent to each tube; reduce the color in tube B with aqua destillata until it matches specimen. Read scale in thousandths and ten-thousandths.

Chlorin: To 4 drops of sample on a white slab add a drop of 5 per cent. solution neutral chromate of potassium (K_2 or O_4). Mix with glass rod and then add a drop of a 1-10 per cent. solution of silver nitrate. If chlorin is present in normal quantities this test will give a reddish precipitate, gradually turning white.

Acetone: In 4 drops of sample dissolve a crystal of potassium carbonate, then add a drop of Gram's reagent. An odor of iodoform indicates acetone. (Care must be taken not to confound the odor of iodoform iodin in Gram's reagent with that of iodoform.) Mount slide and examine with microscope for crystals of iodoform, is best test.

Mucin: Use 10 ccm. of specimen, dilute with equal quantity of aqua, then add 5 drops of glacial acetic acid, and the mucin will separate and can be recorded as Excess, Normal, or Minus.

Albumin: After the mucin has separated, filter, and with the filtrate make the test for albumin. To about one-half a wine-glass of clear saliva add strong nitric acid very slowly, allowing the acid to run down the side of the glass so that it forms a separate layer beneath the saliva. Just above the line of contact note the white line of albumin. Record as Excess, Trace, or Normal.

[II.]

Salivary Analysis.

Name ....Age ....

Time ....Date ....

History of chronic diseases ....

Description of teeth and character of caries ....

Amount of saliva (normal 60 cc. per hour) ....

Consistence ....

Odor ....

Specific gravity (normal 1.002) ....

Precipitate ....

Test for Acid index........Normal........

       Alkaline ....•....

Sulfocyanate ....

Ammonia and organic constituents ....

Chlorin ....

Ptyalin or enzymatic value ....

Acetone ....

Mucin ....

Albumin ....

There being no further business before the section, the Chairman declared Section I adjourned until the next annual meeting of the association.

SECTION II:

Operative Dentistry, Nomenclature, Literature, Dental Education, and Allied Subjects.

Chairman—W. G. EBERSOLE, Cleveland, Ohio.
Secretary—L. L. BARBER, Toledo, Ohio.

FIRST DAY—Tuesday, March 30th.

THE first meeting of Section II was called to order on Tuesday afternoon, March 30th, at 2.30 o'clock, by the chairman, Dr. W. C. Ebersole.

The first order of business was the reading of a paper by Dr. S. D. RUGGLES, Portsmouth, O., entitled "Phases of Improvement in Nomenclature," as follows:

Phases of Improvement in Nomenclature.

By S. D. RUGGLES.

IN the presentation of this paper the writer does not wish to rehearse the long list of terms previously considered by this body, but rather to show some means whereby the achievements of your essayists and committees on nomenclature may be put into use more generally by the profession. Time, however, must always be the meter for the perfection of a great science. When we consider that modern dentistry has but passed its first half-century, what has been accomplished seems little less than marvelous. The kaleidoscopic swiftness with which a crude art or craft has taken on the air of a profession is only appreciated by those among us who have helped to bring this about, and little is the wonder that we become impetuous and restless in this twentieth century, famed for its accomplishments.

The fathers of dentistry were, as a class, not men of culture, but simply artizans, adepts in the use of tools and instruments, and, like most of their kind, of limited education. The dead languages were truly dead as far as these men were concerned, yet their vocabularies were sufficient for the demands of their occupation. As a matter of fact there was no great need for special words or terms until after the trade spirit had passed. When it became obvious that future progress depended upon the exchange of ideas, the workers found themselves hampered by the lack of adequate vehicles of expression. Even at the present time a very large percentage of the members of our profession are not college-bred men, and can scarcely be expected to contribute much in a literary or truly scientific way. Let us not despise, though, the humble toiler, who does well with the means at hand the many delicate and exacting operations intrusted to him, for of men of this sort our state and local societies are largely composed. Men of this type make good listeners, and are usually keen in their appreciation of good essays presented by men better versed in dental training.

During the past ten or twelve years no systematic effort has been made. on the part of the many state and local societies to have their essayists conform to standard and recognized terminology, and therein lies one of the greatest stumbling-blocks to impede universal advancement in nomenclature. Within the past decade there was but one paper published in my own state journal, and what is still worse, no standing committee on nomenclature is provided for by our state constitution. Every state and local society should have an active committee, which might also serve in the capacity of an essay committee, and see to it that all papers to be read before the society, and all published matter, should conform to the system adopted by the National Association. The relation of the latter

to subordinate bodies may well be the same as is maintained by the French Academy to the lesser lights in France.

When we realize that the vocabulary of the high-school student at graduation is something less than fifteen hundred words, and that a man of education uses about double that number, the wisdom of your committee in eliminating terms is better appreciated, *e.g.* cervical has superseded gingival. The tendency is, and should be, one of elimination. Custom and usage establish certain words, and their acceptance has to be acknowledged regardless of fitness, as in the case of model and cast, and the verb cement, which is now pretty generally used as a noun.

Granting that the growth of any science multiplies the number of its terms, the reverse seems to be true after a certain stage is reached. In the older science of music, for example, the tendency is now one of reduction and simplification.

After all has been said, it is quite evident, after reviewing the literature of the immediate past, that the most urgent need is not extension of our present list so much as definite knowledge of and familiarity with it. For instance, the word palatal appears very often in our current reading matter. It is neither anatomically correct nor so euphonious as the more accurate lingual. In proportion as we are careless about tolerating the use of words made obsolete by the eliminating process of those in authority, just so long will progress be slow.

Allow me to call your attention to a few terms that have been accepted, yet do not exactly fill their mission. The word abrasion is defined as "The wearing away of tooth-substance either by attrition or through the action of sharp particles in tooth-powder." There is something lacking in this definition, for the majority of these so-called abrasions are accompanied by conditions so much like erosion that some word is needed to express this process, even if its real cause is obscure. The accepted definition will cover a simple case of abrasion, but some adjective is needed to differentiate between that and the condition just referred to. "Complex abrasion" would at once convey the idea, and is self-explanatory. Since the etiology is not well established, it could serve a temporary purpose at least.

The writer regrets exceedingly that the word substitute was not accepted instead of dummy. Since this is a term used largely before patients, it should express or convey the real idea in question. Either as a noun or verb, the idea cannot be misconstrued if substitute were used.

Approximal is another word in bad form, in spite of Dr. White's efforts to have it accepted. In the formation of compound words it is very cumbersome. Proximal is much the better word, and was recommended by your committee in 1893.

Although the sciences in general favor the Greek language, on account of its multitudinous forms and the delicacy of meaning it is capable of expressing, we do not find the Greek equivalent to some of our terms most commonly used. The Latin has loaned us roots whose use is now well established. Our French and German co-workers have used terms in their language which have become acceptable to the profession in general. Indeed, we have appropriated terms from the Chinese down to the present-day vernacular. Our nomenclature should be broad enough to embrace all useful words, regardless of their origin.

Since this is an era of specializing, and dentistry has joined the procession, cannot these specialists best choose the words for their own particular fields?

Dr. Wilson has made very valuable suggestions in prosthetic dentistry, as have others in orthodontia, operative dentistry, etc. Perhaps no single man has done more toward bringing order out of chaos than Dr. Black, but even he freely admits, in his last work, "Operative Dentistry," the lack of correct expression for certain conditions.

Operative dentistry is, I believe, better equipped with a nomenclature than is any other branch of our work, and yet the majority of essayists will use a blackboard, if one is convenient.

Immediately following the World's Columbian Dental Congress at Chicago, the Northwestern University Dental School had a pamphlet issued for its students, containing a list of twenty-two words, thirteen nouns and nine adjectives. These words constitute by far the best part of our nomenclature to the present day, for there is no limit to their range of application. In 1897 this subject was brought before the Ohio State Dental Society, and three hundred copies of this pamphlet were distributed among its members. For several months after this meeting requests came from different parts of the state for extra copies. This indicated a far greater interest in the subject than was at first suspected. The Institute of Dental Pedagogics has published a glossary of dental terms, under date of January 1, 1909, which is more general than any I have yet seen, but omits the terms used in orthodontia and porcelain work. No mention is made of the nomenclature of instruments. Every practitioner knows the inconvenience occasioned by the arbitrary methods of the manufacturers in the constant changing of numbers. Perhaps one's next order of the same number will bring a different instrument. This subject has been considered by the National School of Dental Technics, and a very accurate and comprehensive system adopted. This is needed more by teachers, no doubt, than by any other class, but will be a great aid to all who appreciate system.

The Transactions of this association have been published at intervals covering a great many years. While an isolated copy of the proceedings of one year occasionally falls into the hands of most dentists, there are few who have access to complete files for reference. I should like to recommend very strongly, in closing, an official publication of the list of terms accepted up to date. A reliable dictionary of medical and dental terms for the dental student might follow. If the present interest in the study of dentistry continues, the next few years should make this possible.

Discussion.

Dr. M. L. RHEIN, New York, N. Y. This subject is one in regard to which I am of the opinion we all are in accord with the essayist, inasmuch as too little attention has been paid to it in the past, and too much attention cannot be given to it in the future. The question of how to reach a general conclusion in regard to some of these disputed points is hard to solve. For example, the essayist took occasion to emphasize his own preference for the use of the term proximal instead of approximal. For my part I could never give my assent to the use of this term, and I believe the reason given by the essayist to be not only a very poor one, but a very contrary one to the principle which he laid down in the first portion of his paper, where he states that terms should explicitly, as far as possible, represent exactly what they state. Proximal, as has been so often said in public, simply refers to something near, while approximal definitely states a fact which we wish to state, i.e. an adjoining surface. I believe that the contention of Dr. White concerning this important word was correct, and I cannot understand why the addition of the two letters in approximal should make it lack in euphony.

I simply bring out this one point in order to show that many difficulties are presented at the present time in regard to the use of different terms. Outside of this particular term referred to by the essayist, I have nothing but words of commendation and approval for the subject-matter of the essay and for the desire there elicited. That is especially true in reference to the suggestion that the committee on essays in all societies should also be the committee on nomenclature. This suggestion seems a most excellent one, for many of the unfortunate errors in nomenclature that appear in print would be avoided, as this committee could eliminate these errors before an essay is published.

Dr. WM. A. LOVETT, Brewton, Ala. I should like to make a correction of one of the statements which have been made concerning the paucity of literature on the subject of the nomenclature of our profession. Several papers or essays published on this subject can certainly be found by searching the records of transactions of this association. If I remember correctly, at the

1906 meeting of the association in Atlanta, Dr. George H. Wilson of Cleveland, Ohio, gave us a very able and lengthy paper on this topic, in which he presented a very full vocabulary of the different terms used in dentistry, their derivation and meaning, recommending in many instances such changes of words as would convey in an intelligent way the exact idea to be communicated by such terms.* I remember this paper very distinctly, because several of the words recommended attracted my attention, as, for instance, the word "substitute" for the word "dummy;" the essayist stated that while the former was a better term, it did not fully come up to requirements. Desiring to aid in the search for definite terms, it occurred to me that the term "dens-replica" would convey the exact idea. In studying the root and full meaning of the word "replica," I found that a substituted tooth would not be an exact reproduction of the lost organ of mastication.

I agree with the essayist that we should have a better system of nomenclature in our operative and prosthetic work. In medical nomenclature the terms used as a rule definitely describe the nature of the disease and its location; in surgery the names of the different operations describe accurately the nature of the operation and the part operated upon, while in chemistry the terminology employed in association with the chemical names gives us at a glance the formulæ of such preparations.

While this is true, dental surgeons as a rule do not comply strictly with medical and chemical nomenclature, as is evidenced by their prescription-writing.

* N. D. A. Trans. 1906, p. 164 et seq. Cosmos for May 1907, vol. xlix, pp. 456-65.

The profession is often brought into disrepute by reason of the poorly written prescriptions of its practitioners.

As far as dental nomenclature is concerned, every dental surgeon is in a measure a law unto himself, and one's failure to grasp a writer's or speaker's exact meaning sometimes may enhance in the estimation of his readers or listeners his ability from the standpoint of education, while in truth he may be using newly coined words of his own making.

I am certainly in hearty accord with the essayist in his effort to establish a better system of nomenclature, and I agree with him as to the several recommendations made in his paper to that end. After we have secured this authentic change in dental nomenclature, we may hope that the profession will use the new vocabulary with more accuracy and greater freedom than it is now using medical, chemical, and surgical terms of known authenticity.

Dr. W. T. JACKMAN, Cleveland, Ohio. I am uncertain whether I understood the essayist correctly when he spoke of the words "cervical" and "gingival." I understood him to say that the word gingival is no longer used, and the word cervical has been substituted in its place. The word "cervix" means neck, and it is correct to use the term if we only wish to indicate the neck of the tooth, but what are we to use to indicate the gum margin? I should like to have the essayist answer that. If he can propose a better word than gingival to apply to the gum margin, I should like to know it, for I know no better word. I hardly think that we are ready to drop the word gingival.

Dr. RUGGLES (closing the discussion). In regard to the use of the words gingival and cervical, I do not wish to be misunderstood in saying that one has superseded the other entirely, because the two words apply to different conditions and should be used differently, but we should no longer speak of a gingival cavity when we mean a cervical cavity. There is a gingival line, the gingiva being a tissue at the cervical portion of the tooth, but we should not call a cavity at the cervical margin of the enamel a gingival cavity, as it is a cervical cavity.

A great many papers have no doubt been written on the subject of nomenclature, but to my knowledge very few such papers have been published in our journals. Dr. Lovett is correct in his remarks about a paper that was read at the Atlanta meeting of the National Association. I know of that paper, for I read it. But I have subscribed for the DENTAL COSMOS for twenty or thirty years past, and have spent considerable time in looking through the volumes for articles on nomenclature. The references to this subject which I found are but short, and I do not consider them properly papers on nomenclature. The principal papers have been read before this body, and they have been few indeed and were chiefly written by members of the committee in charge of that work. As to outside papers, I found one or two in the *Ohio Dental Journal* in the past ten years. This is a subject that has been consistently shunned, and before I had finished this paper I felt very much as if I should

like to shun it myself. An essayist should be able to speak several languages to investigate this subject thoroughly, and should have many years to spend on his investigation. Dr. Black spent probably twelve or fifteen months on his original report to the Columbian Congress. The term which my friend Dr. Rhein finds fault with was submitted at that time and was practically accepted, but for some reason or other it has not been fully accepted by this association. At least one text-book—Black's Anatomy—has adopted the term, and I think others have done the same. It is much easier to say interproximal than it is to say interapproximal. If you will look up the origin of the word, it will not be difficult to convince you that the prefix could well be dispensed with, and the word will be easier for all to handle and it will serve every purpose. We all understand, of course, that Dr. Rhein is a New York man, and probably has a preference for the nomenclature used by the men in his neighborhood, but to my way of thinking, and I believe to a majority of dentists, Black's "Dental Anatomy" is a very good authority.

The next order of business as announced by the chairman was the reading of a paper by Dr. W. T. JACKMAN, Cleveland, Ohio, entitled "The Elimination of Fear in the Practice of Dentistry," as follows:

The Elimination of Fear in the Practice of Dentistry.

By W. T. JACKMAN.

THE bane of human existence is fear. The rich live in fear of losing their wealth; the poor are ever anxious about food and clothing and shelter. If well, many people live in constant dread of becoming ill; if ill, they are fearful that health may never again be theirs to enjoy. Fear is just as real to the patient though wholly imaginary, as it is when caused by a previous experience. People with very sensitive teeth are filled with horror when informed that operative procedure is necessary because of the ravages of dental caries. Many never return to the dentist after the first visit —they would rather lose their teeth than endure the pain. It is with these that we are concerned in particular; yet the humane operator is always unwilling to give anyone pain when it can be prevented. Let us now study ways and means whereby we may eliminate this fear of dental operations.

The title of this paper implies that more humane methods should be employed in our efforts to cure or repair dental and oral lesions, particularly the former. I state the truth when I say that *nearly* all pain inflicted by dentists could be wholly averted if proper and available means were used. This sentence is susceptible of demonstration, therefore is scientific. We have come to the time when cavity preparation may, with only an occasional exception, be made without pain. It would be next to criminal for me to use a bur in a sensitive cavity. This I say after almost

five years of practical experience demonstrating the fact that cavity preparation may be made without fear of pain on the part of the patient. Is this not worth striving for?

Ever since dental operations have been made it has been the study of the best operators to find some way whereby pain might be lessened or eliminated. Other things being equal, are we not or should we not be more interested in this vital question than our predecessors? I am sure that no negative reply will be given to this interrogatory. Then, as we study the prevention of pain, let us first remember that no one ever seeks the professional services of the dentist except as dire necessity drives him to it. How necessary, then, to treat him kindly, gently, humanely. It is understood that the patient will find the office of the progressive, up-to-date dentist neat, tidy, and clean—particularly should this be true of the operating room—with nearly all instruments out of sight.

This leads to one point which I wish to emphasize in particular; it is this: In order that the patient may be at ease while the operation is being performed, there should be fastened to the head-rest a downy feather pillow, size $2\frac{1}{2}$ x 10 x 12 inches, for the patient to rest the head against. The padding of the ordinary head-rest is so hard that it becomes torture for the patient before the end of a two hours' sitting.

Let us now familiarize ourselves with some method or methods whereby we can put our patient at ease and keep her there during the entire visit.

Lest this paper should grow too long, I shall discuss but three phases, viz: First, putting the patient at ease after taking the operating chair; second, the adjustment of the rubber dam, and third, desensitizing the tooth for cavity preparation and pulp removal.

If the dentist concludes that he has a right to hurt his patient in order that a good, saving operation may be made, he is in serious error.

Humanitarian dentistry means, practically, painless dentistry. I do not propose to discuss dental histology, but simply refer to the odontoblastic layer of cells, with their prolongations extending throughout the length of the dentinal tubuli, being the protoplasmic contents of the tubuli, the fibers of Tomes, etc.— and in this connection I wish to remind you that there is sensation from the enamel ends of these tubuli throughout their length to the pulp, and thence to the nerve centers at the base of the brain —but I do wish to discuss with you the fact that just in proportion as we inhibit or prevent painful sensations from reaching the nerve centers we eliminate the dread or fear of dental operations.

In doing this latter, however, the careful operator is always mindful of a possible resultant pathological condition. He consequently makes his clinical tests cautiously, weighing every detail, and from this data forms his conclusions relative to the merit or demerit of any method of practice.

After your patient is seated in the operating chair, proceed at once to allay her fears by assuring her that you will not hurt her. Do not stop here, however, for the chances are that she will not believe you, unless you explain just what you intend to do that she may not be hurt. Having gained her confidence in part, make the operation as promised, and you will ever after have her singing your praises. Now, do not misunderstand me, for I would not lead you to think that one may become so efficient in painless methods as to never cause pain, but what I would emphasize is that more than ninety per cent. of our work may be done without pain, and when pain is inflicted it should be but slight indeed.

In learning to eliminate fear in the practice of dentistry the passing of time must not be considered, for one must have the all-absorbing thought in mind that the patient must not be hurt; then following this the perfect operation can be made, because the conditions make it possible.

It was first discovered that dehydrating the dentin by the use of warm air was a means of no little value in preventing pain; yet in many cases, even though the attempt be skilfully made, it is found to be more painful than the preparation of the cavity after drying with absorbent cotton only. This method, then, has proved to be of uncertain value as a desensitizer.

Next, medication by way of topical application has been much used, and is still being used with considerable success. The chief objection to drugs used topically is their superficial effect—they do not obtund deeply enough, oftentimes, to permit of the removal of a single layer of leathery dentin without giving pain. While warm drugs topically applied have much merit as obtunders, yet they fall far short of the ideal. Following the topical use of drugs came the freezing or cold mixtures. The Van Wyck-Kerr obtunder is probably the best of these. The mixture used is sulfuric ether, with a small addition (5 per cent.) of alcohol. The effect is produced by a small spray of this mixture—operated by compressed air, from fifteen to twenty pounds—being thrown into the cavity, after first placing several layers of cotton over the cavity and throwing the spray on the cotton for a few minutes, then removing the first layer of cotton, and thus gradually removing all the cotton, when the spray is thrown directly into the cavity. This method will obtund, but it has several serious drawbacks. The cavity must be prepared while the spray is being thrown in, for if the spray is removed, sensation will return in about a minute. In preparing a cavity while it is wet the operator is prevented from following the fine lines of decay to their end. Then, again, the smell of the ether is offensive, and lastly, the apparatus is quite expensive. Theoretically, at least, it would seem to produce a condition of the pulp not conducive to its continued health; yet Dr. E. T. Loeffler of Ann Arbor, Mich., tells me that after more than a year's use he has not noted any ill results to the pulp; but this time would seem too short for definite clinical conclusions. There are other cold sprays, such as ethyl chlorid, etc., all involving practically the same objections.

After these came cataphoresis. What a furor this method of procedure created for a time in the dental profession! But this, like many other things which at first gave great promise as obtundents, proved to be inefficient to a very great degree, largely because of the crude apparatus that was available.

My *confrère* and fellow townsman, Dr. Weston A. Price, invented a cataphoric machine that would obtund—the only efficient cataphoric apparatus that was ever put on the market as far as I know. When this was properly used in connection with the milammeter it would do the work; but even the good doctor's apparatus was defective. Although, as stated, it would obtund, this defect proved fatal to its general adoption, viz, too much time was required to obtund, and added to this was the difficulty of properly insulating the tooth to be operated upon.

After the above brief description of what we had in the way of desensitizers up to five years ago, I come to you today with a thing which is not new nor is it old—it is of the tender age of five years; a method that has been of inestimable value to me, and should be to every dentist; a means for obtunding sensitive dentin of which if I were to be deprived I should want to cease the practice of dentistry. I refer to anesthesia produced by a two per cent. aqueous solution of cocain hydrochlorid with the use of the high-pressure syringe. Few dentists, apparently, have had the patience and determination to master this instrument, but when this mastery is once acquired there is no instrument in the dentist's armamentarium of so much value as this, the *proper* use of which will turn your patient's mourning into joy and will relieve you from much nervous strain—consequently you will be less tired at the day's end. It will enable you to operate more expeditiously and perfectly, especially with nervous patients.

This paper is intended to be helpful more particularly from the practical side; therefore I shall endeavor to describe to you in simple terms the procedure that will produce the desired results, viz, the complete obtunding of the tooth, in order that cavity preparation may be made painlessly. Let me say by way of parenthesis that there are many high-pressure instruments on the market, but there are, as far as I know, but two or three that are really efficient.

Let us select, if you please, the typical nervous patient with the blue white teeth that are always sensitive. She comes to the office with fear depicted on every feature, and often we note the tremor of the whole body because of the never-to-be-forgotten previous operation or operations; or perchance it may be her first visit to the office, but fear controls her because she has heard others relate their experience. Let us prepare a cavity or cavities for this young woman of sixteen or eighteen summers. As previously stated, her fears must be allayed, as far as possible, by assuring her that you will not hurt her. After this proceed to adjust the rubber dam, if the teeth and gums do not need prophylactic treatment. Before adjusting the dam, however, a very important procedure should never be neglected, viz, desensitizing the gums with a five per cent. aqueous solution of cocain hydrochlorid. This should be applied for at least five minutes, by grasping a piece of cotton with the pliers, dipping it in the solution and saturating the gum margin, using considerable pressure around the teeth over which the dam is to be placed. Then adjust the dam and proceed as follows, if the tooth to be operated on is a lower right first molar containing a large occlusal and a medium-sized buccal cavity: With a No. 3 round bur make a slight pit in the enamel, over healthy dentin, one-third the depth of the enamel; this pit should be made on either side of the buccal cavity or preferably just below the buccal

cavity, if possible. Then use a No. ½ round bur to slightly deepen the pit already made, but do not drill through the enamel, for this would give needless pain. By running the engine at low speed the operation so far has been without pain. The tooth is now ready for the high-pressure syringe. The syringe I use has forceps handles with a locking device between the handles so that when complete contact is established in the pit with the point of the syringe and the handles closed as far as possible, they remain locked, thus relieving the hand and preventing cramp. Previous to applying the syringe, fill it with a two per cent. aqueous solution of cocain hydrochlorid by placing the point in the solution and opening the handles; this will fill the barrel. Then grasp the handles, dagger fashion, stand behind and to the right of the patient, pass the left arm around the patient's head, place the second, third, and fourth fingers of the left hand under the patient's mandible near the chin with the index finger of the left hand against the tooth to be operated on, for counter pressure. Pass the barrel and point of the syringe, after filling, through the flame of the alcohol lamp to warm the solution. Then place the point of the syringe in the previously prepared pit, press slightly, then close on the handles; if perfect contact be made, the handles cannot be closed far. Remember that perfect contact is not always possible, but the tooth is being obtunded, as to rapidity, just in proportion as the contact is relatively perfect.

We have now come to a point in the operation when the utmost care must be taken, for, with tremendous pressure, water with cocain in solution is being forced into a live tooth. At this point some definite rule must be followed to be successful—no haphazard guesswork will do. The rule is to count by seconds. This knowledge is readily acquired by the study of the swing of the pendulum of a time-regulator; exercise this knowledge in using the syringe. On making the first application thirty seconds are usually required, when perfect contact is obtained, to force the solution through the remaining third of the enamel and a little way into the dentin, which may now be entered with the No. $\frac{1}{2}$ round bur without giving the slightest pain. Then drill through the enamel with the No. 3 round bur. This is done in order that the continued pressure of the syringe may not craze the enamel. In a patient of this age and temperament continue the pressure for one and a half minutes longer, or ninety counts. If there has been perfect contact of the syringe in the pit, or, in other words, if there has been no leakage and the pressure caused by closing the handles has been as great as possible, the pulp will probably have been sufficiently obtunded so that the cavities may be prepared without pain. If, however, there is any sensation, use the syringe a few counts longer, but be very careful not to over-use it. Here is where the careful operator will succeed and continue to succeed, and conversely, the careless operator will fail and continue to fail until in disgust he will conclude that the method is a failure, never dreaming that he, and not the method, is causing the failure.

Let us not forget that even if nothing but water be used in the syringe, it is not difficult to force enough into the pulp chamber in a comparatively short time to strangle the pulp by pressure and thereby cause its death. But our obtunding solution is water plus cocain. Cocain is said to be a protoplasmic poison.* This is true when a high percentage is used. Several articles have appeared in our dental journals in the last four years against the use of cocain by the high-pressure method, because, the claim is made, cocain is a protoplasmic poison. So is strychnin a protoplasmic poison when given in overdose. What would the neurologist do in certain forms of neurosis if he did not have strychnin to depend upon as the sheet-anchor? To be sure, he does not give it in poisonous doses, but when given in 1/120 to 1/60 gr. doses it becomes a nerve tonic rather than a poison. I cannot say that a cocain solution of a strength of two per cent. or less acts as a true tonic when forced into the pulp, and here the analogy fails, but I do claim, after almost five years' clinical test, that I have no proof that it acts destructively on the pulp tissue, but on the contrary, I am sure that I have observed fewer cases of necrosis of the pulp in the last five years under anesthesia produced by high pressure than in any previous five years. There are, I believe, two reasons for this: First, when the pulp is anesthetized it receives no "shock" from cavity preparation—but notice, please, that if great care be not used it may be injured by

* "Cocain is a strong protoplasmic poison, paralyzing all cells with which it is placed in contact. . . . Local application paralyzes nerve cells, fibers, and endings. Sensory nerves are the most sensitive, so that cocain acts as a local anesthetic. . . . It produces a local vaso-constriction at the place of application. . . . On systemic administration it causes an irregular, but on the whole a descending, stimulation and paralysis of the entire central nervous system."—Sollmann's "Pharmacology," 1906, p. 212.

heat generated by running the engine too rapidly while cutting with the bur, particularly if the bur is not removed frequently, although, at the time, the pulp does not respond. Second, it receives little or no "shock" from malleting, for as a rule it does not recover fully until after the operation has been completed.

Reverting to procedure, someone may ask, Do you always get perfect contact in applying the point of the syringe to the pit? In quite a large percentage of cases I do not, yet if we get some pressure, in that proportion, as previously stated, we are accomplishing the work. Some patients are fidgety, and in working on the mandible it is often difficult to get perfect adaptation because of its instability. When one becomes accustomed to the use of the instrument the securing of contact, although it is the most difficult part of the operation, becomes comparatively easy.

For the removal of pulps, use the instrument half as long again as for cavity preparation. This rule must of necessity be a very general one, for the condition of the pulp is always a factor in determining the length of time the syringe should be used. The greater the congestion of the pulp the longer the time required. If congestion has reached the stage of stasis it is impossible to anesthetize by this or any other method. Do you always succeed in obtunding with the high-pressure syringe? This is a pertinent question. The answer is, Yes, and no. I never expect failure and rarely do fail; but occasionally we find a tooth with curly dentin; in such a case, if the pulp cannot be reached at one angle, it may oftentimes be reached from another. Occasionally we find the teeth of an aged person to be very sensitive. Such teeth are usually difficult to obtund, because

the dentinal tubuli are almost obliterated. These two classes are the only ones I ever have any trouble with, when the pulp is in a healthy condition.

These, then, are three advance steps taken in the elimination of fear: First, in the adjustment of the rubber dam; second, in cavity preparation, and third, in pulp removal—three of the most painful operations in dentistry, if made in the old way.

You will have noted that I have presented this plea for a more humane practice of dentistry without superfluous technical verbiage, circumlocution, or rhetorical flourish. It has been stated in plain, simple language so that all who hear and read may understand, and with the one thought in mind that *means are available* for practically painless dentistry.

In conclusion, if you would succeed with the high-pressure syringe, carefully observe the following rules:

First: Never use it in a carious cavity, mainly for two reasons—because (*a*) the mouths of the dentinal tubuli are filled with débris, therefore you will not be likely to succeed, and (*b*) if you do succeed in desensitizing the pulp you will probably force ptomains into it which will be almost sure to cause its death later. If it does not die, it will probably give the patient trouble for which the cocain will get the blame.

Second: Always enter the tooth from some surface point, for by so doing you will have a definite idea as to the relative distance to the pulp. This knowledge is imperatively requisite, for when you recall the case of my patient here you will remember that much more time is required to get the desired result than if you were entering a lower incisor at the gingival line.

Third: Age and temperament must be carefully considered, particularly as to the time required for desensitizing. We know that the dentinal tubuli and pulp in young patients are much larger than in aged ones, therefore much less time is required to obtund their teeth. This is particularly true of the nervous and bilious temperaments as compared with the sanguine and lymphatic. The danger of injuring the pulp by the use of cocain, as suggested above, is so remote that the ultra-conservatism which prevents its use spells injustice to the patient.

If after presenting this paper and demonstrating its teaching I shall have convinced you, or any of you, that fear of dental operations can and should be eliminated, the paper and demonstration will have filled their mission.

Discussion.

Dr. M. L. RHEIN, New York, N. Y. The paper to which we have just listened with so much interest, and almost needless to say with universal approbation, is especially to be commended. The elimination of fear rather than the elimination of pain is the title that the essayist has selected, and without giving his reason for doing so. It is therefore perhaps excusable that I should dwell a moment upon what I believe must have been his reason for choosing this title. It is hard to differentiate between the amount of physical pain and the purely imaginary pain on the part of the patient, which, as the essayist so well said, is brought about by fear. It is hard to estimate in what proportion of cases the latter is present, and we all should give more or less attention to that subject. The essayist has very well started out by dwelling

upon the importance of handling this question skilfully, which is being given a great deal of consideration by the general medical profession at the present time. I have been coping with this question for twenty-five years or more, and I feel that if the patient can be induced to have absolute confidence in the operator a very great part of the battle is won. I have adopted for a great many years the plan of teaching my patients the value of absolute relaxation under operations of any kind. In order to induce patients to assume this attitude, it is essential that they have absolute confidence in everything that you may tell them; therefore you must never tell them anything that you cannot bear out in your practice, for to obtain the condition of relaxation is not an easy task, and the confidence on the part of the patient will not bring about results at the first trial. If you wish to succeed in compelling your patients to absolutely relax, it is essential that you continually call their attention to the fact that they are still far from the point of complete relaxation; but after they have once reached that mental attitude, an almost incredible increase in their comfort is the result. I have known patients who did not begin to relax until after their eighth visit, the stages between partial to complete relaxation being very great.

I have dwelt upon this point at some length, because nothing in the way of general therapeutic agents begins to compare in my mind with the results obtainable from this procedure.

Besides generally commending this paper, I thoroughly agree with its main subject as far as it deals with the use of the high-pressure syringe. The use of this instrument has afforded me most satisfactory results. What I wish to criticize is that the essayist in my opinion has gone to extremes in both directions. He states at the beginning of his paper that no one ever seeks the dentist except when dire necessity compels him to do so. I would take very serious exception to that sentence, because, if this were true, I should be unwilling to continue practicing this specialty. The class of patients that the essayist's remark refers to is very insignificant, because, although patients may first come to us under such circumstances, it should be impossible for them to retain this attitude of mind after we have done our duty in enlightening them as to what dentistry means. The dentistry of today, and much more that of the future, does not mean reparative dentistry except in a few cases of necessity, but preventive dentistry. In this respect it is our duty to so enlighten our patients that they understand that the greatest work which the dentist has to do for them is to take such care of their mouths that they will not require any services that are painful at any time.

I wish to especially commend the essayist's allusion to the padding of the head-rest. For many years I have adopted this, and have found it to be of very great value. I also agree with the essayist's criticism of the Van Wyck freezing apparatus after a very careful trial of it. I consider it useless in the dental office, although I admit that it would produce the desired results. It is similar to an infinitely superior agent that I introduced for this purpose twenty years ago, and it was only because of my inability to procure methyl chlorid that in the last few years I have abandoned its use. No other agent that I have ever used is as valuable as methyl chlorid, which within five seconds is capable of

reducing the temperature to ten degrees below zero. I have used methyl chlorid for a number of years, when I was able to obtain it, without recording a single case of injury to the pulp. The advantage derived from this agent consisted in its instantaneous effect; it produced simply one shock, and then we had complete anesthesia of the parts to be operated upon, and that without any sign of anesthesia in the adjoining parts. It produced local anesthesia, complete and almost instantaneous, the duration of which was sufficient for all of our operations. There was no annoyance of waiting, nor any of the shortcomings as illustrated by the essayist in regard to the cold methods known at the present time. I have endeavored and hoped to induce the manufacturers to again place this article on the market, because I have felt its loss to be a very material one in my practice.

I also take very serious exception to what the essayist has said about cataphoresis. I have in my office today a cataphoric outfit that was first introduced to the dental profession by Dr. Gillett, and I have also had for a number of years the very admirable and accurate instrument introduced by Dr. Price. This instrument has never failed in my hands to produce the desired result, and whenever I hear of the junk-heaps made up of discarded cataphoric instruments I am simply convinced that the men who had those instruments were incapable of properly using them or were unwilling to follow out the suggestion offered in the essayist's paper that the time required is not to be considered in accomplishing such an important result. It is true that cataphoresis is not always possible, but the percentage of such cases is so infinitely small that they are hardly to be taken into consideration. If I were to be compelled today to discard either the high-pressure syringe as spoken of by the essayist or my cataphoric outfit, I should prefer to retain the cataphoric outfit.

With the criticism of the essayist that it is impossible to insulate cavities I do not agree, as a general rule.

Dr. JACKMAN. I said difficult.

Dr. RHEIN. If this insulation is difficult, then it only belongs to the same class as many other operations that we perform. We say continually that it is difficult to put in good gold fillings, but that is no excuse for a practitioner not improving his technique. In the same way there is no excuse for a practitioner not learning how to properly insulate a cavity. I am willing to admit that in certain teeth that contain fillings, cataphoresis is not indicated under certain conditions, because of the possibility of the current passing through the metallic fillings, thus failing to reach the desired point; but aside from such a condition, I know of no cavity in which proper insulation is not possible, if the technique is properly understood and carefully executed.

Although I have taken considerable time in discussing this subject, I would not close without calling the attention of my *confrères* to the fact that we occupy a unique position, inasmuch as we claim to have first introduced the benefits of general anesthesia by means of nitrous oxid, and yet today we find ourselves in the lamentable position of being subject to the criticism of the medical world because our work is so much dreaded and feared by patients.

There is just one other point that is very germane to this subject. I have known of operators who, being filled with that sympathy which all of us more or less have and should have for our patients, have permitted themselves to perform dental operations that do not reflect their own capabilities and are lacking in the accurateness of operative procedure, and who have allowed their patients to pass through their hands with imperfect operations that are bound to be a failure, because of the operator's desire to accomplish the work without inflicting pain. That is an undesirable feature of painless operations which must be condemned as much as every other effort in the direction of humane dentistry is to be commended.

Dr. J. Y. CRAWFORD, Nashville, Tenn. I am very much pleased to appear before you today to discuss this very interesting paper on such an interesting subject.

As to Dr. Rhein's suggestion regarding anesthesia, I do not wish to criticize him, but I simply wish to make a little explanation that I think is due. Dental surgery did not discover nitrous oxid, chloroform, or ether; it simply contributed to the medical world and to humanity the application of surgical anesthesia. That is all that is claimed. We contributed to the world anesthesia, but not anesthetics. When it came to naming this condition, Oliver Wendell Holmes gave us that beautiful, that splendid word, that has perhaps conveyed more comfort to the human family than any other word in our language—anesthesia.

This subject is one of the biggest in dental surgery. I have nothing to offer in the way of criticism as far as the essayist's technique is concerned. In pressure anesthesia as applied to dentin I have very little practical experience. I have tried to apply it a few times, but I did not succeed well enough to warrant continuing my efforts. As to cataphoresis, if you will go back in our literature you will find that the practical idea of the cataphoric instruments was suggested by Dr. Flagg of Philadelphia, in that series of articles on differential diagnosis of the various conditions of the teeth giving rise to pain, in which he suggested a definite treatment for peri-cementitis by the use of electricity in carrying medicines into the tissues. About that time the observation was made by a gentleman in Mississippi, now a resident of Tennessee, that when medi-cines are applied by connecting the posi-tive pole of the electric battery on one side and the negative pole on the other, the acids go in one direction and the al-kalis in another. That was the first prac-tical suggestion of the *modus operandi* by which medicines could be induced to penetrate the structure of the teeth by cataphoresis. Like my friend Dr. Jack-man, I bought one of the first instru-ments of this character, paying one hun-dred and thirty-five dollars for it, but I gave it away, not without feeling, how-ever, that there was something in it. I did not feel justified in condemning the instrument simply because I could not accomplish the feat of complete insula-tion, but I attributed my failure to my faulty technique.

Mr. Chairman and gentlemen, if the essayist will excuse me, I would say some-thing definite which may be worth more than all I may say during this meeting, and perhaps during the balance of my life. There is a theory in philosophy which teaches that if a principle is false in one feature, it is false in all. If in our theory we have one faulty feature we have laid down a bad principle, and if we allow ourselves to be governed by it the whole fabric will be faulty. The subject of dentin has been under consid-eration this evening almost exclusively. If I were to ask the men in this audience to stand up who believe that normal human dentin is sensitive to cutting, what per cent. would rise? Perhaps two or three. Yet there is a misconception. Everybody tells you that the dentist should be an anatomist and a physiol-ogist, and should understand pathology. And here we are talking about the den-tin being sensitive. The dentin is not sensitive to cutting unless it is in a dis-eased, abnormal condition. There is something wrong if, when we attempt to remove the enamel in a tooth that has no cavity, the patient jumps when we touch it; the dentin in that tooth is not nor-mal. With a proper insight into the physiology and the pathology of these conditions, we shall understand that when a tooth is slightly sensitive it is slightly abnormal, no matter whether that sensitiveness arises from a constitu-tional or a local cause. Somebody will say that sensitiveness is due to an irrita-tion of the pulp. Yet you can take a tooth with a large cavity, decayed to such an extent that the pulp is exposed, and as a result of that exposure the pulp may·be injured, and yet on removing the decay you will find that there is no sen-sation at all in the dentin; you may cut *ad libitum* in any direction, anywhere in-side of the enamel shell, and inflict no pain. If there is any pain in preparing the cavity, you can with medication re-store the dentin to a normal condition by one or two treatments, and then cut it without any pain whatever. This is capable of demonstration, and it proves what? That normal human dentin is not sensitive to cutting.

Someone is ready to say, How many people did you ever see that had normal teeth? The first time that I was asked that question I replied: How many people did you ever see that did not have decayed teeth in their mouths? The fact that ninety-five per cent. of the people you see have decayed teeth in their mouths does not indicate that such a condition is normal. It is strange that practically the same percentage of people who have decayed teeth have intensely sensitive teeth, and in proportion as the teeth decay rapidly, they are also sensitive. If the dentin is brought back to a normal condition, we can go along with our cutting, and reduce the painfulness of dental operations. In treating a large buccal cavity in a molar that is sound otherwise, you can put on the rubber dam, scrape off the superficial portion of the decay, dip some cotton on a piece of orange-wood into a four per cent. solution of cocain and apply that to the dentin, and you will find that the sensitiveness has disappeared. That illustrates a principle. I am not advocating that procedure, but I am trying to impress on your minds that by bringing the hypersensitive structure which causes so much pain under the influence of the anesthetic, we shall have a perfectly normal tooth.

Dr. Rhein referred to complete relaxation as a means of affording relief. Yet you may take two persons of the same age, the same temperament, and the same amount of caries, and if possible with the same sensitiveness of dentin; you may put one of these patients in the chair and tell him that you wish him to perfectly relax, and to concentrate his mind on something outside of what you are doing, or to look intently at some object which you indicate, but the moment you touch his tooth he will close his eyes. You may repeat that four or five times, and he will insist on closing his eyes

every time you touch a tooth. You may give the other patient the same instructions, and when he closes his eyes he will fall asleep. In the first patient you may use all the cataphoric instruments you wish, and you may pump all the cocain into his teeth that the dentinal tubuli will hold, and he will continue to the last to keep wide awake. This illustrates the proposition that I first mentioned, namely, that cataphoresis will not affect some people in the same way as it does others, and as I said, a principle that is false in one respect is false in all others.

Dr. W. G. EBERSOLE, Cleveland, Ohio. Dr. Jackman is a very conservative man and one not given to rushing into fads and fancies, but if he is once convinced that a method is proper for both patient and operator, he becomes an enthusiastic advocate of that method.

The doctor has given us a very excellent and yet a very conservative paper. Filled as I am with this subject, I am free to say that it would be impossible for me to present so conservative a paper. And yet to many, no doubt, this paper seems a radical one. To these men let me say that every thought expressed by the essayist is a truth, and every fact stated can be demonstrated beyond the doubts of the most skeptical, if they will but place themselves in a receptive mood and investigate thoroughly the work that Dr. Jackman and others who are following this method are capable of producing.

The essayist says that nearly all pain could be wholly averted if proper and available means were used. With the means at our command at the present time, it is possible to perform practically every dental operation without inflicting any actual pain. It is possible by the use of both general and local anesthetics to eliminate *all* pain from dental operations, but while this is possible, most men find it impractical to use the major general anesthetics. Much is therefore to be accomplished in humanitarian methods before every man in the profession may do practically painless work.

The essayist also made this statement: "We have come to the time when cavity preparation may, with only an occasional exception, be made without pain." In regard to this statement, I would say that it is possible to prepare all sensitive cavities absolutely without pain, if the operator will but take the time, and use suitable anesthetics applied by a proper apparatus. It is impossible to describe here all the methods and means at our command which are necessary to enable one to perform painless operations.

The essayist spoke of the feather pillow for the head-rest. This is a very valuable addition to the comfort of our patients and helps to allay the fear of the hard head-rests. Some years ago Dr. Jackman called my attention to these pillows, and since using them I have had few complaints about my head-rest hurting the patient.

In regard to the Van Wyck-Kerr obtunder, I thoroughly agree with the essayist that no man can use an apparatus of this kind and prepare a cavity thoroughly while any moisture is present.

Cataphoresis, as the essayist states, has created quite a furor, and if properly handled it is a great boon to humanity. I use it almost as frequently as I do the high-pressure syringe.

In many sensitive cavities in the anterior teeth, particularly in small interproximal cavities, cataphoresis is the only satisfactory method of obtunding, unless you are willing either to cut away more tooth-substance than you are justified in

sacrificing, or to make an extra cavity which cannot be included in the original cavity, both of which to my mind are poor practice.

If you attempt to obtund the teeth with a high-pressure syringe, you are compelled to enlarge some cavities beyond all necessity; with a cataphoric machine it matters but little how small the cavity is, it can be successfully and thoroughly anesthetized without unnecessary loss of tooth structure. In fact, there are many cases other than this in which I prefer to use cataphoresis instead of the high-pressure syringe.

If there are a number of cavities in a set of teeth, particularly if they are on different sides of the mouth, I many times open up a cavity on one side and start cataphoresis while I am opening up a cavity on the other side, and by the time I have reached a sensitive portion of that cavity the first one is in such a condition that I can transfer the cataphoric machine to the other side of the mouth while I prepare the anesthetized tooth.

In this way I am able to save time, and I have perfected the system of insulation so that I very rarely indeed have any trouble with the current leaking around the teeth or through a metallic filling in the teeth.

In regard to the use of the high pressure syringe, the essayist says, "Few dentists, apparently, have had the patience and determination to master this instrument, but when this mastery is once acquired there is no instrument in the dentist's armamentarium of so much value as this, the proper use of which will turn the patient's mourning into joy and will relieve you of much nervous strain—consequently you will be less tired at the day's end."

It is really astonishing how few men

have been able to successfully handle this instrument. Some of the best operators in our country have failed owing to lack of patience, as Dr. Jackman says; to which I may add, in many cases owing to lack of common sense.

Not long ago one of the leading dental pathologists of this country took occasion to severely condemn the use of the high-pressure syringe, stating that he had never seen a case in which high pressure had been used in which the pulp did not die within six months. This man was of such high standing and reputation that his statement was calculated to do much damage to the cause of humanitarian dentistry.

Being at that time editor of the Humanitarian department of the *Dentists' Magazine,* it became my duty to reply to this statement. Upon investigation, it was found that this statement was made after the writer had used the high-pressure syringe in five or six cases, in which he had pumped a cocain solution into the tooth for a period of five or six minutes, without giving any heed as to whether or not he had obtunded the dentin. In other words, his method of procedure was about as rational as it would be for a physician to take up a large syringe loaded with strychnin and pump it into the patient until the patient's life was entirely extinguished.

This operator had simply pumped cocain solution into the tooth until he had thoroughly strangled the pulp, and upon the application of such a technique he stood ready to condemn one of the greatest boons ever brought to suffering humanity.

As Dr. Jackman says, it is not the fault of the method, but rather the failure to carry out the prescribed technique, which causes both failure to anesthetize and injury from hyper-anesthesia.

Of the technique described by Dr. Jackman, I have not much to say, for it differs very little from that employed by most men who use the high-pressure syringe successfully.

Relative to the application of a five per cent. aqueous solution of cocain to the gums prior to applying the rubber, I would say that for eleven years or more I have followed that procedure, and rare indeed it is that I find a patient who is afraid to have the rubber applied the second time. In many cases I have seen a patient fairly unnerved by the time the rubber was placed in the old-fashioned way.

I am very glad indeed that Dr. Jackman referred to the fact that it is unnecessary to drill through the enamel before applying high pressure. It was first thought that it was absolutely necessary to drill entirely through the enamel before high pressure could be used.

Some three years ago, I made the statement to some of my friends that it is unnecessary to penetrate the layer of enamel before using high pressure, saying that I was able to force the solution through between the enamel rods, and thus prevent any pain in making the initial pit. These men had been most successful in the use of high-pressure anesthesia. Some of them laughed at me and told me that I was wrong, the essayist being among them.

I made the first public statement of this kind before the Odontological Society of Eastern Pennsylvania, in Pittsburg, November 12, 1907. Six months ago I stated before the Institute of Stomatology of New York city that it is possible to obtund sensitive dentin in a sound tooth without making any opening in the enamel by simply taking a heavy rubber dam, ligating it very tightly around the neck of the tooth and also around the nozzle of the large syringe, and then ballooning the rubber with a cocain solution, allowing the constant pressure of the rubber to compel the absorption of the solution through the unbroken enamel. To accomplish much by this method, however, it is necessary to have the patient under observation for a number of hours.

Dr. Jackman also refers to the fact that it is not always possible to secure perfect contact. The decided difficulty experienced in many cases of this nature may be overcome by placing a few fibers of absorbent cotton over the needle point before inserting the syringe into the cavity. The cotton then acts as a sort of packing around the piston and prevents the escape of the fluid.

To prevent overdosage I prepare that portion of the cavity which is the most remote from the point of injection, and when that can be done without sensitiveness, there is absolutely no necessity of carrying the anesthetic beyond that point, and there will never be any loss of pulp due to high-pressure anesthesia.

In corroboration of what Dr. Jackman says in his paper in regard to the loss of the pulp, I would say that this is a very rare occurrence in my practice in a tooth which I have prepared by either cataphoresis or high-pressure anesthesia.

Dr. Jackman makes the statement that high pressure should never be used in a carious cavity, for two reasons—(a) because the mouth of the dental tubuli is filled with débris, and (b) if you do succeed in desensitizing the dentin you probably force ptomains into it, which will almost surely cause the loss of the pulp.

While it is better many times not to make the initial pit in the cavity, there are many cases in which I make that pit in the cavity, especially if the cavities are at the gingival margins of the labial or the buccal surfaces of the teeth. I have absolutely no hesitancy in making the pit there. In many cavities that were so sensitive that I could not make the initial pit without causing pain, I have set the point of the needle firmly into the carious portion and have forced the anesthetic through it sufficiently to allow me to make the pit painlessly; then proceed as if I had made the initial pit outside of the original cavity. I have followed this procedure many times, and have yet to find a case in which any signs of disturbance followed.

Dr. H. H. JOHNSON, Macon, Ga. There are two sides in our profession, the practical and the theoretical. My position in life and my position in my profession have made it necessary to follow some theory and make a practical application of it, therefore I have studied the practical side from every standpoint and have endeavored to apply it accordingly. There are two sources of suffering in our patients, the mental or imaginary and the actual pain. The subject of anesthesia is a very important one, but in the application of it the fact must not be lost sight of that mental suffering may be increased and intensified unnecessarily by an endeavor to produce anesthesia under adverse conditions. That was the trouble with the application of cataphoresis. Cataphoresis would accomplish the desired purpose, that is, produce anesthesia, but for the very reasons cited above it was impractical. The high-pressure syringe can be made to accomplish that which Dr. Jackman claims for it, but in a majority of cases the use of cataphoresis or the application of the high-pressure syringe will intensify the mental suffering, leaving the patient exhausted to a much greater degree than is occasioned by an expeditious and careful operation conducted without their use. If we study the temperaments of our patients and try to instil confidence in them; if they find that we are endeavoring by every reasonable and practical method to avoid prolonging the operation and inflicting unnecessary pain, they relax, and their mental suffering is diminished. If we use sharp instruments which do not revolve too fast, keeping in mind the fact that fast-revolving instruments produce heat and consequently pain, and if we take into consideration that a bur may be clogged with drill-dust and become a burnisher instead of a bur, and that by cleaning the drill-dust from the blades and revolving the bur slowly the amount of heat is decreased, we will find that sensitive dentin can be cut comparatively painlessly. Just as long as the operation is unfinished, just so long will the dread and apprehension remain with the patient, it matters not how much assurance may be given him.

I have used cataphoresis. I bought three or four machines at a cost of several hundred dollars, but I found them impractical, not because they did not produce anesthesia, but because they exhausted my patients by increasing the nervous apprehension. I have anesthetized teeth and have excavated cavities painlessly, and yet the patient would leave the chair absolutely exhausted. When you string a lot of wires about the room and chair and begin to bind something to the patient's head or cheek, it

gives him the idea that he is to be electrocuted, and in consequence his mental suffering continues until the operation is finished. Expeditious operating, if carefully done, is more practical than any of our prolonged methods of anesthesia. On the other hand, if we wish to produce local anesthesia, why not make an injection in the tissues near the apical foramen. This can be done quickly and with little nervous apprehension. These dangerous looking instruments—like pistols and extracting forceps—when brought in front of the patient cause him shock and mental pain—the very object for which they were intended, the relief of suffering, being defeated by their pretentious appearance.

Dr. A. P. BURKHART, Buffalo, N. Y. This subject is certainly one which should interest every practitioner, regardless of his age or experience in the profession. As I grow older and come in contact with patients day by day, instead of growing rough and indifferent to their feelings I grow more tender, and I find that my attitude is appreciated by both male and female.

Like the speakers who have preceded me, I have spent a great deal of money for various appliances that have been brought to the attention of the profession, yet I never have regretted a single dime that I have spent in that direction, because I recognize that it takes time and experience and money to bring about the very best results. I have used cataphoresis, pressure anesthesia, the cold process, and I am frank to say that pressure anesthesia and the cold process, or the Van Wyck process, have given me the greatest satisfaction. I can say without fear of successful contradiction that with the Van Wyck process, for instance, I can expose the pulp of a molar without causing any pain to my patient, and obtain results which I have not been able to accomplish with other processes. With the Van Wyck process, which in a measure has been condemned by the essayist and by one or two of the previous speakers, I can make a certain sort of crown and bridge work for my patient painlessly, or almost so, which I cannot do by any other known process. I am not able to demonstrate this to you, but in the clinic which I shall give I will show you the particular sort of bridge work which I have in mind.

I consider it the duty of every practitioner to make all operations painless as nearly as it is possible to make them so. One operator may become proficient with ordinary pressure anesthesia and accomplish wonderful results, another with the Van Wyck process, another with cataphoresis—all of which are useful and a boon to humanity.

Many operators have perhaps overlooked the proper adjusting of the rubber dam to the tender gums surrounding the neck of the tooth. In many cases the dam is adjusted without any regard for the feelings of the patient. In every case the gums should be carefully treated, as the essayist has advocated. There is no doubt that the patients' mental attitude is a great factor in our work, and that confidence on their part is very important and necessary. If you can say to your patient, "I can positively assure you that this operation will be performed with scarcely any pain, because I have performed it in that manner time and again," you will gain his confidence, which will aid you in avoiding pain in your operations.

The importance of confidence becomes especially apparent in the administration of nitrous oxid. The patient is seated in the chair, he is frightened, and his heart's action is abnormally rapid, and if the gas is turned on at once, uniformly good results cannot be obtained. That is the wrong way of gaining the patient's confidence or of obtaining the best results from this particular anesthetic. Seat the patient in the chair, then adjust the face-piece, tell him that there is not a particle of gas in the tube or hood, and explain to him how you wish him to breathe, and before you know it the patient will be breathing naturally. He is relaxed, as Dr. Rhein says, and his heart's action is normal. Then turn on the gas, and you will never realize any bad results, and secure a better effect than you would by the rapid method which is too frequently indulged in at the present time.

Dr. W. H. DeFord, Des Moines, Iowa. There are three methods of eliminating pain, one by means of a general anesthetic, another by local anesthesia, and the third by suggestion. In the matter of eliminating pain you must begin first with the dentist, not the patient.

Many dentists are timid about using local anesthetics, many more are afraid of general anesthetics, and but few understand the application of suggestive therapeutics. Consequently more unnecessary pain is inflicted daily by the dentist than by all other medical specialists combined. "Humanitarian dentistry" can never make very much progress till dentists become masters of themselves, and learn to operate with as much assurance when employing anesthetics as they now do without the aid of anesthetics.

Dr. Jackman has shown conclusively that about ninety per cent. of all dental operations can be rendered painless, and boldly states that he would relinquish the practice of dentistry rather than practice without the aid of anesthetics. If Dr. Jackman can operate painlessly other practitioners can do the same, and it is a duty that we owe to those who intrust themselves to our care that we should avail ourselves of these methods.

While I commend all that the essayist has said, and am in hearty accord with the chairman of this section, Dr. Ebersole, who for so many years has emphasized the importance of this subject every month in the *Dentist's Magazine*, I have gone a step farther, and have been raising my voice and doing all I could to show members of the dental profession the advantages of performing all dental operations in a condition of anesthesia by means of such general anesthetics as nitrous oxid and oxygen, ethyl chlorid, and somnoform.

By the aid of general anesthetics everything can be accomplished in the way of eliminating pain that Dr. Jackman has mentioned, and in addition all those painful conditions can be coped with which cannot be overcome by the use of cocain.

A patient presents who has been suffering all night, walking the floor in agony, waiting for the light of day, nervous, trembling, and white with fear. Examination reveals a case of pulpitis; it becomes necessary to remove quite a depth of soft, stringy, leathery, semi-decayed dentin, and at every touch of an instrument excruciating pain results. This is always augmented by mental suffering lest the instrument should enter the pulp, and cocain is not readily absorbed in such cases. Just a few whiffs of one of the general anesthetics referred to and in thirty seconds of time you can enter the tooth, deplete the pulp, making

it ready for an emollient treatment, or remove it completely.

Last May, at the annual meeting of the Nebraska State Dental Society at Omaha, Dr. F. O. Hetrick called me to assist him. He was preparing two cavities in approximal central incisors for fillings. These had become so sensitive that the patient could not endure the cutting. I administered three inhalations of somnoform twice, and in less than two minutes these cavities were properly prepared. This patient, a dentist living at Lincoln, told me afterward that never in his life before had anyone been able to make a proper cavity preparation for him, and at the annual meeting a year previously he sat with the rubber dam on a molar for four hours and only a cavity sufficient to hold cement could be prepared by all methods except general anesthetics. He experienced no pain under the somnoform analgesia, and at no time lost consciousness.

In cases of pericementitis bordering on alveolar abscess, in alveolar abscess where it becomes necessary to enter the pulp-chamber, and especially if a filling must be removed, or in those cases where a pulp has died under a gold crown or a bridge abutment—the most painful operations and the most trying for the patient—cocain is of no value whatever, while a few whiffs of nitrous oxid and oxygen or somnoform render these otherwise long and tedious operations brief and painless.

Two weeks ago, at the clinic of the Des Moines District Dental Society, I saw Dr. Fred Hunt administer nitrous oxid and oxygen, and in two minutes and thirty seconds remove painlessly the pulps of five anterior teeth.

I wish to thank Dr Jackman for calling attention to this subject, and put myself on record as favoring any methods that have for their object the relief of pain in dental operations.

Dr. JACKMAN (closing the discussion). In the first place, I wish to thank the gentlemen for the discussion of my paper, in the course of which nearly all phases of operative procedure were touched upon.

In regard to Dr. Rhein's remarks, I believe, of course, in winning the confidence of the patient, but I do not know of any way that is half as good and takes as little time as the use of the high-pressure syringe. Take the patient mentioned in the paper, or anyone of that character, no matter how fearful she may be, I can generally gain her confidence in but a few minutes by proceeding with the operation in the manner suggested in the paper, and when she comes back the next time she simply relaxes, because she knows from previous experience that she will not be hurt. After you have thus won the patient's confidence, she will ever be your friend, providing you do first-class dental work. The old way of obtaining the patient's confidence by inducing her to relax by thinking about something else, looking out of the window, etc., has its place and is of some use, but we have far better methods than that. In three or four minutes you can have the patient's confidence, and you do not have to go through the same procedure every time she comes to your office.

I spoke of the patient coming to the dentist only driven by sheer necessity, and I think that is true. Of course, as Dr. Rhein suggests, we should teach patients the benefits of oral hygiene to such an extent that there will be little or no need for large painful operations, but that is largely missionary work, and we

are far, very far from such an ideal now. We have to meet conditions as we find them. We are finding cavities in teeth, and we have to fill them. Of course I teach my patients to take care of their teeth, and I hope that the day will come when we shall not find so many carious teeth; but I should like to know how many patients come to Dr. Rhein or any other dentist before there is any necessity for dental operations? Very few indeed, I assure you. Dr. Rhein spoke of methyl chlorid, but the shock that he speaks of seems undesirable to me. When the shock is over, of course one can go on with the work painlessly, but I think we can employ better methods than that.

Dr. Rhein spoke of the Gillett cataphoric apparatus. There were a few men in my city who used this apparatus for a time and did good work with it, but most of the machines were defective. I do not use cataphoresis. I have an apparatus that cost me one hundred and thirty-five dollars, but I have not used it more than two or three times since I began using the high-pressure syringe.

I said in the paper that time was not to be considered in gaining the confidence of the patient, but in using cataphoresis several minutes and sometimes hours are consumed in desensitizing the tissues, and then when we begin to work on the tooth the tissues may not be desensitized deeply enough, and we have to go all over the same procedure again, thus unnecessarily consuming a great deal of the patient's time, which may be worth more than our own. This is eliminated by the high-pressure syringe; a second application may be necessary for a minute or two only, to again desensitize the tissues.

I disagree with my friend Dr. Ebersole in the use of this instrument. I do not believe in making useless cavities, but when I find cases in which I cannot reach good sound dentin at the cavity margin I do not hesitate to make a little cavity on the buccal or lingual side of the tooth, and inject into the dentin from that point. How easy it is to fill a cavity not larger than a pinhead and in a location where a filling will last just as well as if there had been no cavity. The results being so satisfactory, I do not see any objection to that procedure at all. Personally, I encounter trouble in trying to use this method in the cavity; I therefore apply it only in healthy dentin.

As to Dr. Crawford's remarks, I thought the time gone by when anybody would maintain that healthy dentin is not painfully sensitive. If I am correctly informed, the latest teachings of Black, Williams, and others is that the contents of the dentinal tubuli, while they are not organized like nerves proper, yet exhibit symptoms of the presence of nervous sensation.

Dr. CRAWFORD. What is that sensation—is it ductile or sensory?

Dr. JACKMAN. It is sensory. When grinding a normal tooth for a bridge we find almost invariably that the tooth becomes very sensitive as soon as the dentin is reached. I am aware that the theory has of late been advanced that this sensation is ductile, but I believe this to be theory only, without proof.

The high-pressure syringe will desensitize a tooth without the patient experiencing pain. Dr. Crawford told you that normal healthy dentin is not painfully sensitive, but that of course has nothing to do with the paper. We have to meet the conditions as we find them, and when a patient comes to you complaining, you have to deal with a pathological condition.

I am surprised that Dr. Johnson should have spoken as he did. I do not see how he can in any sense feel justified in hurting his patients. He spoke of scaring the patient with the instrument. One of the first things I do is to show the instrument to the patient and explain to him its purpose; that usually removes all fear.

Section II then adjourned until Wednesday afternoon, at 3.30 o'clock.

WEDNESDAY—Second Session.

THE second session of Section II was called to order by the chairman, Dr. W. G. Ebersole, at 3.30 P.M., Wednesday, March 31st.

The first order of business was the reading of a paper by Dr. G. S. VANN, Gadsden, Ala., entitled "Dental Science a Part of Universal Literature," as follows:

Dental Science a Part of Universal Literature.

By G. S. VANN.

THE word literature is used in two distinct senses. Its first and literal meaning is, something written—from the Latin *litera*, a letter of the alphabet, an inscription, a writing, a manuscript, a book, etc. In this general sense the literature of a nation includes all the books it has produced, without respect to subject or excellence.

By literature in its secondary and more restricted sense we mean one special kind of written composition, the character of which may be indicated but not strictly defined. Literature of this nature is occupied chiefly with the great elementary feelings and passions which are a necessary part of human nature, such feelings as worship, love, hate, fear, ambition, remorse, jealousy. These feelings are common to man, and through them men separated by education or surroundings are able to sympathize with or understand each other. Literature expressing and appealing to such feelings shares in their permanence and universality. In the poetry of the Persian Omar Khayyam, of the Greek Anacreon, of the Roman Horace, and the English Robert Herrick, we find the same familiar mood. Each is troubled by the pathetic shortness of human life, each shrinks from the thought of death and tries to dispel it with the half-despairing resolve to enjoy life while it lasts. Neither time nor place prevents us from entering into the work of each of these poets, in many respects so widely separated, because they express a common human feeling,

which we can understand through imagination or experience. So the Œdipus of Sophocles and the King Lear of Shakespeare, though written centuries apart, appeal to people of all classes and climes, treating as both do of that elementary feeling of love between parent and child, and while that feeling lasts those immortal portrayals of it will be admired and understood.

Works of literature in this limited, higher sense, therefore, are like music, painting, or sculpture, mainly concerned with the feelings—that is, they aim to please, to awaken thought, feeling, or imagination, rather than to instruct—and in this are distinguished from the books of knowledge, or science, whose first object is to teach facts. This distinction between literature and science was laid down in a famous passage of DeQuincey: "There is, first, the literature of knowledge (*i.e.* science), and secondly, the literature of power. The function of the first is to teach; the function of the second is to move. The first is a rudder, the second an oar or a sail. The first speaks to the mere discursive understanding or reason, the second speaks ultimately, it may happen, to the higher understanding or reason, but always through affections of pleasure or sympathy." In a word, then, to ascertain, and communicate facts is the object of science; to quicken our life into a higher consciousness through the feelings is the function of art. Yet, however good this distinction may hold as a rule, much that is literature in the strictest sense does deal with facts, whether of history or of science—that is, being expressed in a form of permanent beauty or value it is lifted out of a special department of knowledge and made of universal interest. Shakespeare's historical plays, Carlyle's French Revolution, or an essay of Bacon, DeQuincey, or Macaulay, while they tell us facts, are, as we well know, strictly literature; also many of the works of science—political, professional, and otherwise—fulfil these conditions and are included in this class.

Fortunately for us who are present here as members of this organization, and for the profession at large, the men in whose minds was conceived the idea of dentistry as a profession held this high standard of literature. That the divine energy should incarnate itself and find expression in the form of men, and that these men should inspire each other to think and write, to do and dare, is a subject the contemplation of which should make us stand uncovered. It was in this spirit that the first dental college was established, the first society organized, and the first journal published. Let us bear these facts in mind—not primarily, however, because they were the first, but because (and this is the great reason) here was the beginning of a change of spirit as well as of method, a change from a trade always mindful of self, accumulative, afraid of competition, exclusive, gaining knowledge only to hoard it, to a profession with broad fraternal feelings and with intellectual culture.

Thus was created an atmosphere in which professional life began to live and move and have a vigorous being, and bring forth a literature that was a fitting complement to the great fabric of scientific thought and expression that was built up during the first half of the last century, the dental phase of it taking on a compact and permanent form when Chapin A. Harris issued the first edition of his "Principles and Practice of Dental Surgery." This was successively followed by Garretson's "System of Oral Surgery," Burchard's "Dental Pathology," and Gray's "Anatomy"—three works which have a philosophic insight into truth, and are set forth in a most satisfying literary form. The French writer Magitot, and the scholarly Tomes of England were also writing at this time, both producing standard works; the former a treatise on "Dental Anomalies," the latter a "Manual of Dental Anatomy, Human and Comparative," which for precision of thought and finish of style is possibly not excelled by any other single production of a scientific nature.

While these men were removing the stigma of empiricism from dentistry by discovering the principle of rational connection between a vast assembly of disjointed and inco-ordinate facts and theories, in which what was sound and true was often linked to what was false and contradictory, the younger members of the profession were hastening their day by working along individual lines. Conspicuous among these are E. H. Angle, V. H. Jackson, and Calvin S. Case, specialists in the field of orthodontia. Each of these men has a different story to tell, and each has told it in his own way, bringing many rubrics of thought to bear upon the subject, and proving by the incontestable logic of results the soundness of their respective theories. Together they have lifted the department of orthodontia from a dependency to a secure partnership with dental science and literature.

However interesting the later subjects

may have proved to the general practitioner, the soul of the profession, with all its growing powers, from its inception has been centered upon the solution of the great problem of dental caries. Not only the leaders of thought, but even the lives and struggles of the mass of men who toiled daily at the dental chair, were pregnant with the question, until, within the last few years, through the labors of the great triumvirate—G. V. Black, W. D. Miller, and J. Leon Williams—the question has been settled. These men each approached the subject from a different point of observation, and with intellectual proceedings calm, patient, and regular, they mastered the subject, pursuing cause and effect with a steady tenacity through multitudes of details that would have checked other men with less mental ardor and lacking the same invincible persistence. As a consequence, each one of these men has made the profession his profound debtor by recording the result of his researches in a brilliant series of essays that are not only a restrained, lucid, and logical exposition of the subject in hand, but from a literary standpoint are the peer of any from the time of Bacon to the present. That is to say, these men in the treatment of their subject are no longer merely dentists, operators, scientists— they are pre-eminently thinkers, able to rise above purely contemporary interests and stand out alone, each in the genius of his own individuality: Black, the direct and forceful logician; Miller, the subtle metaphysician, and Williams, the master of a rational style that approaches prose poetry in its harmony of thought and expression, wealth of illustration, and inexhaustible fertility. To some degree the unprecedented enthusiasm with which their work was received within profes-

sioual ranks may, of course, be attributed to the subject upon which their writings are engaged; but beyond this, and speaking broadly, it is due also to the fact that they brought to the discussion of that subject distinctive literary gifts, and feelings for style which enabled them to express their thoughts in a form of lasting value and literary interest.

In an exhaustive review of dental literature other standard contributions might be added to the list, but a sufficient number have been noted to emphasize the point that the works of dental literature have a beauty, power, and individuality of expression that is all their own, and that help to make them both permanent and universal. Not only is there value in the thought contained, but there is a distinct and added value in the special form in which the thought has been embodied. Each writer has his own style or manner, his characteristic way of addressing us. This style is the expression of his personal character, and we have learned to know him by it, as we recognize a man by his gait or by the tone of his voice. Thus through this personal element in their work the great writers of dentistry have expressed to us a part of their inner selves—indeed, have been impelled to give us, as best they could through written words, the most they have gained by experience. In the poet's verse we have long been accustomed to read the lesson of the heart which he has learned from living; it is warm and alive for all time with his sorrows, exaltations, hopes, and despairs. And now, in the essay of the scientist, we are coming to read the innermost thoughts of his mind gained from toil of research and from experience. It is in this sense that literature is born of life and we come to look on the works of each great writer as an actual part of a human life mysteriously preserved and communicated to us.

But we must go still farther, and realize that each nation as well as each individual has a distinct character and inner life; that in generation after generation men and women have lived who have embodied in literature not their own souls merely, but some deep thought or feeling of their time or nation. Often thousands feel dumbly what the great writer alone can express. Accordingly literature is not only personal but national. The character of a nation manifested through action we commonly call its history; the character of a nation written down in its books we call its literature. For more than twelve hundred years the English nation has been revealing its life, and way of looking at life, through its books; to study English literature, therefore, is to study one great expression of the character and historic development of the English race.

What is true of national life is particularly true of professional life; and, as we have seen, for nearly a hundred years the makers of dentistry have been setting forth its advancement in its literature; in such a manner has the progress of the last century been crystallized for thought and study. But with the passing of the century a change has been apparent. Whereas a decade or so ago the profession was judged by the individual efforts and achievements of a few representative men, today the demand is being made that every man measure up to the standard, fill his place with skill and genius, and share the general responsibility. The cry is being heard on all sides, and although at present the superior tasks —the finishing and molding of nearly all great undertakings—are still delegated

to the comparatively few, yet the thinking element has already begun to regard the higher fields of achievement as too great territory for sole occupation by the minor portion of the profession, and are beginning to provide for the development of that spark of genius which, barring the idiotic and hopelessly insane, resides in every man's bosom. This, however, is but in keeping with the progress of the age, which through the industrial activity of the nineteenth century has given man a new material environment, upon the plane of which the twentieth century must develop for him a higher intellectual and spiritual surrounding. This is the proposition before the world, in the presence of which it might well stand agape were it not for the fact that the way of advancement is already opened up through the evolution of the public school system, with its departments of mental, manual, and artistic training, out of which the candidate steps into a college for higher intellectual and special development, from which he is graduated into the organized ranks of his chosen calling.

This is the cycle of progress that has been begun, and the question that confronts the dental profession today is, whether as a whole we are keeping abreast with its advancement. To my mind the question resolves itself into two phases, that of education and that of organization. With regard to the first, listen to the outline defined by President Eliot of Harvard of what constitutes a liberal education—"A clear conviction in discovering and recognizing the truth, a development of the imagination, and a literary power of expression"—and be encouraged that, with the prerequisites being established by the dental colleges and boards of examiners, it is possible for the student body of the next generation to reach this degree. This leaves the question of organization with *us*—in consideration of which may I call attention to the Illinois State Dental Society's postgraduate study course, promising as it does to be far-reaching in its effect upon associational work and in the dissemination of the knowledge of dental literature; which, together with the plan providing for inter-related membership of the local with the state society, and the state with the national body, may attain to the ideal basis upon the platform of which every member of the profession may be led to stand in the reorganization of associational work as a whole.

Here, again, as in the beginnings of dentistry, we see that the standard of progress is broader fraternal feeling and higher intellectual culture. And that the latter may be as great as possible, let us not confine ourselves to the study of dental literature entirely, or works of a scientific nature, but also surround ourselves with books of general literary interest; not, however, as did Peter, czar of Russia, with the big volumes at the bottom and the little ones at the top, upon which the accumulating layers of dust marked the passing years, but with books chosen as you would a friend—books of history, that you may learn to read the future by the lessons of the past; books of poetry, the great epics, dramas, and lyrics, for inspirational value; and the literature of the essay, Bacon's, DeQuincey's, Burke's, Descartes', Spinoza's, and our own Emerson's. Never fear, there is no danger of knowing too much! Something, indeed, has been said about the spark of genius being smothered by too much learning, yet that can be but error, for experience shows that knowledge is the fuel of genius and that no blaze could be made without it in some form. Every genius has knowledge—to be a genius means that one has studied more than his fellows—not necessarily books altogether, but good, constant, honest, hard thought given to the thing in hand. Everyone who has a normal mind can become a genius by the same process, but right there comes the difficulty: Every mind seems to naturally adopt the views of others. It is so much easier, so much less trouble, in fact, to fall into the habit of doing and thinking as others do. The genius gets above this. He studies and thinks for himself about some particular thing. He gathers information from every quarter possible, and learns from experience and observation and the failures of others, and finally the solution comes to him, not by accident, not by intuition, but as the natural result of his diligent, honest, untrammeled thought and labors. Merely to know books, then, or to fill the mind with their contents, is not the object in view; but rather to use them to get at the best that is known and thought, which in turn gives to the student inspirational form for the expression of his thoughts and ideals in clear, convincing English.

Would that every member of the dental profession would get this working knowledge of literature and books. Then no longer would the general practitioner be simply an operator of ability, but he would become the scientific and literary exponent of his calling, capacitated to do something toward enriching the human mind, really adding to its treasure—perhaps be enabled to take a step farther and discover some unequivocal truth in a region where it seemed that all was known and explored, and being prepared to produce this thought, observation, or invention in some form great, large, acute, reasonable in itself, could thus speak to his profession, to the world, in a style that is all his own, yet a style that finds itself the contemporary of all ages. Take such a man as the type of the individual practitioners of dentistry, advancing as an organized body the world over, and you will get the twentieth century ideal of professioual progress measuring up to the world standard, and revealing itself in a literature that is at once both permanent and universal.

Discussion.

Dr. F. L. HUNT, Asheville, N. C. You will all agree with me that Dr. Vann has presented to us an extremely interesting paper on a most difficult subject. Most of us could write possibly on some subject pertaining more especially to dentistry, but when it comes to writing on such a subject as Dr. Vann has selected, we should hardly be prepared.

The essayist has so fully covered this subject, in my opinion, as to leave but little to be said by way of discussion. Following the line of thought as suggested by the paper, I am very glad indeed that Dr. Vann's paper will be recorded in our literature. The essayist takes us out of our everyday work and carries us into the poetry of living; he shows that the members of our profession have built literary monuments, which will reflect credit upon the writers individually and upon our profession. These works will endure for all time; they will aid us in carrying out our greater plan of living by appealing to our mentality and instructing us so that we are better prepared to bring about that physical harmony so essential to our highest type of living. While the skilled operator deserves the greatest credit for his work, it does not compare at all with the work done by these great authors, whose writings have inspired our operators of ability. I am inclined, however, to think that the essayist has placed our works on dentistry on rather too high a plane from the purely literary point of view. A purely literary production is generally conceded to be interesting to many classes of readers, while our works on dentistry are interesting to dentists especially, because they teach principles and facts inherent to dentistry. Notwithstanding this, the highest credit and honor is due to our writers in dentistry.

In this connection might be mentioned the attitude of our teachers in the colleges at the present time. At one time I expected to write a paper on the subject of dental education, and to that end I wrote to the deans of our dental colleges in the United States and Canada, among other questions asking for information as to the educational requirements for admission, the graduation requirements, and their opinion of the present preliminary educational requirements. I wish to thank these gentlemen very heartily for their interesting replies, and I hope in the future to be able to use the information which they gave me. Nearly all of them made a plea for higher educational requirements, believing that to be essential to enable the students to become most proficient and to reflect the greatest credit upon themselves and their profession. To these teachers, also, high credit is due for the very excellent work which they are doing toward lifting up the dental education of today.

Dr. J. Y. CRAWFORD, Nashville, Tenn. I cannot possibly forego the pleasure of giving my high commendation to this excellent paper. I was strongly impressed with the timely *morale* of the paper in its general scope, and particularly with one portion of it, where the essayist referred to some of the living contributors to our splendid literature. Not all of us have had the advantages of the younger men in regard to literary preparation. I would therefore make a most earnest appeal to the young men in the profession to go to the archives of the world, and particularly to those of this great country, whose shelves contain monuments that will last longer than any memorials that may be erected by hands. Make it a rule every day of your life to write down some fact, some truth, however short, that will be a contribution to the volumes of our literature, because on that we depend for the perpetuation of the reputability and honorable history of our profession.

Cultivate your memory and compare your thoughts with those of the writers of the present and the past, and try to contribute to the literature of your profession truths that will last forever.

Dr. G. V. BLACK, Chicago, Ill. I did not expect to partake in the discussion of this paper, which I consider to be especially opportune and befitting the time and place (if I may bar what has been said about myself), and one that is very much needed. Without wishing to censure, it is commonly said that the dental profession is not a reading profession, and I have been looking forward to the time when the stimulation of the reading habit would become characteristic of the profession. This paper has that aim; we should stimulate the young men of our profession to read more and to write more. Especially do

we badly need more good English writing in dentistry.

It should be the first object of every young dentist, no matter what his preliminary education may have been, to master as well as possible the English language both in writing and speaking. You may not have had great advantages in your early training, but do not let that deter you. Lincoln had no advantages in early training, but he became one of the greatest masters of English. After that, if you can, make yourselves master of one or two of the modern languages. A review of the old French writers on dentistry affords a wonderful insight into the history of dentistry. They are among the very best writers from the literary standpoint. A review of the German will also be of great benefit. These writers are wonderful aids in the mastery of what has gone before. That information every man should gain for himself. If I may be allowed to allude to myself for a moment, which I seldom do. I would say to these young men here who may not have had excellent advantages in early training, that I had none. Two or three months in the common country school in the winter for five or six years was all. What else I have done I have accomplished since, and you can do the same, if you work with a will. There is no reason why many of you should not do just as much and perhaps more than I have done, for the time in which you live is better and is more stimulating; there is more to be done, there is more insight to be gained in dentistry now than ever before.

Dr. VANN (closing the discussion). I am very grateful to the association for the kind reception accorded my paper. I have set forth my views as clearly as I could, and I have nothing else to add, except to express my appreciation of the honor conferred in my being requested to prepare a paper on this subject.

The next order of business was the reading of a paper by Dr. J. R. CALLAHAN, Cincinnati, Ohio, entitled "Root-Canals," as follows:

Root-Canals.

By J. R. CALLAHAN.

"OF the viscera responsible for the more obscure cases of nervous, and mental derangement, I have no hesitation in designating the teeth as the most important, the two most important lesions being impaction and abscess.

"The object of dentistry is the conservation of the tooth for mastication and ornament. Pulpless teeth were formerly filled, the main pulp-chamber being plugged and the roots left open. It was found that abscess was practically invariable in the course of some years at the roots of such teeth. Modern practice is to fill to the end of the roots as nearly as may be. To estimate the proportion of success and failure of this procedure it will be necessary to consider in brief the course of events in these cases. The process is in effect a battle between the germs and the blood.

"The germs, practically always present in spite of the greatest care and skill, march down the hollow of the tooth by multiplication, often requiring several years to cover the distance to the end. Once out of the opening and in the jaw-bone, they are like a squad of soldiers with their backs against a wall. The forces of serum or the white blood cells can only attack in front with an effectiveness diminished by half, and even if successful for a time, more germs are

always lurking in absolute safety in the dead tissues of the tooth. If to prevent this condition filling material is pushed to the end of the root and a little of it forced through into the jaw, an irritant is in contact with the tissues, and in most cases bacteria accompany it. If, on the other hand, it falls a thousandth of an inch short of the opening, the tiny germs find ample space for lodgment.

"A man is as old as his arteries, and his arteries are approximately as old as the combined action of suppurative and other toxins has made them in the preceding years. Oral sepsis is not all superficial. Its most important location is usually deep in the jaws. In probably no other part of the body can purely irritative lesions be studied in contrast with suppurative ones and toxemia, and the symptoms of each condition be followed with accuracy. Impactions result in pure irritation; dental caries in irritation with a minimum of toxemia; abscesses begin in irritation, and result, when large and multiple, in chronic intoxication. The preservation of dead teeth is of doubtful value. Suppuration may occur about well-filled teeth, and even about teeth that are unfilled and undecayed; it is almost inevitable about bad teeth, and the one sure method of treatment is extraction—which may, however, in many cases be reserved until after the trial of conservative measures. The ominous conjunction of multiple abscesses with the triad of cardiac, renal, and vascular diseases is casually noted in several of the cases reported in this series and in some others. To exclude suppuration as a factor in these cases skiagraphs are absolutely necessary.

"Many other lesions are potent in causing irritation. Fillings which encroach upon the soft tissues or bones are often revealed by skiagraphs, and thus can be remedied. It is only possible for me at present to make the broad statement that irritation and septic poisoning should be removed in every case, and that local results of dental lesions are trifling in comparison with their profounder effects on general health."

The above is taken from a recent medical work on insomnia and nerve-strain, and is made use of here as a text to show that the dental profession is to be held to account, by both the medical profession and the laity, for the deplorable suppurative conditions to be found in the mouths of many of our patients.

This quotation tends to disprove the statement so often made on the floor at many of our meetings that the medical man knows nothing about dental conditions. It also serves notice that the forceps are to return to a prominence that will be distasteful to many of us, unless we can show better results in the treatment of the class of cases referred to.

I believe that every thoughtful dentist will agree in part at least with Dr. Upson when he says: "Of the viscera responsible for the more obscure cases of nervous and mental derangement I have no hesitation in designating the teeth as the most important"; and, personally, I believe that suppurative conditions of the mouth play an important rôle in various forms of intestinal toxemias.

If half of what has been said be true, no apology is necessary for bringing the old story of root-canal treatment before so dignified a body as the National Association. It is hardly necessary to say that the present results of root-canal treatment are not always satisfactory.

Since the time of Pierre Fauchard (1733) up to the present time we have been hammering away at this subject, but notwithstanding the immense amount of commendable and scientific progress that has been made, we seem to neglect or evade or fail to recognize, or give up in despair, the key to the situation. I refer to the extreme or last one-eighth of an inch of canal near the apex of the root, or that portion of the canal that passes through pure or almost pure cemental tissue.

In the normal mouth we may expect to find about fifty-six canals. Twenty-eight of these are usually large, straight, and easy of access, seldom constricted, open as a rule, so that fifty per cent. of the roots, if occasion require, should with comparatively little effort be thoroughly treated and successfully closed, showing no subsequent inflammation, if the teachings of Dr. Buckley are followed closely.

In cases of tortuous small canals, with single or multiple foramina, and an apex covered with cementum or abnormal growth, it is many times seemingly impossible to find the canals; yet it will be found that by somewhat complicated procedures and in two or three sittings these seemingly impossible cases can be successfully treated.

In order to develop the technique that I wish to consider, we select a lower left first molar, from which we grind the buccal surface of crown and roots sufficiently to disclose the pulp-chamber and canals. (See Fig. 1.)

Let us say here that the skiagraph would be of inestimable value at this time, and should be made use of at almost every stage of root-canal treatment; but this is not yet practical except in a very few offices, and consequently I shall make no further mention of this important aid.

I should add that we are not discussing putrescent conditions, further than

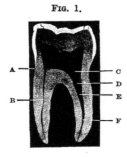

to say that as a rule I would not begin opening these canals until the preparatory treatment as advocated by Dr. Buckley has been followed out.

The anterior buccal canal presents an abrupt or square entrance, and therefore is not easy to locate or easy to enter when found. (Fig. 1, A.) A No. 5 Donaldson broach is finally passed as far as B on the diagram, where it meets with a constriction. Below this point, we have reason to believe that the constricted canal contains fragments of dead pulp tissue or a minute blood-clot in a more or less disintegrated condition, which even though mummified to the best of our ability and sealed in this position, will finally, in from one to five years, under the influence of the secretions of the body, become food for some itinerant

microbe. These pulp fragments should be removed and the canal be put in such condition that drugs and filling materials may reach the apical foramen with the greatest degree of ease and accuracy. To this end the mouth of the canal should be enlarged, constrictions and curves made easier, and its general shape should be that of an attenuated funnel. With a Gates-Glidden drill as large as conditions will permit, we start the funnel shape at the mouth of the canal (c), being careful to have the canal as dry as possible, for it is in the wet canals that the drills lock and break. Be careful to allow the drill to go only far enough to make a pocket, say, of a depth equal to half the length of the head of the drill.

A smaller Gates-Glidden drill will then go a little farther into the canal (D), the operator being careful to stop short of a curve. Then place a drop of forty per cent. sulfuric acid in the pocket; next, with the largest Donaldson broach that will enter the canal at the extremity of the pocket thus made (E), begin pumping, enlarging the canal to the size of that broach as far as possible. Then repeat the process, using this time a smaller broach (F), keeping fresh acid in the canal and continuing the gentle manipulation of the broach until an obstruction is met with.

Then, with cotton or a small syringe, introduce into the cavity a saturated solution of sodium bicarbonate, and note what happens. If there be sufficient acid in the canal, enough carbonic acid gas is manufactured to cause a series of rapid and easily noticed explosions, coming from the very end of the canal, carrying every particle of débris out of it, leaving it cleaner than it can be made by any other practical procedure.

The obstruction met with consists either of cementum at the apex of the root or of pulp tissue rammed ahead of the broach. At this point it may be pertinent to inquire as to what has happened to the minute fragment of pulp tissue in the remaining twentieth of an inch of the canal at the apex. It is reasonable to suppose that the acid by the time it reaches this point is neutralized a little at least, and that the pulp fragments have been changed somewhat, carbonized slightly and somewhat hardened, but are still freely soluble in the presence of sodium-potassium.

The enlarging, straightening, and smoothing of the canal, as above described, enables us to carry on a worn No. 5 Donaldson broach small particles of sodium-potassium to these pulp fragments with a reasonable certainty that they will be dissolved or broken up by the strong alkali. Then the soapy residue should be gotten rid of, lest, if left in the apex or apical space, it would in time be so changed that it would become attractive to germ life. Such is the uncertainty of getting water to it with sufficient force that I have made a second application of sulfuric acid followed by a sodium bicarbonate solution, with the idea that the liberation of the resultant carbonic acid gas would free the canal of every deleterious substance.

Then seal a mild or light dressing of Dr. Buckley's cresol and formalin in the canal for a day or two, when most likely the canal will be ready to be filled.

The opening of the anterior canals will of course be more difficult or perhaps impossible, but persistent and patient effort will often bring the desired results, by the use of sodium-potassium whenever pulp tissue blocks the way, and of sulfuric acid when bony tissue interferes

with easy access to the apex. Twenty years of constant use of the acid method has convinced me that the dissolution of a small portion of bony structure surrounding pulp-canals is not only harmless to the tooth, but is an absolute necessity, to the end that a direct and unobstructed smooth passageway to the apical region may be obtained, thus facilitating and rendering certain the penetration of medicaments and canal fillings to the end of the root.

During the years that sulfuric acid has been used in root-canal treatment but three objections have been brought forward that deserve discussion. First, it is said that many broaches are broken off in canals owing to the action of the acid on the steel. It is true that the broach does become brittle, but breakage is usually the fault of the operator. Most likely he has been punching at the canal at an angle, instead of in line with the canal, when such an accident does occur. If the canal be filled with acid at once and the soda solution thrown in, the fragment of the broach will be forced out of the canal by the gas explosion, provided of course that the broach has not been rammed deeply into the canal by extreme force. In this case it will be well to pack the canal over and about the broach with crystals of iodin and to seal it tightly for a day or two, when the steel will be converted into iodid of iron, which can be removed.

The second objection offered is that the acid destroys the bone-matrix. This it seems to me is just why we use it, with the qualification, however, that its solvent action is practically self-limiting, or sufficiently so that it is easily kept under control.

Thirdly, it is said that sulfuric acid in 40 per cent. solution, if allowed to escape through the foramen, will set up a state of violent irritation. Yet the very men who raise this objection apply 2 to 50 per cent. formalin solutions to canals, or sodium dioxid, sodium-potassium, or carbolic acid. If we place a liberal dose of any of the above drugs about the necks of teeth on one side of the mouth, and treat the other side in like manner with 40 per cent. sulfuric

the two canals are connected by a flat narrow space filled with dead tissues of one kind or another that need to be cleansed away. In Fig. 2, B, the root has been treated with instruments alone, such as drills or broaches, and has possibly been opened clear through to the apex; yet the walls and the thin flat space between the canals are still packed with dead tissue. (See Fig. 2, B; also

FIG. 2.

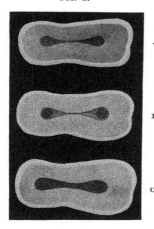

A

B

C

FIG. 3.

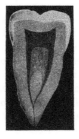

Fig. 3, longitudinal section.) The figure shows that a hole has been drilled through the mass of substance that should have been removed. It is impossible to remove this clinging mass in any other way than by the use of sodium dioxid, sodium-potassium, or sulfuric acid and soda solution. (See Fig. 2, c.)

acid, we shall find that as an irritant H_2SO_4 is not in the race for a minute. In fact, the stimulant, astringent effect makes H_2SO_4 in 40 per cent. solution a valuable remedy in highly inflamed and congested areas for starting granulation. As an available antiseptic it has no superior.

The removal of all débris from the canal is a point that I feel has not received the attention which it deserves. In most of the broad flat roots, the anterior roots of lower molars or the root of the upper first bicuspid, where we find both a buccal and a lingual root-canal, close inspection will show that nearly always

The H_2SO_4 treatment has the advantage of removing bone spicula, of being less caustic to delicate membranes, of consuming about one-tenth as much time in its application, and of leaving the walls of the canal smooth for filling. (See Fig. 1, c to F.)

Having the canal prepared, and taking the posterior canal as shown in Fig. 1 as our ideal, it is plain that any liquid or semi-liquid substance that may be placed in the funnel-shaped mouth of the canal at c will find its way to the spot which we are trying to reach. In an upper tooth, of course, it will need some assistance.

Dr. Broomell of Philadelphia has recently given us a most excellent and helpful book under the title of "Practical Dentistry by Practical Dentists." In chapter viii, under the heading of "pulp-devitalization," we find seventeen different ways of destroying this wee bit of anatomy. Under "pulp-extirpation" we find thirty-six plans for the removal of the corpse. Under "root-canal treatment" we find fifty-one different procedures, any one of which may be thought the best. Under "root-canal filling" we find seventy-one methods for sealing canals and keeping them forever sweet and clean. And yet we are not happy! Under the head of "treatment of pulps and pulp-canals," miscellaneous, we have sixty-six preparations, each one more potent than its predecessor. Under the heading of "root-canal treatment in deciduous teeth" we are given thirty-nine different ways, and the author intimates that he may have overlooked a few. Total, 280 prescriptions and procedures for one poor sick little tooth!

With all this advice, is it to be wondered at that the busy practitioner frequently changes his mode of root-canal treatment? Of the seventy-one methods for the filling of root-canals, is there any one that can be said to be perfect? I think not.

Like many others, I was attracted for a short time by one of the zinc oxid, formalin, and other ingredients—cement compounds that are so extensively advertised for root-canal filling. A brief trial has convinced me that they are not so good as they look. They do not show clearly in the radiograph. They are porous, they disintegrate in the presence of moisture, and are more or less irritating to the tissues beyond the foramen. The canals of some twenty extracted teeth were filled with several of these compounds and white gutta-percha cones, and after letting them set or harden overnight, the teeth were covered with hot wax except at the apical foramen. They were then placed for two hours in water colored with anilin pigment to a bright red. The teeth were then ground with a carborundum wheel until each canal was exposed. This showed the cement canal-filling substance to be stained well into each canal, proving, in my opinion, too great a porosity to be trusted in a root-canal for any length of time.

These same teeth were placed overnight in a moist chamber, the moisture being supplied by a piece of wet cotton about the bulk of a molar tooth. The cement substance showed a decided softness. This simple test, along with other conditions noted, caused me to return to my old favorite, chloro-percha and red gutta-percha cones in the apical third, as nearly as possible, of all canals with open foramina; the pulp-chamber and the remaining portion of the canals, including canals that are not open through, being filled with zinc oxychlorid. After placing the gutta-percha, the cone should be packed in the canal with a cold instrument, after softening the gutta-percha with hot air.

All medical and surgical treatment should be varied or adjusted to meet the requirements of the numerous idiosyncrasies and physical conditions of the individual patient. This, however, is "another story."

Discussion.

Dr. A. H. PECK, Chicago, Ill. Dr. Callahan has covered his subject so thoroughly that there is little of value to be said in addition. In fact, if I were to follow my own personal inclination, I would simply adopt the rule which so many follow in discussions, and compliment the author on the thoroughness with which he has treated his subject and take my seat. There are, however, two or three minor points which I think it will be well to refer to again. I would voice just a word of caution in connection with the use of sulfuric acid which I believe will be of some value, not especially to the older practitioners, but to the younger and more inexperienced men who may read this paper. You will observe that the essayist in presenting this subject has carried throughout the idea of success, and if his paper were to be left with us without further comment, we would gather the idea that he is uniformly successful in his efforts to enlarge root-canals by this method. Maybe he is—I hope he is. I have had some trouble with this method and have found root-canals which I was unable to successfully or satisfactorily enlarge by this or any other method.

In regard to the use of sulfuric acid, even in a forty per cent. solution, the statement was made that no special trouble can result in this connection, because the acid is self-limiting in its action on the tooth-structure. That statement without qualification I believe may mislead the younger and inexperienced practitioners, because we all know that this acid is not self-limiting in its action on tooth-structure. It may be more comprehensive to say that the self-limiting action of sulfuric acid on tooth-structure depends on the quantity of the acid used. Of course a comparatively small quantity is applied in this work, and probably in the great majority of in-

stances not enough of the acid is used to result in any damage, but I have experienced trouble in its use in this connection. It does not require very much sulfuric acid, even of a forty per cent. solution, when it comes in contact with the soft tissues, to bring about a very considerable irritation, and any irritation produced in the soft tissues about the apical space is not always easily abated.

The use of an alkaline solution in connection with this work was not sufficiently emphasized. It is my habit, when using sulfuric acid in this work, to apply an alkaline solution—sodium bicarbonate or something equally effective—afterward, in order to be on the safe side. This does not take much time, and especially after the last application of the acid I think it well to use the alkaline solution as thoroughly as possible. For carrying the acid I use an iridio-platinum broach, which can be procured from the dealers. These do not corrode from the action of the acid and are very much less liable to break in the canals than the ordinary steel broaches.

Dr. J. D. PATTERSON, Kansas City, Mo. A paper upon root-canals is in my opinion always timely. Often, when the topic of the treatment and filling of root-canals is suggested at dental meetings, immediate objection is raised to the discussion of a subject so trite and threadbare. As the essayist suggested, the average success in this operation has been alarmingly inadequate, and has brought upon our profession merited as well as unmerited criticism. Therefore suggestions for an improved technique and therapy in root-canal treatment are of vital importance.

Dr. Upson, in the extracts cited by the essayist, has made observations which demand the careful consideration and study of every member of the National Dental Association.

He is not the first of prominent medical specialists who have criticized the ordinary and accepted procedures in respect to what the medical profession and the laymen are pleased to call "dead teeth," and advocated their elimination. Some years ago Drs. Sexton and Theobald of Baltimore, specialists in diseases of the eye and the ear, gave similar warnings to the dental profession. The closing paragraph in the essayist's quotation, viz, "It is only possible for me at present to make the broad general statement that irritation and septic poisoning shall be removed in every case, and that local results of dental lesions are trifling in comparison with their profounder effects on general health," leads us to the inevitable proposition that, if we cannot divorce infection and irritation from dead teeth, they should be removed by the forceps.

Is it possible that we too often, in our zeal for the preservation of dental organs, trust too much to the kind efforts of nature? In our belief that the tissues will absorb irritations, mechanical, chemical, or resulting from micro-organic life, without too great a strain, are we asking too much? When with all mechanical ingenuity, and with the aid of therapeutics, we have placed the root of a tooth in what we consider a promising condition, and are disheartened to see chronic inflammation and discomfort supervene, do we properly consider what may be the outcome of such confidence in the germicidal qualities of the tissues and strain upon the organism? In our longing for bridge supports do we not too often build upon toxic supports? Does

the orthodontist, in his strenuous claim to never sacrifice a dental organ for the sake of occlusion, properly consider what may be the result of his ill-advised fight for a hopeless first molar? Does the pyorrhea specialist who "saves everything" (?) ever turn his thoughts to the strain which he is placing upon the *vis medicatrix naturæ?* I think not. Therefore the question brought to our minds by the essayist, no doubt prompted by careful clinical observation and perhaps incited also by the pungent criticism of Dr. Upson in the extracts quoted, contains a note of warning.

What is the lesson to be learned? It certainly behooves us to use every energy and to test all methods by which root-canals can be placed in better aseptic condition.. Dr. Callahan presents to us a method introduced by him some years ago, and demonstrates to us that his continued success in so treating root-canals prompts his belief in its efficacy. Other practitioners, too, have introduced this method in practice and speak favorably of it. If it will lower the percentage of failures and preclude the harrowing effects of nerve-strain which may result in mental derangement, it must greatly appeal to all of us. I fear that we have allowed ourselves to drift into treating root-canals and subsequently filling them in the "easiest way," with little conception of the risk, and when irritation and chronic abscess appear, we dismiss it with the remark that "no harm will result," especially so when the delinquent tooth furnishes anchorage for a valuable piece of bridge work.

The essayist tells us that the "key to the situation is the last one-eighth of an inch of the canal at the apex of the root." We must agree with that statement, as clinical experience confirms that success or failure depends upon the treatment of that portion.

What the essayist says respecting this treatment should be most carefully tested.

When I received the first draft of the paper, the advice regarding the filling of the root-canals had not yet been embodied in it; and to leave the subject at the point of root-preparation ready to receive a filling seemed to me totally wrong, for it is my belief that subsequent irritation depends very largely upon how the root is filled after having been properly prepared. Therefore the description of the technique of filling roots which was added later to the paper was very welcome.

The essayist mentions the various methods of root-filling, and expresses the opinion that in the apical third chloro-percha forced to place with a red gutta-percha cone should be used, and that in the pulp-chamber and the remaining portion of canals zinc oxychlorid is most satisfactory.

I am certainly pleased to be in accord with his belief in zinc oxychlorid as a root-filling material. I was taught its value first by the late Dr. W. W. Allport of Chicago, who used it for that purpose, and pressed it to place with cones of No. 4 non-cohesive gold foil rolled upon a fine broach.

Many years ago I made numerous experiments with gutta-percha, chloro-percha, oxychlorids, oxyphosphates, shellacs, and amalgam in root-canals of freshly extracted teeth, and in glass tubes simulating the form of tooth-roots, which were afterward subjected to aniline solutions. I found that the oxychlorid root-filling was the most impermeable of all, with the exception of dry amalgam. (Amalgam for general use is of course only permissible if sufficient space is present.) Chloro-percha, reinforced with gutta-percha points and pressed to place when the solution is hardening, still shrinks so that the anilin solution freely permeates it. Shellac in solution, or heated, is finally permeated. Oxyphosphate, while shrinking slightly as compared with chloro-percha or warmed gutta-percha, still shrinks so as to allow the anilin to penetrate between the dentin and the filling material. Tin foil or gold foil alone cannot be placed in a root so as to prevent penetration. Oxychlorid does not shrink nor exhibit such objectionable characteristics as the above materials; it is penetrated more slowly by the solution than any other material tested—with the exception of amalgam. While it is certainly true that different cases demanding root-fillings require different treatment, I am strongly of the opinion—my opinion having been gained from the removal of all kinds of root-fillings exhibiting a variety of irritations and odors, and also from the experience of others—that a root-filling made as perfect as possible with zinc oxychlorid is the best root-filling known today, and will best prevent the leaving of a space where moisture may penetrate and where germs may produce toxins, bringing about the dire results noticed by Dr. Upson.

I confess that I am so suspicious of chloro-percha as a root-filling that no such solution is in my office. If I desire a solvent, I use preferably oil of cajuput in very small amount, and generally I seal the apical third (or rather fifth) with a gutta-percha point of the white variety, because it shrinks less than the red, surrounded with zinc oxychlorid, preferring the risk of going a little beyond the apex to the *certainty* that if

11

chloro-percha is used leakage will ensue.

I also confess that in cases in which inflammatory conditions have been continued so long that we may judge that the apical territory is very weak in resistance and that future trouble may ensue, I sometimes fill permanently with white gutta-percha points surrounded with a smear of zinc oxid, cresol, and formalin, as found in the preparations known as "oxpara" or "triolin." They may disintegrate, as our essayist has told you, but I have not found that they irritate, and besides, in suspicious cases the filling may be subsequently removed for additional treatment.

In closing, I would emphasize again that this subject is of great importance, and let no one believe that even our best methods of treatment are not susceptible of correction and improvement. Dr. Callahan deserves our thanks and appreciation for his effort.

Dr. A. J. COTTRELL, Knoxville, Tenn. I do not care to enter into a very lengthy discussion of this paper, but would like to state the results of my own clinical observation and experience. Dr. Callahan suggested this treatment to the profession about fifteen years ago. I was at that time laboring under the need of an effective method, and at once adopted Dr. Callahan's suggestions. His statements have been ultra-conservative; he has exaggerated nothing, rather he has not told all the possibilities of this method. I do not believe that any more valuable suggestion was ever made to dentistry than that of sulfuric acid treatment for root-canals. Dr. Peck's assertions to the contrary notwithstanding, there is not the slightest danger of any permanent injury resulting from the use of sulfuric acid in root-canals. I am not basing this statement on scientific analysis, but on actual experience extending over a period of fifteen years.

. Dr. RICHARD L. SIMPSON, Richmond, Va. In my opinion, Dr. Callahan has done more than all the other members of our profession to stimulate the successful manipulation of root-canals. His work has inspired my own in this line. For this reason I feel like repeating here the adage, "Fools rush in where angels fear to tread." But duty to my convictions demands that I tell you that in my opinion the advocates of the sulfuric acid method (Callahan's) derive most benefit from the acid as a lubricant and antiseptic, just as oil or soapy water is used in drilling iron. Let someone, unknown to Dr. Callahan, substitute any liquid antiseptic for his fifty per cent. sulfuric acid, and he will open canals just as successfully. The mental effect lends him courage and gives him confidence. Dr. Callahan is also deceived in thinking that he is enlarging the canal, when in reality the broach is being made smaller by the acid, also more brittle and thus more liable to break.

My technique is different from his to some extent, and if you will pardon me for a moment I shall illustrate on the blackboard what I mean [illustrating]:

(1) Antisepticizing the canal contents by allowing the liquid antiseptic (Buckley's) to reach the apex by means of capillary and vacuum force, induced by a smooth and slender explorer made from a worn-out barbed broach.

(2) Enlarging the canals by "extra fine" barbed broaches and "medium" Fellowship twist broaches, to be used with an in-and-out movement, facilitated by the liquid antiseptic, which acts as a lubricant. The twist broaches can also be twisted, as their name implies.

(3) Absorbing the milky débris formed by the above action with shreds of cotton wound around smooth and slender cotton carriers. This cotton acts like a washrag.

Dr. S. D. RUGGLES, Portsmouth, Ohio. This very excellent method of root-canal treatment has saved my life, so to speak, several times, and perhaps that of the patient. I do not care to discuss this paper, but I wish to say that this body has recognized the necessity for a definite nomenclature, and yet we have heard the speakers and the essayist use terms that are not in conformity with that recognized nomenclature. So I should like to suggest that the term "nerve" be dropped hereafter, and that the word "pulp" be substituted. Apropos of this subject, the word "fang" is also obsolete, and the term "sixth-year molar" should be dropped.

Dr. M. L. RHEIN, New York, N. Y. I cannot allow this opportunity to go by without emphasizing the splendid method which Dr. Callahan presented to us several years ago of using sulfuric acid in breaking down osseous constrictions, so to speak, in the canals. I also wish to emphasize my approval of his technique in filling and sealing root-canals. All the difficulties which I have encountered owing to pathologic conditions arising from imperfect root-fillings and root-fillings of zinc oxychlorid at the end of the root have in a large measure been due to the powerful irritating effect of this substance after penetrating the foramen, and I have come to the conclusion that we have nothing so compatible with the soft tissues around the end of the root as gutta-percha. In my opinion it is advisable, if we go to any extreme, to have some of the gutta-percha protrude.

If my understanding of the technique is correct, the chloro-percha is used only as a sort of gluey substance, the cone of gutta-percha being the real filling substance. For some years past Dr. Dunning of New York has been experimenting with paraffin and subnitrate of bismuth as a root-filling material, and while the work is only in the experimental stage, I believe that we may look forward to a most promising root-canal filling material. I do not wish to leave the impression that zinc oxychlorid has no place in our work. I thoroughly agree with the essayist in attributing to it so much importance—after the end has been sealed with some non-irritating substance. Make that substance as small as possible, but place the zinc oxychlorid above it.

It has been my good fortune for some years past to demonstrate a scientific technique for this purpose, and I am pleased to see that Dr. Callahan has adopted the use of sodium and potassium for destroying the organic substances in the canals, which make up the major portion of the canal contents.

In closing, I wish to say that the difficulty in root-canal treatment is due to the lack of willingness on the part of the operator to devoting sufficient attention to diagnosing the irregularities of the roots, and to the means of obtaining a straight line toward the end of the root, also to give time to getting to its end. If he follows that course he will succeed, admitting of course that there is a certain percentage of roots that we cannot succeed in filling properly; but that percentage is so infinitesimal that it is not worth considering.

Dr. L. A. SMITH, Port Gibson, Miss. I should like to ask the essayist if he has ever used hydrochloric acid in this connection? It will attack the inorganic tissues more vigorously than sulfuric acid, and as it is only slightly caustic to the soft tissues, I have for some time given it preference in the treatment of pyorrhea.

Dr. CALLAHAN (closing the discussion). I wish to say in the beginning that I specifically stated in my paper that there are many roots which it is absolutely impossible to fill properly, thus answering the question raised by one of the gentlemen.

One of the speakers took exception to my method of locating the point of constriction. The diagrams are not anatomically correct, but are simply drawings made from specimens to convey the idea.

One gentleman spoke of the method of opening root-canals by the use of the Buckley solution. Very possibly he has lost sight of the principal reason why I wrote the paper. The most beneficial action in the whole procedure is the explosion of the carbonic acid gas. I wish I could put this idea in more impressive words, but I believe that it is the explosion of the carbonic gas that cleans out the canals and carries the tissues with it.

Dr. SIMPSON. Is that explosion ever directed back toward the apex?

Dr. CALLAHAN. No. This has been tried by the experiment of placing a tooth in a cork, and the cork in a bottle filled with water; after the explosion there will not be a bubble in the water, showing that the explosion was not directed toward the apex. The action of the sodium and potassium can readily be demonstrated by experiment. If you extract a pulp with a broach, place it on a glass slab, and apply a small portion of the sodium and potassium to the end of the pulp, you will see the sodium and potassium eat it up, so to speak. You will be astonished how quickly that tissue will be destroyed, which proves the action of the sodium and potassium in the pulp-canal.

As to the formula, I have refrained from putting chemical formulæ in any paper written on this subject, as I do not care to pose as a chemical expert. I know a little chemistry, but I have not made any attempt to discuss this subject from the chemical standpoint. I think the formulæ communicated to me by Dr. D. Stern of Cincinnati in a letter on this subject are of sufficient importance to be included in the record. Dr. Stern writes as follows:

I should like to say a few words in regard to the chemical changes which take place as a result of the 40 per cent. sulfuric acid treatment. Analyses have shown that dentin, on an average, contains 77 per cent. and cement 67 per cent. of inorganic matter. The organic matter in these analyses has been removed by combustion, and the remaining ash has been found to have the following constituents:

	Ash.	Calcium phosphate.	Magnesium phosphate.	Calcium carb.
	Per cent.	Per cent.	Per cent.	Per cent.
Dentin . .	76.8	70.3	4.3	2.2
Cement . .	67.1	60.7	1.2	2.9
Enamel . .	96.9	90.5	traces	2.2

I have given the figures for enamel, although it is not under consideration while introducing H_2SO_4 into the pulp-chamber.

It is not probable that any serious results will follow after the organic matter has been destroyed by the acid, neutralized by an alkaline chemical, and washed out thoroughly. Some of the calcium phosphate might be converted into the calcium sulfate (insoluble in water), which in its desiccated state is plaster of Paris. Chemically stated the reactions are as follows:

$$CaH(PO_4) + H_2SO_4 = Ca(SO_4) + H_3(PO_4)$$

| Calcium phosphate | Sulfuric acid | Calcium sulfate | Phosphoric acid |

The phosphoric acid produced is neutralized by sodium bicarbonate:

$$H_3(PO_4) + 2NaH(CO_3) = Na_2H(PO_4) + 2CO_2 + 2H_2O$$
Phospho-   Sodium   Sodium   Carbon Water
ric acid   bicarbonate phosphate dioxid

The sodium phosphate is soluble in water and the carbon dioxid gas is violently liberated, and forces all small particles of solid matter out of the pulp-chamber. A very small percentage of the magnesium phosphate may be converted into magnesium sulfate, but the quantity is too small to have any significance:

$$MgH(PO_4) + H_2SO_4 = MgSO_4 + H_3PO_4.$$

The phosphoric acid which is formed is also neutralized by the sodium bicarbonate. The calcium carbonate is converted into the insoluble calcium sulfate, as follows:

$$CaCO_3 + H_2SO_4 = CaSO_4 + CO_2 + H_2O,$$

with the liberation of CO_2.

The formation of insoluble salts prevents any excess of sulfuric acid entering into the tubuli and doing any damage whatever, and any trace of the acid going through the apical foramen will probably do more good than harm in destroying diseased tissue and perhaps starting a process of granulation to build up healthy tissue of repair. I frequently use aromatic sulfuric acid to accelerate the healing process after having treated an alveolar abscess, and I think that the cure is sometimes hastened by its application. This is to demonstrate that sulfuric acid, judiciously applied, may be as efficacious in assisting in building up as it is in tearing down.

I am particularly interested in this part of the paper, for the reactions can be shown by chemical equations, which are absolutely controlled by immutable laws of nature, and I should be glad to discuss this part of the paper, could I be at the meeting.

[At the request of Dr. Callahan we add Dr. Stern's reply to the question in regard to the use of hydrochloric acid in place of sulfuric acid.]

Referring to Dr. Smith's suggestion in discussing your paper, as to the use of hydrochloric acid in place of sulfuric acid, there should be no doubt in giving the latter the preference. Hydrochloric acid attacks organic matter slowly, and acts violently upon calcium salts. It is most liable to enlarge the opening at the apices of the roots, and also rapidly transform the calcium phosphate and calcium carbonate of the tooth structure into calcium chlorid, which is extremely soluble in water and is used by chemists for desiccating purposes.

The following are the chemical changes that take place:

$$Ca_3(PO_4)_2 + 3H_2SO_4 = 3Ca(SO_4) + 2H_3(PO_4)$$
Calcium   Sulfuric   Calcium sul- Phosphoric
phosphate   acid   fate (plaster of acid
              Paris, insoluble
              in water)

$$Ca(CO_3) + H_2(SO_4) = Ca(SO_4) + CO_2 + H_2O$$
Calcium Sulfuric (Plaster of Carbon Water
carbonate acid   Paris, insol- dioxid
           uble in water)

If HCl is used:

$$Ca_3(PO_4)_2 + 6HCl = 3CaCl_2 + 2H_3(PO_4)$$
Calcium   Hydro- Calcium   Phosphoric
phosphate   chloric chlorid (very acid
          acid   soluble in
             water or saliva)

$$CaCO_3 + 2HCl = CaCl_2 + CO_2 + H_2O$$
Calcium Hydro- Calcium Carbon Water
carbonate chloric chlorid dioxid
        acid (very soluble
           in water)

These formulas speak for themselves, and show how much sulfuric acid should be given the preference over hydrochloric acid. In my humble opinion it is only justifiable to use hydrochloric acid for heroic treatment when the tooth fails to respond to the use of sulfuric acid.

————

At this point Dr. Joseph Head, Philadelphia, Pa., was granted the privilege of the floor for a few minutes to speak on

Tartar Solvent.

Dr. HEAD. At the National meeting held in Boston last summer, I presented a paper describing the use of bifluorid of ammonium as a tartar solvent. This solvent was considered so novel that a committee was appointed by the association to investigate the properties and action of this preparation. The committee presented a report stating that a tooth dropped in the solvent was unharmed after six hours, but that the tartar had become softened. I wish to reiterate that for three years I have had a continued series of successes in the use of bifluorid of ammonium, with the exception of those roots in which absolute necrosis had set in. As I have said before, this solvent will not dissolve large lumps of tartar that are to be found on teeth, because we are not able to use the solvent in the mouth in sufficiently large quantities, but it does seem to have the faculty of breaking up the attachment between the cementum and the lumps of tartar, so that the tartar either falls off or is so much loosened that after one or two applications a scaler will absolutely remove that which before the application was so strongly adherent that it was impossible to remove it.

I expect tomorrow to give a clinic on the use and application of this solvent, and so I shall not go into the technique of its use at the present time. I wish to say that it has more than fulfilled my wildest dreams. I can also say that this is not only my experience, but the experience of many of my friends who have for the past year been using it. That my friends get the same results as I do is a source of great satisfaction. This solvent seems so revolutionary in its action that I have felt at times that I was suffering from a sort of pipe-dream, that I was deceiving myself, that I did not really get the good results that I thought I seemed to get.

Another thing I would especially like to mention: Last summer I had to make this material in small quantities, one or two teaspoonfuls at a time, and when I tried to make it in larger quantities I very nearly poisoned myself, or at least thought I did, from the fumes of the hydrofluoric acid. I therefore went to numerous chemists to see if I could get this solvent made in large quantities, and right away they would ask if it was a perfectly safe thing to make, and I was compelled to admit that I felt there might be a certain amount of risk concerning it. None of them would make it. I was therefore compelled to face the possibility that this valuable discovery would be lost to the profession, because the material could only be made in minute quantities. I was asked by many members of the association last summer and by my friends to see if I could not find some chemist who would provide them with a standard solution of the material, and after much hunting around I succeeded in getting Mr. Adamson, a member of the firm of Baker & Adamson, the great hydrofluoric acid manufacturers, to take the matter up, and when I explained to him what I wanted, after some experimentation he told me that he would have no difficulty in making it in any quantity desired. He explained that there were great difficulties to be overcome, but that he was a sufficiently expert chemist, and had a sufficient knowledge of hydrofluoric acid to overcome these difficulties, and that in addition he had the wax apparatus for handling the material that ordinary chemists did not have. He, however, positively refused to have the handling of it, but said that if I could get the S. S. White Company to act as wholesale agents for it, he would supply any demand that the profession might make. And so the S. S. White Company now has it, under the name of Tartar Solvent, and anyone wishing to obtain it can do so in any quantity desired.

I wish to state further that I was extremely unwilling to go into the supervising and looking after the manufacturing of this material, but having done so, I wanted to see that it was done in such a way that the material would be of a standard quality. I, however, wish to say that in the light of the Taggart suits and in the light of the suits of McKesson & Robbins on Calox, there are no restrictions on the making of this material; it is given to the profession without a string. My wish is that some day this can be made by various firms so that I may be relieved of the responsibility of looking after it and seeing that it is up to standard, but until that time comes I assure you that for the sake of the discovery and for the sake of the very great value that it will be to the profession, I intend to see to it that it is kept up to standard quality, and I do hope that you will all have as good results and as much success with its use as I have had.

Section II was then declared adjourned until the fourteenth annual meeting, 1910.

SECTION III:

Oral Surgery, Anatomy, Physiology, Histology, Pathology, Etiology, Hygiene, Prophylaxis, Materia Medica, and Allied Subjects.

Chairman—C. CHANNING ALLEN, Kansas City, Mo.
Secretary—J. W. HULL, Kansas City, Mo.

FIRST DAY—Tuesday, March 30th.

THE first meeting of Section III was called to order by the chairman, Dr. C. Channing Allen, Kansas City, Mo., at 8 P.M., Tuesday, March 30, 1909.

The first order of business was the reading of a paper by Dr. TRUMAN W. BROPHY, Chicago, Ill., entitled, "Recent Progress in Oral Surgery," as follows:

Recent Progress in Oral Surgery.

By TRUMAN W. BROPHY.

IN presenting to you a report on the progress recently made in oral surgery, I desire to call your attention, in the brief period of time that is allotted me, to some important procedures which may be advantageously employed in practice. Among them I will include—

(1) Intra-oral operations.

(2) Prosthesis following operations.

(3) Deformities removed by cosmetic operations. Plastic surgery, including paraffin injections.

(4) Anesthetic agents.

(5) Bismuth paste in the treatment of chronic suppuration.

If the subject of dental pathology and modern ideas of oral surgery were better understood by students of medicine, if the curricula of the medical colleges included these subjects, which they unfortunately do not, with very few exceptions, there would not be so many unsightly scars exhibited as the result of operations performed in a manner unwarranted. Every practitioner has observed conspicuous scars and disfigured faces due to surgical operations performed by men who did not understand the pathological conditions which they were attempting to treat. I exhibit to you photographs of patients who have been treated in this manner (see Figs. 1 and 2) by surgeons of good repute, who presumed that such operations were indicated, but did not know the real cause of the morbid condition present. Diseases of the teeth are more prevalent than any other diseases known to mankind, and when we are impressed with the fact that medical students are not given an opportunity in the regular course of instruction to acquire a knowledge of the many pathological conditions to which the teeth are subject, it is not at all surprising that so many serious errors are made by them, as practitioners, in caring for oral diseases which afflict their patients.

The photographs which I have passed to you show the effects of incisions made by surgeons, presumably for the treatment of caries or necrosis of bone, but which in fact were operations for the cure of sinuses leading from dento-alveolar abscesses. The treatment of necrosis and caries of the maxillary bones never calls for external incisions. The entire mandible may be removed within the mouth; so, too, may the bones of the maxilla be removed without external incisions. Tumors of enormous size, involving the maxillary bones, may be removed without dividing the external soft parts.

Operations for treatment of trigeminal neuralgia which involve the second and third divisions of the fifth nerve may be successfully treated without external incisions, and the nerves removed at the foramina through which they pass at the base of the crania. It is not necessary to state, however, that intra-cranial operations for the purpose of removing the Gasserian ganglion call for external incisions. Such operations are rarely indicated. They are not made as frequently as formerly.

PROSTHESIS FOLLOWING OPERATIONS.

An interesting article recently appeared from the pen of Dr. Carl Beck of Chicago, entitled "Plastic Reconstruction of the Lower Jaw," which reads in part as follows:

The removal of a portion or of the whole mandible has its effect on the functions of the jaws and the form of the face. The effect on the functions of the removal of a portion of the jaw will depend greatly on the part of the bone removed and its size. If a small portion of the middle part of the jaw is removed the function may not be disturbed at all. If half of the ramus is removed, the mastication and the speech may be greatly impaired, and if the whole jaw is removed, the function of the lower jaw will be entirely abolished. Even a small resection, however, will have an effect on the shape of the face, which as a rule will be shown by disfigurement or deformity.

The jaw plays such an important rôle in the formation of the face through support of the cheeks and the prominence of the chin that the symmetry of the face and the esthetic effect is greatly disturbed if a part is missing. This is shown in those cases in which, through lack of or asymmetry of teeth, or through atrophic changes, the face becomes disfigured.

These points have to be taken into consideration in cases of operation on the lower jaw, more especially on account of the possibility of preventing such deformities by the proper treatment during operation.

There are many indications for operations on the mandible which call for a partial removal of the bone. Inflammatory conditions which lead to necrosis of the bone, and especially tumor formations, are the main causes for such operations. If a resection is made it is the duty of the surgeon to see that the part removed is in some way replaced by some resistant tissue which will give support to the soft structures and which at the same time will allow motion. It will be necessary to replace the removed bone by some material which will give to the face normal expression and shape. The best

to give to us a method of removing the jaw without causing disfigurement or impaired function. Although he was not the first one to expound the idea, he was the first to apply the method practically, and a large number of patients operated on with good results are a proof that his method is practical and successful. He prepares a prosthetic appliance before he removes the jaw, or part

FIG. 1.

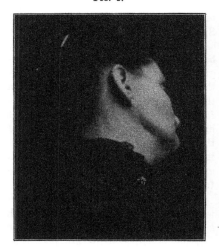

FIG. 2.

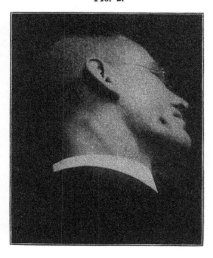

method at present is the replacement of the removed structures by foreign bodies in the shape of dental plates. A plate which holds the teeth and imitates the shape of the jaw is well borne within the mouth, ordinarily causes very little irritation, gives to the soft structure a support, and restores the shape and symmetry of the face. Many surgeons, among them Bardenheuer of Cologne, have tried to restore a jaw by autoplasty, but the results are not very gratifying. The majority of experienced men have decided in favor of the prosthesis. Difficulties arise, however, when the prosthetic appliance is to be put in place some time after the operation, because the deformity and impairment of function takes place immediately with the removal of the bone.

Dr. Claude Martin of Lyons, France, a dental surgeon of great ability, was the first

of it, and implants it at the time of the operation in the cavity remaining on the removal of the jaw. The appliance is made of hard rubber, with a complicated system of channels through which the cavity, which naturally secretes a great deal of pus, can be irrigated and kept clean. This hard rubber prosthesis is only temporary, and is replaced later by the permanent dental plate with teeth—which can be removed for cleansing purposes and carried in the same manner as the ordinary plate after the removal of the teeth—which hinges on the alveolar process. Each individual case requires an individual plate, so that no such plate can be bought from a manufacturer. Some operators have objected to this method in some particulars, although they accept the principle of it, namely, that a prosthetic appliance is necessary, but as material they have used metal instead of hard rubber. Boennecken and Partsch of Breslau have suggested the use of metal splints; the former suggested a wire splint, the latter a plate which can be cut to a desired size and fastened into the jaw when needed. Of course this means that the splint can be applied only in median resection, but when one-half of the jaw is resected clear up to the joint, the metal appliance is out of the question. Martin's method, however, allows even in these cases, or in cases of total removal of the mandible, the appli-

FIG. 3.

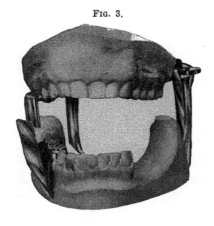

cation of a prosthetic appliance. The accompanying illustration [shown] is from photographs of two models which I received from Claude Martin, through the kindness of Dr. Carrel, and which represent the average case of a central and lateral resection.

In my experience in the treatment of patients for whom I have removed a portion of the mandible, I have learned that even when half of the bone was removed, if the remaining half be held in place so as to prevent it drawing over toward the opposite side, which always occurs by muscular contraction, the normal occlusion of the teeth of this remaining half with the upper teeth may be preserved, providing the surgeon holds the teeth of this part in occlusion with the

upper teeth until cicatrization of the wound is completed and well set. It is necessary to hold the remaining part of the lower jaw so that the teeth will occlude with the upper ones at least two months in order to make their permanent occlusion certain. I exhibit to you a cast (Fig. 3), a counterpart of which was first brought to my attention by Professor Martin of Paris at the Fourteenth International Medical Congress at Madrid, Spain, in 1903.

Horse-hair sutures, which may hardly be regarded as of recent origin as surgical sutures, are highly appreciated by those who have employed them. In their use in hare-lip work I have found that no suture scars are left. I have found, too, that if the surface of the lip be kept dry and free from dressings, the wound . heals, usually with greater satisfaction, and we have not so frequently interruptions of union.

I exhibit a form of *adhesive plaster* which has *hooks* adjusted in it, in such a way that in the adjustment of the dressing adhesive strips are placed on both sides, and then the two strips are laced together after the fashion of lacing a shoe. These strips admit of removing the dressings, if used, without removing the adhesive plaster, the act of which often repeated is painful, as it will irritate the skin and excoriate it.

DEFORMITIES REMOVED BY COSMETIC OPERATIONS; PLASTIC SURGERY, INCLUDING PARAFFIN INJECTIONS.

Since the introduction in 1900, by Professor Gersuny, of paraffin for the purpose of removing depressions of the face which have occurred as the result of surgical operations or loss of tissue from any cause, leaving a depression that will change the facial contour, this agent has been extensively utilized. I have used it quite generally, and have succeeded in restoring the facial contour in patients for whom the half of the mandible was removed, bringing out the angle of the jaw and the depressed tissues anterior to the ear so perfectly that the loss of the bone would scarcely be recognized. This paraffin may be advantageously used, with most happy results, in cases of deep depressions at the ala of the nose in aged people following the loss of the cuspid teeth or whenever occasion requires restoration of facial contour.

It is absolutely essential in the use of paraffin that the skin be made as thoroughly clean, by means of an antiseptic solution, as possible, and that the greatest precaution be observed in having everything attending the procedure most carefully sterilized, as an infection within the tissues following such an injection would be most disastrous.

ANESTHETIC AGENTS.

Nitrous oxid, as you all know, was the first anesthetic employed. When Dr. Horace Wells introduced it to the profession he conferred upon humanity its greatest boon. The dental profession is justly proud of his remarkable achievement. The popularity which was accorded to nitrous oxid in general surgery for a brief period was to a great extent supplanted by the introduction of ether, and subsequently chloroform. Nitrous oxid was thought to be useful for operations requiring only a little time; it was therefore lightly regarded for major operations. Within the past few years nitrous oxid administered with oxygen has been employed for prolonged operations, with marked success. Surgeons have been drawn to it by reason of its comparative freedom from danger to life.

The new methods of administering nitrous oxid with oxygen by nasal inhalation have made it possible to maintain anesthesia sufficiently long and satisfactorily to perform any operation. Recently Dr. F. K. Ream of Chicago administered it for me in an operation in the mouth requiring an hour and twenty minutes for its completion. Prior to this administration, I was of the opinion that nitrous oxid and oxygen might serve the purpose for other than oral operations, but that operations within the mouth could not be performed by its use, since the inhalation of atmospheric air would counteract the effect of the gas and render complete anesthesia impossible. It was gratifying to me, however, to perform this long and difficult operation while the patient was under the influence of nitrous oxid.

The experiments recently conducted by Drs. Walter H. Hamberger and Fred E. Ewing of Chicago—presented in the Section on Surgery and Anatomy of the American Medical Association at Chicago, 1908—on the blood changes incident to surgical anesthesia, with especial reference to those induced by nitrous oxid, resulted in bringing out the follow conclusions:

(1) In an analysis of the blood changes incident to nitrous oxid anesthesia in a series of clinical and experimental observations we find that—

(a) The hemoglobin is not permanently reduced nor is anemia produced.

(b) Hemolysis is not increased.

(c) The changes in the readings of the hemoglobin and erythrocytes are transient and of no surgical significance, and are most likely to be explained on the basis of capillary stasis. The production of reduced hemoglobin is not a result of the anesthetic itself, but is due to the accompanying asphyxia.

(*d*) The changes in coagulation time are not constant, but in general there is an increase in the time required for clotting, most marked about the third day.

(2) In an analysis of the blood changes incident to ether anesthesia in a series of experimental observations we find that:

(*a*) The hemoglobin is slightly reduced and therefore a slight anemia is produced.

(*b*) Hemolysis is not materially increased.

(*c*) The changes in hemoglobin and erythrocytes are to be explained on the basis of blood inspissation.

(*d*) It causes a marked decrease in the coagulation time, most marked from the seventh to tenth days.

(3) In an analysis of the blood changes incident to chloroform anesthesia in a series of experimental animals we find that:

(*a*) The hemoglobin is reduced, and therefore an anemia is produced.

(*b*) Hemolysis is increased.

(*c*) It causes a slight decrease in the coagulation time, most marked in the seventh to tenth days.

(4) In a comparison of the three anesthetics from the standpoint of the blood changes, we conclude that nitrous oxid causes no permanent effects of any significance; that ether causes more harmful changes (slight anemia and marked decrease in coagulation), and that chloroform causes the most harmful results (hemolysis and production of distinct anemia).

BISMUTH PASTE IN THE TREATMENT OF
CHRONIC SUPPURATION.

It is to the credit of Dr. Emil Beck of Chicago that the profession has been put in possession of a most valuable therapeutic agent in the form of bismuth paste. It is well known that subnitrate of bismuth is an opaque substance; Dr. Beck conceived the idea that if subnitrate of bismuth were injected into a sinus it would enable him to make a

skiagraph, and thus clearly outline the course of the sinus, with its origin. To his gratification, following these injections into the sinuses the suppuration ceased and the wound healed, and within a short time the patient was cured. Since this time he has been employing bismuth paste extensively in the treatment of chronic suppuration wherever found. His brother, Dr. Rudolph Beck, taking up the work of treating pyorrhea alveolaris, has found that suppuration will cease in a very short time and the tissue surrounding the pockets will change from a congested appearance to a normal color. It seems to be necessary, however, after the suppuration has ceased, to stimulate the surfaces of the tissues so as to promote the formation of granulations, thus closing the pocket with new tissue. I exhibit to you a syringe and some of the paste. I have found bismuth paste especially desirable in the treatment of the antrum of Highmore.

I have been in the habit for many years of making a large opening in the antrum through the canine fossa and removing the polypi which are usually present in chronic cases; then, after keeping it open and well cleansed for about a week, I fill the cavity completely full of bismuth paste and let it so remain about a week, when it will again require refilling, as I have found that the paste will be more or less contracted. In the presence of the bismuth, suppuration will cease, and the walls of the cavity, except in malignant cases, will assume a normal condition.

In the January 1909 number of the *Dental Review*, Dr. Rudolph Beck published a preliminary article on the use of bismuth paste in the treatment of pyorrhea alveolaris. This method consists in injecting a warm liquefied bismuth-vaselin paste into the pus pockets of the teeth affected with pyorrhea alveolaris. For this purpose an all-metal syringe is employed, holding about a half-ounce of the paste, provided with a flexible, tapering, blunt point, made of pure silver, platinum, or gold. The paste consists of: Bismuth subnitrate, 30 per cent.; vaselin, 60 per cent.; paraffin, 5 per cent.; wax, 5 per cent. It is prepared as follows: The vaselin, paraffin, and wax are boiled, and the bismuth subnitrate is added and stirred in as soon as it is taken from the flame. The syringe is then charged with the liquid paste, the point of the needle introduced into the deepest part of the pus pockets by gentle and steady pressure, and the paste is so injected that it reaches all diseased crevices of the pocket. Dr. Beck says:

I do not remove any of the deposits previous to the first injection. At the next sitting I remove all deposits and useless teeth, also remove or correct all obstructive materials, such as ill-fitting crowns or fillings, cleanse and polish the teeth to be retained, and ligate them with strong non-elastic material. Then I make a second injection and have the patient return in two days. The injections hereafter are repeated every other day until the discharge stops, and the tissues resume a healthy condition. The frequency of the injection varies according to the pathological condition present, and is determined in each case individually. This method of treatment has been employed by me in a large number of cases of pyorrhea alveolaris, and the results hereby obtained are far superior to those obtained by any method I have heretofore employed, so that I do not hesitate to recommend it to the profession. Among these cases are many of long standing which had resisted former treatment, and which after a few injections of bismuth paste entirely cleared up. The results were not at all surprising to me, since I knew what could be accomplished with the paste, having for several years observed its application by my

brothers in chronic suppurative sinuses, and I desire to quote their explanation of the factors which produce these favorable results. Dr. Joseph C. Beck states in a paper published January 2, 1909, in the *Journal of the American Medical Association*, the following: "Either the metallic bismuth or the nitrate coming in contact with the diseased tissues produces a local leucocytosis and changes in the connective tissue cells, both of which destroy the vegetable organisms. When the bacteria are destroyed, the disease process undergoes resolution, provided no foreign body—sequestrum—or necrosis be present."

In general surgery, where large quantities of this paste are injected, there is a possibility of its being absorbed, causing symptoms of chronic intoxication similar to those of lead poisoning. This can hardly be considered a danger in dentistry, where the paste is used in such small quantities and is not liable to absorption. Experience with this paste has certainly proved very gratifying, and I trust the dental profession will give it an earnest trial. Although not sufficient time has elapsed to form final conclusions as to the permanence of the cure, the method should be tested and then given its proper place in the treatment of pyorrhea alveolaris.

*   *   *   *   *

CONCLUSIONS.

(1) The injection of the thirty per cent. bismuth-vaselin paste into the pockets of pyorrhea alveolaris is a remedy far superior to any thus far employed.

(2) The same paste injected into the fistulæ of chronic alveolar abscesses or sinuses of the jaws produces a rapid closure of the same, provided every recess of the sinus has been reached, and no sequestra are present. Tubercular sinuses are no exception.

(3) The secretions of the sinuses change their character after injection; they become serous and the micro-organisms gradually diminish and finally disappear.

(4) Bismuth subnitrate is a bactericidal and chemotactic substance which is slowly eliminated.

(5) By its retention in pus pockets and not being acted upon by saliva, it prevents further infection and decomposition.

(6) No serious complications due to bismuth absorption need be anticipated, since 100 grams of the paste are rarely used. In larger doses it may produce symptoms of ulcerative stomatitis with black borders around the gums.

(7) As a dressing in cavities it is preferable to any other, inasmuch as it promotes healing of chronic suppurations and rapid formation of granulations.

(8) Where systemic disease is the underlying cause of the pyorrhea, the general treatment in connection with the local is imperative.

Discussion.

Dr. J. D. PATTERSON, Kansas City, Mo. It is very little that I have to say upon this admirable paper. The methods and appliances described are almost entirely new to me. What the essayist has said in regard to the treatment of pyorrhea with vaselin and bismuth subnitrate especially appeals to me, and having much to do with the treatment of pyorrhea, I certainly shall avail myself immediately of the treatment recommended so highly by Dr. Brophy and which has been proved to be valuable by Dr. Beck. In some cases we are annoyed by the slow healing of very advanced pockets, and a paste which is non-infectious and bactericidal with which we can fill these pockets for a time will be very valuable for us.

There is another feature that especially appeals to me in regard to the treatment of the antrum after the operation. When the disease has been of long duration the polypi which are usually present must be removed, and the surfaces curetted, and usually, after curetting and cauterization, the cavity is packed with iodoform gauze and left in for from twenty-four to forty-eight hours; then the gauze is removed, and the wound dressed again. I have

very often been annoyed with the irritation that results from packing of that kind, and am very glad to find some remedial agent which will take the place of the iodoform gauze, and will remain antiseptic, be germicidal and non-infectious, and give relief to the patient; for we cannot for many days keep the antrum packed with iodoform gauze or any of the usual surgical dressings. If we can fill the antrum with the medicament suggested and allow it to remain there without its becoming infectious, a great advantage is gained with scarcely any risk of irritation.

Adhesive plaster with eyelets is novel and very good indeed, as are the other appliances illustrated, especially the splint for a broken jaw, which obviates many of the difficulties experienced heretofore.

In the beginning of his paper Dr. Brophy spoke of the possibility of making an operation upon the bones of the mouth without cutting from the outside. You and I have often seen a common dental alveolar abscess treated in that manner, prominent scars being the result, which are hard to get rid of finally, and we have wondered why a physician or a surgeon when any complication of that kind arises does not at least seek the advice, if nothing more, of an intelligent dentist. I have known physicians who appreciated perfectly well the fact that the dental surgeon should be consulted when any growth appears upon the jaws, any necrosis, or any swelling, but still they would go on with treatment and often make incisions from the outside of the face. I am not criticizing the physicians and surgeons, but it seems to me that while we know that "knowledge comes," "wisdom lingers" in their treatment of such cases.

I speak of this more particuarly, because only a short time ago a very vivid illustration of this negligence on the part of the surgeon was brought to my notice. A young man was held up in Oklahoma and robbed; his jaw commenced to swell very rapidly, and he came to our city and was placed in charge of a surgeon, who diagnosed that the jaw was broken. There was considerable swelling; an incision of about an inch and a quarter was made at the ramus where the break was supposed to be, and the surgeon treated that every other day for five weeks, when I saw the case. Upon close examination I found that there was no fracture. The young man was very much surprised at my diagnosis, but on being questioned he gave the following history: Before he was knocked down and robbed, he had a sore jaw, which did not give him much trouble, but after this experience his jaw commenced to swell rapidly, and he came to our city. The patient would not believe that the jaw was not broken, so I sent him to two of my *confrères* to obtain their judgment in regard to this case, and their opinion was that the jaw was not broken. I found upon further examination that an unerupted third molar caused the trouble. After some consultation with the patient's relatives the tooth was extracted, immediate healing ensuing, and in a short time the discharge ceased—there had been a discharge from the outside, kept up probably by curetting the bone—and the jaw is now perfectly well.

To obviate this practice, so common among physicians and surgeons, we need not criticize them so severely, but whenever the opportunity offers suggest to them in a friendly way that whenever a pathological condition of one or both of the jaws is presented to them they should

at least consult an intelligent dentist. The case cited is only one of a score or more that I have seen, resulting in a bad scar on the face and in a great deal of unnecessary pain.

Dr. T. P. HINMAN, Atlanta, Ga. The paper presented tonight has interested me intensely for various reasons, one being that it has been my pleasure and privilege to be a student of Dr. Brophy's. I can therefore substantiate what he has said tonight in regard to the use of bismuth subnitrate, which I have used in my own practice. But before going into that, I wish to say a few words in regard to the removal of the maxilla intra-orally. If anyone has seen the operation done extra-orally, and observed the large scars which such an operation leaves, he can appreciate what it means to the patient to have the portion of the maxilla or mandible removed intra-orally. The four or five cases of this kind which have come under my observation have been mostly extra-oral operations. In the first case of this kind that I operated upon I was unfortunate enough to remove half of the mandible extra-orally, and while the operation was a success, and the man is today in good health, still large scars were left as the result of the operation. I feel a certain amount of remorse every time I see that patient for not having made the operation intra-orally. At that time, however, these methods were not at our command. In several of these cases I had only to make an artificial appliance in place of the portion of the maxilla that had been removed intra-orally.

The appliance which Dr. Brophy showed for keeping the mandible in line fills a long-felt want. I have had great trouble in making appliances for such cases, and two patients, in whom infection had taken place at the age of about six years following the extraction of the second premolar by a physician, and in both of whom the mandible on one side had subsequently been removed intra-orally, presented to me for an appliance which would bring the mandible toward the median line. An attempt was made by covering the upper teeth with a vul-canite plate on which an inclined plane was placed against which the lower teeth could strike, and in this way the jaw was brought back to the median line to a moderate degree. In another case upon which I operated, the distortion was not so great and treatment of the same kind was not so difficult. I readily appreciate the admirable instrument de-signed by the essayist, which will greatly add to the cosmetic effect in cases of re-moval of portions of the mandible.

Paraffin injections, especially in the posterior pharynx, as applied in one case mentioned, have been used to a great ex-tent by practitioners of dermatology, but the essayist did not speak of the fact that in certain cases subsequent serious trou-ble has arisen from embolism, the par-affin being carried into the bloodvessels and producing an embolus. This method does not seem to have stood the test, and is not now being used to so great an ex-tent as it was at one time. These com-plications may have been due to an excess of paraffin injected, and if that is the case I should like to know it, as in cer-tain cases we can get admirable results with this material.

I have used bismuth subnitrate to a considerable extent, and am familiar with the article by Dr. Beck which appeared in the *Dental Review,* but the results that I have obtained in the treatment of pyorrhea alveolaris have not fulfilled my hopes. My trouble is, that when the

pockets are injected with the bismuth subnitrate paste, it will not stay in the pockets. If it can be kept in the pockets I believe we can obtain good results, but I have been unable to keep the solution in the pockets, although I have tried very faithfully in several chronic cases. In the treatment of fistulæ, however, I have had practically uniformly good results with this paste. The paste is placed in a platinum-pointed syringe, and after the fistula has been washed out with a boric acid solution, the point of the syringe is inserted into the canal, and after a piece of soft rubber or cotton has been packed tightly around it, pressure is brought to bear on the syringe, and the bismuth subnitrate is forced into the fis-tula. When the paste comes out, the excess is wiped off, a finger is placed over the fistula, and under pressure on the syringe the paste is forced to all the ramifications of the abscess. I have had, as I said, practically uniform results in these cases, in some of which the necrosis was fairly extensive. In cases where there was considerable destruction, two treatments were necessary, and in one case, where both the lateral and central· teeth were abscessed, it required three injections of the bismuth subnitrate to effect a cure, undoubtedly because the paste did not completely fill the necrotic area.

In cases of chronic antral trouble, this paste seems to be the panacea for which we have so long searched. I wish to ask Dr. Brophy what would be the possibility of filling the antrum with bismuth sub-nitrate in chronic antral cases where the patient wears a metal plug. I have two cases in which the patients would not consent to a radical operation, and I thought of filling the antrum with the subnitrate solution, with the hope of effecting a cure in that way. The antrum in these cases may contain polypi, as there is a continual slight muco-purulent discharge. It is my practice now to take X-ray photographs of injected cases to ascertain the ramifications of the paste in the fistulæ, and in a few cases which have been treated for a considerable length of time I expect to again take radiographs to see what results I have obtained by the subnitrate injection. This solution has appealed to me particularly in the treatment of fistulæ in the mouths of children. Frequently children present a fistula on one of the deciduous teeth, and my practice is to thoroughly cleanse the fistula, also the pulp-chamber, place a quantity of the paste in the pulp-chamber and force it—by pressing on a small piece of unvulcanized rubber large enough to fill the pulp-chamber— through the tooth and fistula, and then make my filling in the cavity, leaving the solution in the root-canals. This treatment has so far proved to be very satisfactory, the fistulæ healing up and the teeth remaining comfortable.

The appliance which the essayist has shown for the adjustment of fractures of the mandible is a very admirable one. My experience with gold splints in such cases has not been very satisfactory, especially when a portion of the mandible is movable. The best results I have obtained by drilling through the mandible and wiring the broken ends together with a No. 20 gage silver wire.

I wish to thank Dr. Brophy for his very admirable paper. It makes us appreciate more and more our duty toward our patients in regard to oral surgery.

Dr. A. G. FRIEDRICHS, New Orleans, La. I have had some experience in regard to the treatment of fractures, and can appreciate that when the teeth are

present Dr. Brophy's appliance is admirable, but I should like to ask him how he would manage a case if there are no teeth present behind the fracture. I have had no difficulty in forcing the fragments into position and keeping them there by means of the teeth locking in the splint, which is made similarly to the one presented, only making it in one piece; I then force the jaw into position, allowing the teeth to lock and hold the jaw in correct position. But how would Dr. Brophy treat an edentulous case of fracture at the angle of the jaw?

Dr. M. C. SMITH, Lynn, Mass. I should like to ask Dr. Brophy if he would use the bismuth subnitrate solution if a pocket or a sinus is affected by actinomycosis?

Dr. H. C. FERRIS, Brooklyn, N. Y. In reference to the splint used and recommended by the essayist in this case, the size of the material and the forces that work behind the apparatus, it would seem that the movement of the teeth in the alveolus would counterbalance the force active from the other side of the arch. In orthodontia practice, in reducing a case coming under a division of class III of Angle's classification, we utilize the reactive action by such movement of the teeth with the use of intermaxillary elastics, thereby supporting the lateral action and these teeth, and the contraction of the masseter muscles on the affected side, by this cross action of the elastic from one side of the face to the other. I should imagine that in the case under discussion the teeth on one side of the jaw or the other would move buccally.

The bismuth subnitrate paste recommended has been used in my hands in a number of cases, and like Dr. Hinman

I have found a great deal of difficulty in getting the mixture into the pockets. There has also been some irritation in the lower pockets, from some unknown cause.

I should like to ask if this bismuth paste is introduced in cases where the tissues are broken down around the apex of the tooth. We sometimes have a sharp piece of bone, or the tooth has become affected at the apex, leaving the latter very sharp; will bismuth paste overcome that trouble, or is it necessary to excise the end of the root?

Dr. HINMAN. My experience in this work is so recent that I cannot answer that question except by saying that in the only case where the X ray has shown such a condition the bismuth paste has been used, and a cure has been effected. The radiographs of these cases show the end of the tooth completely encapsulated by the paste.

As bismuth subnitrate, paraffin, and wax are all insoluble, the only soluble portion of the paste being vaselin, I should like to ask whether there is any virtue in the paraffin or wax, and whether bismuth and vaselin alone would produce the same results?

Dr. BROPHY (closing the discussion). The use of the Roentgen ray seems to be the chief feature of this discussion. Dr. Beck's object in using the bismuth paste, as stated in the paper, was to place some opaque material in the tissues, so that he might by the use of the X ray discover the course of a fistula, and he found that following these injections suppuration ceased. I cannot say too much in favor of the X ray. It would seem to me impossible, after our experience with it, to get on without it. It clears up many obscure conditions, and enables us to make a diagnosis in a case about

which, prior to its use, we were in doubt. With it we have the way cleared regarding the actual condition of a part, especially if we have diseased bone, necrosis, malposed teeth that may be centers of neuralgia, spiculæ of bone, excementosis, foreign substances in the tissues, etc.; I cannot name all the conditions that render it necessary to employ this agent as a means of diagnosis.

In the use of paraffin in the restoration of the symmetry of the jaws and face, I have not had any of the bad effects mentioned by Dr. Hinman. If such trouble appears, it may be accounted for by the solution having been too thin. A solution used in a tooth might pass into the circulation, but if the paraffin is used in the form of a paste I think you need have no fear of its causing a thrombus or of disturbing the circulation.

I do not blame the young men of the medical profession for making errors in regard to an operation which they have never had an opportunity to learn. But I do find fault with the schools of medicine which do not give the student the chance to study pathology in all its phases. We know that a very large majority of the medical schools in this and other countries have no men to teach the morbid anatomy of the teeth and all the pathological conditions caused by diseased teeth, and we see the sequelæ of this lack of training. We could not reasonably expect anything else. If the medical school did not teach the treatment of cutaneous diseases, should we wonder that the young physician made errors in attempting to treat them? If they did not teach ophthalmology, should we wonder if the physician passing out into practice made errors in attempting an operation of the eye or in treating the ordinary everyday lesions of that organ?

Certainly not. I am not finding fault with the medical men for making errors, but in my opinion they should not attempt operations which they do not understand. At the meeting of the American Medical Association held in 1907 at Atlantic City, a report was made by the Committee on Schools in which the statement was made that fifty per cent. of all medical colleges in the United States are so poorly equipped and are so imperfectly organized and have such meager facilities, that it would be better for the profession if they were discontinued. I do not know whether that report was absolutely correct or not; but we cannot expect so poorly educated physicians to be well-qualified practitioners. We make errors, and yet we study hard with the view to preventing them; the most successful man is the one who makes the fewest errors. I have seen the entire symphysis of the lower jaw removed from molar to molar by a surgeon who thought that the patient had carcinoma, and there was nothing wrong with him except that a dento-alveolar abscess discharged lingually and lifted up the tissues forming the floor of the mouth. The patient was a vigorous young man, a student in one of our great universities. He came to me to see if I could adjust some artificial appliance to compensate for the loss of bone. As Dr. Patterson says, these errors are being made all the time by men of great repute, not by men of meager capacity—because of the lack of knowledge of that important subject, dental pathology, which medical students do not learn.

I might state in passing, that in cases where it is expedient, and where the patient must lose a great portion of the bone—necrosis of the mandible following eruptive fevers, such as scarlet fever or measles, etc.—I have frequently kept the sequestrum in place while removing the bulk of the bone until the periosteum would throw out new bone, thus preserving the contour of the face. I had two patients that were damaged in this way. Instead of removing the sequestrum when it seemed proper, after the line of demarkation formed, the necrotic bone was kept there until the periosteum formed a shell of bone surrounding it; then, by taking the bone out piecemeal, the normal balance and contour of the face was preserved.

In the case of a patient for whom I removed half of the lower jaw last year, I did not make use of the appliance exhibited, but wired the teeth together and in that way succeeded in obtaining a perfectly normal occlusion. The principal thing to do after the loss of a portion of the mandible is to hold the teeth in position until cicatrization takes place, and when that is complete, all the tissues will set and harden and the normal occlusion will be preserved. This appliance, which I will pass around later, will hold the jaw, until cicatrization is complete, and the patient can continue to chew on one side. I wish to state that in some cases the necrosis is aggravated by the injudicious use of oxygenated waters, such as hydrogen dioxid. In these waters the gas is liberated and must come out somewhere, in the same way as a cannon will burst if the powder charge cannot get out of the muzzle of the gun. If you put these waters in contact with pus or blood the infectious material will be forced beyond the territory to which it would otherwise be confined, producing necrosis of the bone.

I hardly agree with Dr. Hinman that paraffin is not being used as much as it was formerly. Many people are greatly benefited by its use in the restoration of disfigured features.

To make the bismuth paste stay in the pockets, just a little more wax or a little more paraffin is added to make it harder.

I do not think much of metal tubes worn in the antrum. I formerly used them, but have abandoned them. I cannot understand how any man can tell what is in the antrum without making a big opening and looking into it. We may as well try to see what is in a barrel by looking in the bung-hole—it is all dark in there, and we cannot see anything. But if a sufficiently large opening is made in the canine fossa we can easily see what is in the antrum, and I venture the assertion that in chronic empyema the antrum is nearly if not quite full of polypi. I tell every student, when we open an antrum that has been diseased for six or eight months, that we shall find polypi, and I have never failed yet. I operated upon two such cases last week, and in both the antrum was filled with polypi. An opening was made large enough to disclose the inner walls of the antrum, through which I could curet the polypi. Next week these antra will be filled with the bismuth paste. If a tube is put in the antrum for drainage, it will drain, but of what use is draining? The tube will simply drain the pus that is forming around the polypi as long as the polypi remain. But we need to get at the bottom of the trouble, remove the cause of the disturbance, and effect a cure.

Dr. Friedrichs remarked that he had encountered trouble in splinting the fractured ends in fractures occurring back of the teeth. I wish therefore to say that this appliance is not applicable in all cases, but only when the teeth are present. When a fracture occurs back of the teeth or at the angle of the jaw, other means have to be employed, the wiring together of the ends of the bones being the simplest and most reliable method. Sometimes we can adjust the interdental splint in these cases, but we have to use judgment, and call upon our ingenuity to work out something that will meet the conditions presented.

The moisture, which is troublesome in putting the splint in place and fastening it, is very easily overcome by adjusting the rubber dam.

Dr. Smith asked about bismuth paste in the treatment of actinomycosis. Upon returning I shall try it in a case that has just presented. About two years ago I presented a paper on the subject of actinomycosis before the National meeting held at Minneapolis, which you will find published in the Transactions. I there described a method of treating this disease which I have used successfully in a number of cases. Actinomycosis is curable if the patient is treated with potassium iodid and sulfate of copper before any bone has been destroyed. In one case that I now have under treatment I shall try the bismuth paste and report my results.

Dr. Ferris spoke of the application of force on the splint. I know of no better splint that exerts equal force on both sides. It conforms very well to all the irregularities of the lower teeth, so that when the patient closes the mouth it exerts equal force on both sides. It is often necessary, however, after adjusting this splint and allowing the patient to try the occlusion, to now and then touch off a little spot with the stone where the occlusion seems to strike a little harder than anywhere else, and in this way we enable the patient to go on using the jaw. This splint offers the advantage that as soon as we adjust it we enable the patient to use the jaws, which is much better than fixing the jaws by some appliance which must be sometimes accomplished by wiring the teeth and holding them still. This appliance offers an ideal way of securing proper occlusion, and the chief object in treating fractures after union has taken place must always be to secure proper occlusion. If we succeed in securing normal occlusion after a fracture, we have attained the highest degree of success that is possible in the treatment of such cases.

In conclusion, I wish to say that I feel indeed grateful to my audience and to the gentlemen who participated in the discussion for the very courteous appreciation of my hurriedly composed paper.

The next order of business was the reading of a paper by Dr. A. H. THOMPSON, Topeka, Kansas, entitled "The Evolution of Tools," as follows:

The Evolution of Tools.

By A. H. THOMPSON.

"THE tool was man's first scepter: It asserted his royalty over Nature."—*M. de Pressensé.*

NATURE is both prodigal and niggardly in her dealings with man. Prodigal in furnishing for his use many simple things that are necessary for the maintenance of his existence, and niggardly and reluctant in surrendering the more secret materials and forces that have contributed so much to the wonderful advancement of civilized man. Primitive man utilized the simple things that nature furnished ready to his hand, and they were sufficient for his wants, while civilized man, by his intellectual powers and scientific knowledge, wrings from her reluctant hand the means for producing the wonders of this marvelous age. But from her great storehouse, nature supplies both savage and civilized man with the indispensable means of gratifying his requirements. Her manifold products are his resources, and her mysterious forces are harnessed to do his will. Nature was a benefactor to primitive man, but civilized man has made her his slave. Without the simple resources she placed in the first men's hands, life would

have been impossible, and the new race would have perished from off the face of the earth. It would have been a catastrophe akin to that which overtook whole groups of animals in past geological ages.

The primeval industrial life of the human race must therefore be considered first in the light of what nature provided ready-made for existence against antagonistic conditions. These simple things placed the balance of power in his hands, and he lived. Without them he would have perished, and the earth would have remained the wilderness of animal and plant life that it was before the advent of man. We must therefore contemplate the capability of that primeval troglodyte, that man-ape who was utterly incapable of creating implements and weapons from the materials around him. He was capable of using in a simple simian way the gifts of nature as they came from her hands, without any artificial modification whatever. Kindly nature gave him these resources to supplement the waning powers of his natural organs, which were being rapidly modified in the process of his psychic evolution. Having lost valuable weapons in the reduction of his teeth and claws, he must needs adopt external aids to enable him to survive amid the hostile conditions in which he found himself placed. What the primeval man-ape was losing in physical organization as compared with other animals, he more than equalized in the development of ability to utilize the materials that nature supplied ready to his hand. From that point the departure of man from his simian ancestors began.

Among the important gifts with which nature aided struggling primeval man may be noted first those which were furnished by the vegetable kingdom. Like his near relatives, the quadrumana, simian man was probably arboreal in his habits, or partially so at least. Many of man's rudimentary structures point to the fact of such an existence. The apes of today furnish examples of the transitional stage, such as that when primeval man gradually became a terrestrial animal in the process of his evolution. This primitive arboreal life first taught him the use of such products of the vegetable kingdom as the limbs, fruits, etc., of the trees, which might be employed as tools and weapons without modification. These were the missiles and clubs ready to his hand. The development of the grasping powers of the hand checked the growth and caused the reduction of the jaws and the teeth as prehensile and fighting organs. The hands were evolved by climbing, and an accidentally broken limb left in the grasp would suggest its use as a missile or a club. This is the natural automatic action as observed in monkeys. The club, therefore, either for striking or throwing was a natural weapon. Nature kindly placed this most effective and typical weapon in the hands

of primeval man at the very first and most critical stage of his existence. His survival as a species probably depended more upon his discovery of the club and its use at this time than upon any other agency. It gave him a new resource, and placed the balance of power in his hands. It enabled him to dominate over other animals, and we probably owe our preservation as a species to the discovery of the club and its subsequent modifications. When we consider the reduction of the jaws and teeth as weapons in man, and recognize that without such external resources to supplement his waning powers he would probably have succumbed in the struggle for existence, we must admit the importance of the timely discovery. The first pithecanthropus who broke off a limb and used it for a missile or a club was the genius who saved the race from extinction. With this weapon he became a formidable enemy and more than a match for the destructive animals which menaced him. The evolution of the club down to our own times, with all its modifications, is a most interesting history, and shows the eventful rôle that this weapon has played in the development of the race.

Next to the club came the stick for throwing, which would early suggest itself by accidental discovery in the first place, in the first struggles with wild beasts and wilder men. From this were evolved the boomerang, the knobkerry, and other throwing-sticks which are constructed upon such scientific principles as are surprising among the very primitive people with whom they are found. Primitive man would soon discover the difference between a sharp stick and a blunt one. With a sharp stick he could better pierce animals to kill them, and dig in the ground to reach roots and grubs. With a very slight advance in intelligence he learned to sharpen the stick, but that important step placed him beyond the stage of the man-apes, and he became a man. With still further advancement he hardened the point of the stick in the fire, and later on attached still harder points of stone or bone. From this simple weapon was developed the spear and arrow and their relatives, but all originated from the sharp stick found ready to his hand. In this category belongs the sharp thorn, from which was developed the awl, the needle, and the pin.

In the mineral kingdom, we again find nature's kindly provision most fruitful. Stones of various forms and densities were furnished ready to the hand of primitive man, which could be used for pounding or for missiles. With the stone as a hammer, he reduced refractory food substances, such as nuts or bones, and thus secured food. As his teeth and jaws had been much reduced, the stone hammer came as a saving resource. The stone also served an important purpose as a missile for defense or to kill animals for food. As a missile the stone did not undergo as great an evolution as it did as a hammer in early savage life, but in modern warfare the missile has become by far the most important and efficient weapon. These ready-made weapons were necessarily adopted at a very early stage, as we know of the quadrumana throwing stones as missiles. When man attained the stage of modifying and shaping stones to make them more effective as implements and weapons, he began to sustain life more easily, and even to acquire some luxuries. When we consider the multifarious forms of stone implements and their innumerable uses, we must acknowledge a debt of gratitude to old Mother Nature for her beneficence in placing

such a very useful material in the hands of primitive man. Without the indispensable mineral substances, he could have progressed but little beyond the merest savagery. If the vegetable kingdom supplied the first resources for the preservation of his life at the first emergence of man from the animal stage, then did the mineral kingdom supply the means for the next step, the advancement to the stage of improved savagery.

The stone as a hammer developed great possibilities in the process of its evolution from the mere natural pounding implement. With the birth of inventive and mechanical powers, it was early modified to meet various purposes by chipping and grinding into many and varied forms to serve the demands of life. The hammer is still important as a tool in reducing substances that contribute to the wants of man, but with all its modifications its relationship to the primitive pounding-stone can be readily traced. As Tyler states in "Early History of Mankind," "Mere natural stones, picked up and used without any artificial shaping at all, are implements of a very low order, yet from this lowly origin all hammering tools were derived." That stones as simple pounding implements were long in use unmodified by man is demonstrated by such savage tribes as yet survive which are without artificially formed stone implements, but use cobble stones for pounding for all purposes. This is illustrated by the customs of the Seri Indians of Sonora, Mexico, on the Gulf of Lower California. Of them Prof. W. J. MaGee says (Bureau of Ethnology Report): "The Seris lack essentially the tool sense. Practically, they have but a single tool, which is applied to a remarkably wide variety of purpose —the natural cobble, which is used for crushing bones, severing tendons, grinding seeds, rubbing face-paint, or for weapons, etc. This many-functioned tool is but a water-worn pebble, and is artificially shaped only by wear, or use, and is summarily discarded when a sharp edge is produced by fracture. Cobbles and similar stones are found in quantity on their range and in their ancient shell mounds, with an occasional rudely shaped arrow-head, but not a single knife of stone or other wrought substance has been found." The offices of the pounding-stone in cracking nuts, in breaking bones, crushing shell-fish, etc., quite early revealed new food resources and thereby extended the possibilities of life and of survival. These possibilities stimulated invention also, and led to the attachment of a handle to a well-adapted stone, and thus to other methods of increasing usefulness. It is interesting to note also what the lowest degree of savagery is in the manufacture and use of stone implements. This is furnished by the Tasmanians, who were in the beginnings of the stone age when discovered. Mr. H. Ling Roth says of them in his "Aborigines of Tasmania": "Fragments of rock, either natural or artificial, are treated in one way only, by striking off small flakes all along the edge on one side only. This is, however, done with such skill as to keep the edge straight and sharp. None of the implements were furnished with handles, but were made to hold in the hand only. None of them were even ground." Mr. Tyler says, in his preface to Mr. Roth's book: "If there have remained anywhere up to modern times men whose condition has changed little since the stone age, the Tasmanians seem to have been such a people; they stand before us as a branch of the negroid race illustrating the condition of man now in his lowest stage of culture. The workmanship of their stone implements repeated the condition of paleolithic man. The round cobble stone with one side chipped to an edge is a typical implement, which makes it appear that the Tasmanian was at a lower cultural stage than the primitive man of Europe, who was a skilful chipper of flint, as evidenced by the implements found in the drift and in the caves. An extraordinary ignorance of tool-craft thus prevailed among the Tasmanians previous to their discovery by the whites. On the whole, the life of the Tasmanians may give us some idea of the condition of earliest primitive tribes of the old world, for there is no record of the Tasmanians having made a needle to sew skin, or drawing or carving like the primitive men of Europe."

The so-called "eolithic problem" has been a greatly discussed question among anthropologists of late. It refers to some rudely chipped flakes found in deposits before the age of the oldest known chipped implements, and antedates in history of workmanship the oldest artificial forms. These rude implements were described by Prof. George G. MacCurdy in the *American Anthropologist* for 1905 as "Roughly hewn pebbles and nodules and naturally broken stone showing work, with thick lustrous patina, found in early geological deposits. The discovery, in pliocene deposits, of incised bones first led to the finding of flints thought to have been chipped intentionally. The retouches and marks of utilization were most convincing." Other authors declared that they are mere natural chips, and that all of the marks could have been produced by natural causes. But they have been found in many places in the tertiary formations, and the evidence that they are artificial is generally accepted. They are often found with the remains of extinct animals of the tertiary age. The objects consist of chipped flakes, scrapers like spokeshaves, rude awls, daggers, etc. Prof. MacCurdy continues: "The hammer and knife were the original tools. Both were first picked up ready-made. A sharp-edged natural flake served for one and a nodule or a fragment for the other. They were produced by chipping so as to be held comfortably in the hand. The stock of tools increased with the slowly growing needs. As these multiplied the natural material was supplemented by the manufacture of artificial flakes. The marks are often the result of use. A natural sharp edge was used till it was dulled and was then cast aside. The signs of use were unmistakable. Thence accidental chipping led to the suggestion of artificial chipping, and tool-making began. There are three groups of eolithic implements: First, thin flat fragments of flint, natural flakes with chippings and notches along the margins, producing at times rude points. Second, thin flat pebbles with edges chipped to serve as scrapers. Third, flints trimmed to be of dagger or poniard shape, with rimmed hand-part. These were mere natural fragments chipped ever so little to adapt them to an apparent purpose. At the next stage of culture, however, paleolithic man took large stones and nodules and made from them such implements as he desired, but eolithic man merely adapted such chips as he found ready to his hand. The transition from eolithic to paleolithic tools in some deposits is well marked, both kinds being present. The eolithic culture precedes the paleolithic culture in point of geological time, and thus pushes the age of man farther back into the ter-

tiary, and evidences human existence at this early period."

A most important tool and weapon, the knife, was also the gift of the mineral kingdom. A flint chip picked up on a hillside where an accidentally broken rock had produced it was probably the first knife. Another accident disclosed how it could be made, and thence its evolution was assured. The discovery of the cutting flint was a great boon to primeval man. It opened up a vast field of resources, not only of means of procuring necessities, but for comforts and luxuries as well. Man could skin animals to make clothing, cut up flesh for food, and do many other things that were not possible before the discovery of this useful tool. As his inventive powers developed, many modifications of the knife arose. Here, again, the resources of nature supplemented the diminishing powers of jaws and teeth. Unlike the carnivora, he was not armed to procure and reduce flesh for food, but the knife came in to supply this deficiency, and gave him command of a new source of food supply. It is indeed probable that while man was originally a vegetarian, like most of the quadrumana, the discovery of the knife was the means of extending his diet and increasing his nourishment.

Archeologists divide the prehistoric period roughly into three principal epochs, according to the material from which man made his tools and weapons. These are as follows: First, the stone age; second, the bronze age; third, the age of iron. The *stone age* is again divided into two principal parts, depending upon the finish given to the stone implements as an indication of culture. These are (*a*) the paleolithic, the period of rough or chipped stone art, and .(*b*) the neolithic, or polished stone period. The paleolithic or rough stone age was of the greatest extent, for it reached far backward into the limitless past, while the neolithic was comparatively recent. As has been said, "The first long chapter in the history of human effort and progress was written in stone." The paleolithic implements were merely chipped without polishing, and are found in glacial drift and cave breccia, as precious relics among living savage tribes, or as strays on the surface of the ground in all parts of the world. They are often worn or fractured by water action, and show surface matrix stains or the oxidizing of the elements, producing that vitreous appearance as evidence of antiquity called the patina. They have also sometimes tree-like markings, called dendrites, which are dear to the heart of the archeologist as indicating great antiquity. These markings are especially conspicuous on the implements found in glacial gravels or in the cave-earth with the bones of extinct animals under the thick stalactite floors where they have lain for untold thousands of years. Many rude implements of the paleolithic type have been found on the surface in this country which were probably not made by the recent Indians, as they were in the polished or neolithic stage. The Indians say they were made by their forefathers or their gods, and left for them to use. They were regarded with veneration and were often employed for ceremonial purposes; by ignorant Europeans, even, they were believed to be thunderbolts.

The neolithic, or polished stone age was characterized by the grinding and smoothing of implements, of which so many thousands have been found in all parts of the world. This came on gradually, of course, and laps over into the bronze and iron ages, and even down to our own day, for stone implements, as hammers and knives, are still used for simple purposes. It indicated an advanced stage of culture, for the people of this age had attained many comforts and even some of the luxuries of life. The American Indians, at the time of the discovery of America, were in the neolithic stage, for they ground their axes, although they used rough implements and weapons as knives and arrow-points as a matter of economy. The numberless stone implements found all over this country attest the industry of the Indians in their manufacture, and that they answered well for all the purposes of their lives. The wonderful carvings and sculpturing of stone of the temples of Mexico and Central and South America show the value of stone for such purposes, and obsidian knives and hatchets were not entirely superseded by the iron of the conquerors. But though still in the age of stone, the Indian was just emerging into the age of bronze, or rather copper. But he treated native copper and iron as stones, for he did not smelt the ore till the coming of the whites. He forged native copper but probably did not melt it. The neolithic culture is also illustrated by the remains found in the mounds, barrows, and lake dwellings of Europe, associated with the bones of recent animals. The Marquis de Nadaillac, in his "Prehistoric People," says: "To the paleolithic age succeeded one of a very different kind, to which has been given the general name of the neolithic age. The extinct fauna had disappeared and in their places we find the bones of the ox, the sheep, the goat, and the dog. Man had ceased to be a hunter and had become an agriculturist and a shepherd."

There are indications everywhere of new ideas and new modes of life. This progress is especially seen in the industrial arts. Metals, it is true, are yet unknown, but side by side with roughly chipped tools we find for the first time hatchets, celts, small knives, and arrowheads admirably polished by long continued rubbing with stone polishers. Much-worn polishers are quite numerous." Some of the implements are of most beautiful workmanship, especially those of Scandinavia and Mexico. Implements and tools of bone, finely made, such as fine needles, awls of bone, and carvings on bone are characteristic of this period. Baked pottery also appeared, as it was unknown in paleolithic time. Civilization in many of its phases took great strides in the neolithic age, much of which was due, as in all ages, to the better workmanship and effectiveness of the tools employed.

The next period was the age of *bronze,* "during which," says Mr. J. A. Worsaae in his "Antiquities of Denmark," "a greater degree of civilization was introduced into the country, and by this means all previous relations were completely changed. The people were now in possession of two metals—bronze (a combination of copper and tin) and gold. They possessed woven cloth, handsomely wrought and ornamented weapons and shields, and bronze tools gradually supplanted implements of stone, which, however, continued for a long time to be used by the common people. Hunting and fishing gave way to agriculture, and cremation of the dead prevailed. Bronze implements have been found in great numbers over nearly the whole of Europe in barrows, lake dwellings, bogs, etc. Instead of the simple and uniform implements and ornaments of the stone age,

we meet suddenly with a great variety of splendid weapons, implements, and ornaments of bronze, and sometimes with jewels of gold. The transition is so abrupt that from the antiquities we are enabled to conclude that the bronze period must have commenced with the eruption of a new race of people having a higher civilization than the earlier inhabitants. As the bronze tools and weapons spread over the land, the ancient and inferior implements of stone and bone were naturally superseded, although the general change was gradual." Mr. Paul du Chaillu, in his "Viking Age," says: "From the finds of beautiful and often costly antiquities of the bronze age and their great numbers, the fact is brought vividly to our mind that even before iron was discovered there existed throughout Europe a remarkable culture. They had attained a great proficiency in the art of casting. The models were sometimes made of wax and a clay matrix made around it. The wax was melted out, and the molten bronze was poured into the cavity, and the matrix broken to take out the sword or other object. Some of the daggers are marvels of casting, and large swords were made in one piece. These weapons often had their hilts ornamented or twisted with threads of gold." Hatchets, axes, chisels, awls, and all of the common implements took the same shapes that have come down to us, and attest the advance made in the improvement of tools during this age, and their adaptation to a great variety of work. Many of the tools were the models of those which succeeded in the iron age. The tool sense was highly developed, as is demonstrated by the well-wrought objects, which were made with a skill that is quite equal to the productions of today in some instances. The Indians of North and South America were just emerging into the age of bronze at the time of the discovery of America. They were in the neolithic or polished stone age and were just beginning to use copper. That they had a means of tempering copper is generally believed, for chisels of hard temper have been found. Still it is probable that the stone carvings of Mexico and Central and South America were made with stone tools, flint or obsidian. The latter stone was of universal service and effectiveness for all purposes. The native copper of Lake Superior was hammered into axes, chisels, knives, etc., which were of hard enough temper to be useful. The Indians had not yet discovered the art of casting or of making bronze alloy, but were probably just on the eve of it, and with such a resource their civilization would have taken on great advances in every direction.

The age of *iron* ushered in the historic period. Iron was probably brought from the East by the ancestors of the Scandinavians. Worsaae says: "The difference between the bronze period and that of iron is that they made use of iron for those objects which they had previously made of bronze, except the use of the latter metal for trinkets, jewels, etc. But the character of all the works of the iron period, both as to material and efficiency, and workmanship in general, is completely changed. The bronze period was in all probability supplanted at a comparatively modern date, since all the objects of the iron age exhibit the influence of a more modern civilization. The close of paganism is clearly reflected in the iron period. Weapons of iron, swords, battle-axes, spears, arrows, armor, etc., were highly developed, and continued down to our own time in similar patterns. The common tools were mul-

tiplied, and shapes originated which we have today. Ornamental trinkets of gold and silver were highly developed, as well as glass and enamel."

The iron period develops into the historic era, our own period, and from those that have gone before we have inherited the weapons and tools that we have in use today. Modern machinery was not known, of course, but the most elaborate tools of today can trace their genealogy back to those of the primitive savage. With a club, a cobble stone, and a flint chip, he met the problems of life bravely, and planted the seeds of civilization that made life for us possible. As we boast of our greatness in art and industry, let us not forget our debt to primeval man, who first discovered the modification of natural products to adapt them to his wants, and laid the foundation of the industrial achievements of humanity. We are the cultural heirs of a long line of artizan ancestors, reaching back through the ages of iron, of bronze, and of stone, far back to the first dawn of human handicraft.

Discussion.

Dr. L. G. NOEL, Nashville, Tenn. This paper, and especially the essayist's reference to the ingenuity of apes, has interested me very much. Naturalists have said that man is the only animal capable of reasoning. Yet when we study Darwin and Thompson, we come to the conclusion that the lower animals have a somewhat similar power of reasoning. Darwin, for instance, tells us of an ape that soon learned to take a stone and crack cocoanuts in order to get the milk from them, and would then hide the stone, which showed the idea of property. He also tells of another ape that had the ingenuity to take a stick to pry the lid off a box, to get something out of it. He also relates instances of elephants that used the foliage of the trees to fan the flies away with their trunks, and mentions a great many other instances of ingenuity in the lower animals.

We all have no doubt seen many of these curiously shaped stones picked up in Alabama, Tennessee, or Kentucky, and I have myself picked up flints of considerable length, carved in the shape of arrow-heads, that may have been used as implements. Prescott tells us of stones with exceedingly sharp edges which the priests used for sacrificing their victims. With a piece of this stone, which they called *itzli* and which we know as obsidian, they would cut out the heart of an animal and offer it to their gods. Dental writers also report the finding of wonderful inlays in Yucatan, and in one of the Boston museums, I am informed, there are preserved inlays of some mineral that are more ingeniously done than we could make them today with the tools at our command. There we have evidence of lost arts. Dr. Guerini, in his interesting history of dentistry, which I hope will appear soon, tells us of the Etruscan, the Grecian, and the Egyptian dentistry, taking us back four, five, and six hundred years before Christ, when successful workers in gold made bridges and introduced crowns, and in many instances soldered gold substances together in such a way that the loosened teeth were held fast in the mouth. That is another evidence of lost art, and yet, when someone in the nineteenth century found a method of making crowns, he immediately rushed to the patent office, and formed a Tooth Crown Company, although such dentistry is nothing new!

Some of the older gentlemen present have probably heard Wendell Phillips' lecture on the lost arts and tell of his researches in ancient languages, which furnished strong evidences that many implements and tools employed at present are old and were well known to past and forgotten civilizations. He was sure that the ancients knew the art of making glass, and that they had constructed microscopes and other optical instruments. In many arts and sciences the Egyptians excelled our workmen of the present day, and we know that in the city of Damascus, hundreds of years before the Christian era, they were familiar with a way of tempering steel that was very effective, and that has become one of the lost arts.

We also know that the paints of the old masters have stood the test of time better than any manufactured today. The works of the old Venetian masters, when cleaned up, exhibit very bright and beautiful colors today, but our modern painters produce works that fade after a short time.

From these lectures of Phillips we gather that we have probably lost many achievements of dentistry, and Dr. Thompson tells us that the ancients could cast before they had learned to make tools by forging, which indicates that we are going backward, for we are just now beginning to make castings.

Dr. G. V. I. Brown, Milwaukee, Wis. The reading of Dr. Thompson's paper suggested to me quite a number of important thoughts that might be valuable in the discussion of the subject, but are not sufficiently interesting to keep you longer at this late hour.

I desire to say, however, before passing the subject, that I personally feel, as I am sure you all do, a sense of indebtedness and gratitude to Dr. Thompson for the very great work which he has done. His unselfish effort of so many years has helped to secure the dental profession a place among the other scientific branches. He has done much to preserve the bond of union between dentistry and the other sciences, thus securing for us due recognition. His work in anthropology and allied subjects has been unselfish, as it has not brought him personal benefits or aggrandizements as some other more lucrative and better appreciated research would, and we all owe him a great debt of gratitude for his efforts.

Dr. F. O. HETRICK, Ottawa, Kans. After Dr. Thompson has been dead for a hundred years or so, the members of the dental profession will appreciate his work more than they do now, when everyone is much more interested in getting rich than in the foundation of our present modern ideas.

The use of tools in our work, as mentioned by the essayist, reminds me of an anecdote of Dr. Atkinson. Dr. Atkinson was giving a clinic before one of our meetings, and on his operating table lay an elaborate set of very beautiful instruments. One gentleman, in looking over these instruments said, "Anybody could do such work with those instruments." Dr. Atkinson immediately announced that he would give another clinic the next day. He then prepared a cavity for a gold filling with a single excavator, and when he had finished the preparation of the cavity, he broke off the point of the excavator and filled the tooth with gold, and very few men could insert a better gold filling with modern instruments than he did with that broken instrument. This illustrates that it is not so much the tool as it is the man behind the tool.

Dr. Thompson has done a great deal of valuable work in the study of evolution, comparative anatomy, anthropology, etc., carrying on scientific work for years at his own expense in Arizona and New Mexico.

With all of our modern equipment, we have not yet gotten past using the club, which was the first tool used by man. The dental profession has been progressing in the matter of tools, which fact is making our work easier; but is our work really better than that which some men did years ago with only three or four tools?

I am afraid that the men who are devoting their efforts to bridge and other work are too intent on gain to give thought to the scholars who laid the foundations of their work. Dr. Brophy, Dr. Brown, Dr. Patterson, and others have taken up some specialty, working out a tool or a method for it, leaving it to the dentistry of the future to reap the results of their labors. Shall we therefore not honor the men who as pioneers blazed the way for us?

Dr. C. C. ALLEN, Kansas City, Mo. Dr. Thompson by his unselfish work has made a name for himself as an anthropologist which will live after him for many generations. There is more in the world than the mere practice of dentistry, and to me one of the great compensations of the art and science of dentistry is the fact that a man who has his practice properly ordered may keep up well in his specialty and still have time to devote himself to some extraneous subject. To me that is the greatest reward of the profession. There is certainly no great financial remuneration to be gained in dentistry, and while every man may make a living in that calling, if he is ambitious for worldly goods he had better keep out of it. But any man who so desires may devote himself to some of the collateral sciences, and do work that will stand as a monument in his honor and will be a source of pleasure to him in his declining years.

The subject was then passed.

Section III then adjourned until Wednesday evening at 8 o'clock.

WEDNESDAY—Evening Session.

THE second session of Section III was called to order by the president, Dr. Turner, who introduced Dr. J. P. Corley, chairman of the Committee on Oral Hygiene, to preside, at 8 P.M. Wednesday, March 31st.

The first order of business was the report of the Committee on Oral Hygiene, which was presented by Dr. J. P. COR-LEY, chairman of the committee, as follows:

Report of Committee on Oral Hygiene.

By J. P. CORLEY.

Mr. President and members of the National Dental Association:

The importance of a profession is measured by its possibilities in the service of humanity. Its progress is determined by the class of men who constitute it.

The dental profession have but recently learned that immunity from dental and gingival disease is not only possible but practicable, with all which that means to the human race. The larger task remains of producing a dental staff that will practice and teach this doctrine of immunity. This is the crux and *bête noir* of the situation.

The few men who are fired by a zealous enthusiasm find their efforts thwarted and their energies paralyzed by the apathy and opposition of the official leaders of the organized profession.

Your chairman has persistently besought the National Dental Association to take the matter up in an official way in an effort to enlist the co-operation of all the dental societies in the country in a general crusade for education both of the profession and the public. We have proposed plans whereby the National body, maintaining a strong central committee, could induce each state and local

society to create an auxiliary committee, thus covering the territory from the Lakes to the Gulf, but our petitions have fallen on deaf ears.

A few state and local societies have taken up the work in a systematic and practical way, organizing lecture bureaus and creating and maintaining free dental clinics. If these scattered and unassociated forces were corraled, and united into one coherent and well-managed organization, backed by the influence and under the auspices of the National Association, the potential momentum thus acquired would carry the work forward, and make popular dental education an accomplished fact.

Every Chautauqua platform, every teachers' institute, every summer school, every normal college, every educational association, every superintendent of education and every school board in the United States should be memorialized by the National Dental Association on the importance of instruction in oral sanitation and dental prophylaxis.

Every orphan asylum, every indigent home, every penitentiary, every reformatory, every city school system should have a dental staff; and who, may I ask, could more gracefully

13

request or more strongly influence the introduction of such a *régime* than the National Dental Association?

The work of Koch and his immortal collaborators has demonstrated to the world that the "great white plague" is not only curable but preventable, and the scientific element in the medical profession have so arduously preached the doctrine of pulmonary hygiene that scarcely a child of the United States does not know the value of fresh air and the danger from infected sputum.

The systemic prophylactician is learning more and more to appreciate the dangers from a diseased oral cavity, and the time has come for the application of sanitary science to the gateway of the human body.

The publication of a treatise on the Care of the Teeth by the National Dental Association is a substantial encouragement. We indorse this work and heartily recommend that officers of state and local dental societies be supplied with sample copies at the expense of the National body, and that they be urged to bring the matter before their organizations for the purpose of putting the pamphlet in the hands of the public. Its publication shows that this body is waking up to the work, and will perhaps serve to open the way for a more aggressive and substantial advance in the field of popular dental education.

If a nation's health is her greatest asset, and if a diseased and unsanitary condition of the mouth and teeth is the most common cause of lowered vitality predisposing to systemic decline; if immunity from oral disease is the highest purpose of dental science, if a popular knowledge of the laws of hygiene is a prerequisite to a prophylactic regimen, and if, as we suppose, the National Dental Association represents the *summum bonum* of the dental profession, then in the name of deductive logic and in the common interest of humanity, why does not this association put her shoulder to the wheel?

Discussion of the report was postponed until after the reading of the succeeding paper.

The next order of business was a paper by Dr. F. A. JOHNSTON, Sheffield, Ala., entitled "Oral Hygiene in Alabama," as follows:

Oral Hygiene in Alabama.

By F. A. JOHNSTON.

As some of you know, a verbal report of the work done by the Committee of Oral Hygiene was submitted to the Southern Branch of this body last year, and we beg your indulgence for repeating a part of that report in this paper by way of elucidation.

As was stated in that report, we have fallen far short of what we had hoped to accomplish, and we might have long since given up but for the many letters of inquiry and approval received from all over the United States.

It seems that many dentists are fully alive to the importance of oral hygiene, but have been waiting for some plan of campaign to be suggested which they might follow. We are not prepared to say that our method of procedure is a very good one, but it is the best we could find, for as far as we know no one had suggested a successful way of procedure, consequently we were compelled to follow such plans as suggested themselves to us.

We are sorry to say that the dental profession of Alabama has been very indifferent, especially the leading men, from whom we naturally had a right to expect the most encouragement.

Our first efforts were directed toward arousing an interest in oral hygiene among the entire profession. Various means of reaching the public were suggested, the most important path of publicity being through the public schools and colleges.

Dentists were asked to send the names of teachers in whose schools they would lecture, if invited. The committee would then write to the teacher urging him or her to have oral hygiene taught, and suggesting that he invite this same dentist to lecture. By this means no one would be a self-invited lecturer, yet would have pledged himself to lecture when invited. Few dentists complied with our request, but most of the teachers to whom we wrote replied promptly, though no reply was asked for, and expressed themselves as heartily approving our ideas. This was especially true of the presidents of the various colleges of our state.

Of the few dentists who favored us with a reply, some suggested the public press as the best means of educating the public, some thought that the chair was the only place, some could not lecture, and a few others agreed to lecture. All except the few who consented to help forgot the truth of the saying that whatever reforms are to be introduced in a nation they must begin in its schools, that the schools are the only place where all classes can be reached, and that at a time of life when the most lasting impressions can be made.

How many present would now have nearly perfect dentures instead of crippled ones had they only had the proper teaching as to the care of the oral cavity when between the ages of six and sixteen? Damage has been done that no hand, be it ever so skilled, can repair. And who shall say to what extent contagious and other diseases have flourished because of unsanitary mouths?

It has been an exception when a teacher has failed to manifest a lively interest in our work. Teachers are always eager to accumulate useful knowledge for themselves and their pupils, and so we have expected nothing less than a hearty welcome from them.

In every school in which we have lectured, we have been given a hearty welcome and the best of attention, and in some of the schools we learn that an examination was given, and questions were asked so as to bring out all the important facts that had been taught.

This year a directory of the schools was secured through the kindness of the state superintendent of education, and a circular letter setting forth the importance of oral hygiene and urging teachers to invite dentists to teach in their schools, was sent to each teacher, five hundred in all. Owing to unavoidable hindrances, these letters were not sent out until recently, but we trust that they will do much good.

The greatest obstacle we have to overcome is the indifference of the dental profession. While we would not discourage other means of reaching the public, we fully believe that the greatest good can be accomplished in the schools. Fossils neither in the profession nor out of it can be reformed. How many of you ever taught an old man or woman to brush the teeth?

That the general public is wofully ignorant of the importance of oral prophylaxis must be apparent to all when we remember that more than fifty per cent. of the most intelligent people of our country do not take sufficient care of the teeth to avoid the loss of some of them in early life, and often give no attention to the teeth of their children until an ugly dark spot is seen on the child's tooth, or what is worse, the little one complains of pain.

Who in the dental profession has not observed the expression of surprise on the intelligent mother's face when informed by the dentist that the first permanent molar in the child's mouth is not a deciduous tooth but a permanent one, and should not be removed, though she has brought a little one to the office for that purpose?

Who of you have not seen the intelligent man or woman, faultlessly dressed, with perfectly kept hands, face, and hair, and who could discuss intelligently almost any topic of the day, but whose mouth was a very cesspool of filth, and whose breath was so repulsive as to almost stagger anyone who came within its range? Yet this particular class always has far-reaching powers. Such a person has not swallowed a clean mouthful of food for months, or probably years, and the air which they inhale is always contaminated. We speak of this, not in order to condemn those who are thus afflicted, for they are usually unconscious of the existence of such a condition, but rather to show where the fault really lies. No thoughtful person would willingly tolerate such a condition about him. The fault lies with the dental profession, and we as dentists should wake up and teach the people of the danger to the general health from such oral conditions.

If such a condition exists in the mouths of intelligent cultured people, what must be the condition of the mouths of those too ignorant to seek the services of our profession? Will our brother practitioner, the physician, ever wake up to the importance of seeing that his patient's mouth and teeth are well cared for while confined to bed, or will he continue to allow his patient to believe that strong medicines ruin the teeth? Of all times in life when the mouth and teeth should be well cared for, the most important is when people are sick.

It is with shame that we confess that a great many dentists, some of them standing high in the profession, go about their work daily with mouths as unsanitary as those which we have tried to picture to you. What is precept worth when such an example is set? We do not contend or believe that a sanitary oral cavity is a panacea for every ill, but we do believe that it plays a very great part in the health, the happiness, and the longevity of the human race, and that there should be a general awakening as to its importance, first among dentists, then among physicians, and last, but by no means least, among the laymen.

Who in the dental profession who has studied the development of the face and jaws and the effects of adenoids, arrested development, etc., on the entire physiognomy, does not daily see one or several persons, as he meets them on the street and at public gatherings, the beauty of whose face is spoiled by imperfectly developed jaws, by a twisted or otherwise imperfect nose, by irregular teeth, or some other imperfection that might have been prevented by the co-operation of dentist and rhinologist, had the child been treated at the right time.

When dentists do their full duty, children will find their way to the dental office early in life. When all these imperfections are observed early in life, the parents' attention called to them and proper treatment instituted, then faces that would have been deformed and weak will be made to grow strong and beautiful.

We earnestly appeal to all who love

humanity and wish to render the best service possible to their patients to enter heartily into this work. When you practice preventive dentistry as enthusiastically as you now do reparative work, there will be far fewer crowns, bridges, and plates to be made, and yet you will never be without work to do.

When we can get dentists to take as much interest in preventive dentistry as they are taking in inlays and crowns and bridges, we will have no trouble in teaching the public.

We wish to make an earnest plea for the hearty co-operation of the entire profession in advancing knowledge on oral hygiene, thus adding to the health and happiness and longevity of the human race.

[After the presentation of Dr. Corley's committee report and of Dr. Johnston's paper, Dr. P. G. White's paper was read, prior to conjoint discussion. Dr. L. C. Taylor's paper was later introduced and was also embraced in the discussion. Closing remarks by Drs. Johnston and White on their respective papers will be found at page 216.]

The Chairman here announced the reading of a paper by Dr. PAUL GARDINER WHITE, Boston, Mass., entitled "What We Have to Give," as follows:

"What We Have to Give."

By PAUL G. WHITE.

THE wealth and general prosperity of a nation or people depends largely upon a condition of healthfulness in both body and mind, both assets of great value. Whether mankind has deteriorated in these valuable attributes with the advancement of civilization and our modern methods of living is now a greatly discussed subject. Evidently the pioneers of this country of ours, those who cleared the vast forests and developed a great wilderness into this beautiful and fertile land as it is observed by us today, were a class of men with a physique and health with which the present generation is unfamiliar. And the women of that period, who shared in the hardships incident to those times and cared for the large families of children which were of common occurrence, must have required the best possible physical condition. If this is a fact, we must acknowledge that civilization and modern methods of living have something to do with our physical development and the general state of being healthful both in body and in mind.

Observations have led us to believe that human beings will pay attention to almost anything under heaven rather than to their own bodies and health, and in the work which we have in hand our advice seems perhaps to fall on deaf ears. The great majority have been taught along old-fashioned medical lines such as these: "Eat what you like, everything that tastes good; live as you want to, and then when you are sick, as of course you will be about so often, call on me and I will open my pill-bag and 'cure' you at so much per."

Millions today honestly believe that if drugs, chemicals, medicines cannot cure them, it is the will of a loving Father that they should die. To offer to these millions a means of perfect health which is entirely removed from drug superstition is to speak to them in a new language. To point out to them their errors and try to set them right without giving them something in the shape of drugs is considered useless, and one is put down, I suppose, as being somewhat queer.

We must sympathize with this ignorance. It is the stone wall against which truth and health dash themselves to pieces, and this wall *must* be torn down. We must not adopt the easy "let alone" policy, for mental, moral, and physical degeneration is sure to come just as soon as mental, moral, and physical advancement stops. It is for those who know to say whether humanity shall advance or retrograde. That is the question we must answer; it is ever before us. What shall we do? We have the possibility of teaching the young, because we know that perfect health depends upon neither pills nor prayers, but upon an intelligent following of the rules of correct living. Each of us becomes a little center of light out of which gleam the rays which will eventually enlighten the world, now in darkness. Shall we hide our light? is the old question. The answer is: *No!* let that light shine, whether it be only one candle or an immense arc-light—it will do much to dispel the gloom.

We must talk to the people. When a man stops talking, he is soon forgotten. The same is true with a cause. Few great names or great causes rest upon one message to the people. Whether they be embodied in a book, a poem, a speech, some of the world's greatest truths are great because of their repetition. For people forget; each day begins anew, and the story told yesterday must be told to-day, differently, perhaps, but nevertheless told again. It is the story told day after day that makes its point felt.

The public learns like a child, by repeating a name, a phrase, a sentence over and over until it is known. Let us start the public on its lesson now. Let it see our cause exploited daily, every other day, twice a week, until it is learned. Let the light shine on!

As the oral cavity has been fittingly called the gateway of life, so·may oral hygiene be correspondingly styled the gateway to health, or the key to all personal and domestic hygiene. As personal and domestic hygiene are closely related to sanitary science, this same key may open the way to a larger and broader domain of state and municipal hygiene. Oral hygiene may be defined as that subdivision of general hygiene which treats of the care and proper use of the mouth and teeth. As the healthy body depends upon the air which it breathes and the food which it assimilates, and as both of these are directly affected by the conditions existing in the oral cavity, it is not an exaggeration to say that three-fourths of the ills of mankind would be —nay, will be—banished as soon as the mouth and teeth receive the care and attention they require.

The great important question which arises here is, How is this care and attention to be brought about? The answer is, By educating the public. And then again the much-mooted question arises, How?

Since the mind of the adult is not as susceptible as is that of the child, even if the instruction be given properly, and since it seems almost hopeless to attempt to reform the adult, our entire efforts should be directed to looking out for the future generation. Inasmuch as it has been convincingly demonstrated by statistics that the family cannot be relied on to safeguard what may be considered one of the most vital physical functions, it devolves on the schools to inculcate habits of oral hygiene. As Dr. Grady says: "Is it not the duty of the school to arouse society to intelligent thought on the importance of better modes of life? Is it not the duty of the school to train people to live better—is not this the true purpose of the schoolroom? The logical place to begin is with the physical life of society—the one phase of life that has been most ignored by our educational methods."

We must stop at its source all this mischief. There are more than 20,000,000 school children in this country, one-fifth of the entire population, and hardly a child among them that has no defective teeth; and among the other four-fifths of the population there is scarcely one man or woman who has never had need to employ a dentist. These same conditions prevail throughout the civilized world. Dental caries is a disease of civilization, and how to check the havoc which it is working upon humankind is one of the serious problems of the day.

The presence of bacteria within or upon the human body, the transmission of disease germs from the sick to the well, is but one of the factors which tend to cause disease. A lowering of body resistance is the first step, and here disease finds its opportunity. The healthy body has the power of resisting disease, but a body cannot be healthy with a foul and neglected mouth.

It would be a waste of time to repeat to you, who know them so well, all the complications which are often ascribed to dental disorders; suffice it to say that too great stress cannot be laid upon this question. There is not a disease to which the human body is liable that is not aggravated by an unhealthy condition of the mouth; in fact, many diseases are originally caused by neglected teeth. Health is impaired, beauty marred, happiness destroyed, and life shortened by the deplorable ignorance of the hygienic laws governing the preservation of these important organs.

In my opinion, it can be said with perfect truth and without serious fear of contradiction that our public schools have served as an incubator for the developing and the disseminating of more disease than any one single cause known. The number of deaths due to such causes, if the truth were known, would certainly be appalling.

In some states compulsory education is a part of our public school system, and tardiness and irregular attendance are not tolerated. To compel a child to attend school, and to subject it to infection that may result in sickness or death, if such conditions are known to those in authority, is absolutely unjustifiable—is nothing short of a crime.

There is yet a weightier reason for legal insistence upon proper instruction in the care of the teeth in the schools. Many thousands of dollars are expended each year for systems of school ventilation, and the people cheerfully bear this burden of expense because they are convinced of the need of keeping the air of rooms in which children are brought together as pure as possible. But, strangely enough, school authorities have thus far overlooked the important fact that the pestiferous odors issuing from neglected mouths are rendering the problem of ventilation almost impossible of solution. How much money, and what is of greater importance, how much health might be saved by intelligent attention to the laws of oral hygiene!

If there is any country in the world where such conditions should not have been permitted to exist so long without being detected it is our country, where state laws declare that whatever else is done with a child's time in school he shall be taught hygiene and physiology. To these subjects alone is given right of way for so many minutes per week, or so many pages per text-book, or so much of each chapter. For failing to teach this subject with the frequency prescribed by law, teachers may be arrested, fined, and removed from office. Yet in spite of laws in every state and territory, and in spite of the army of publishers' agents ready at a moment's notice to jump to the defense of these laws, physical defects and unhygienic living are quite as common here as in countries where opposition to alcohol and tobacco is not strong enough to influence legislation. The chief purpose of school hygiene has hitherto been not to promote personal or community health, but to lessen the use of alcohol and tobacco, and there is not a single physiology or hygiene book used in the public schools today that contains a chapter on oral hygiene, which should be the longest and most important in the whole book.

Although it has been repeatedly denied, we are all aware that a feeling of jealousy exists between the physician and the dentist, which will continue just as long as these professions are taught separately.

This fact strikes us as being more natural than that there should exist a feeling of jealousy between the dentists themselves. In a certain section of this country—and I suppose the same applies to other sections—when a petition was being circulated to establish oral hygiene in the schools, dentists repeatedly refused to sign it, always raising the question, What are you trying to get out of it? or, Your theories are all right, but not for me; I am not going to ruin my business. This movement did not stop here, however, but continued and increased, until a feeling of jealousy sprang up and became more evident between the colleges. Many refusals came in the form of an answer similar to this: It is a very good idea and surely ought to go through, but as you are not a member of our college (as my college is doing work along this line), I cannot sign your petition. I believe in loyalty to our alma mater, its interests and advancement, but I believe that our first consideration should be given to our profession. Just as long as this petty jealousy exists, just as long as our profession is divided, just so long will our advancement and interests and the welfare of humanity progress slowly, but if we are once united, working for each other's interests and a worthy cause, success is ours. It will come about, perhaps slowly at first, but surely, as the truth dawns upon us, that every board of health shall have its dental member, every hospital, prison, and reformatory its dental department, the army and navy its dental surgeons, and every school its inspector and instructor in oral hygiene; and better still, the mortality rate will be decreased over fifty per cent.

It has been said that organization makes the vast difference in effectiveness between a mob and an army. The dental profession in the United States is a mob. It lacks the inspiration, the discipline, and the unity conferred by a thorough and effective organization. Its many associations interest but a moiety of the profession. They are independent units, each going its own way with but little regard or concern for its fellows. Our dental profession has no controlling or directing head. It has no mouthpiece. It has no systematic means or methods for reaching its scattered members or those who newly enter its ranks, to interest them in matters concerning the profession.

Specialists in medicine are prone to overestimate their importance, but dentists seem to be an exception. The far-reaching relations of dental health or disease to health or disease in general are as yet very little appreciated. How, then, may they be appreciated? Will dental examinations bring this about? Perhaps, but with the best result? No! Cities and towns are not as a general rule in position financially to undertake the proper care of school children's teeth, and even if they were, it is a mooted question whether that would be the best way out of the difficulty.

In the model dwellings built for the indigent poor of London, a tour of inspection, six weeks after the tenants moved in, revealed the use of porcelain bathtubs as coal-hods, the plumbing stopped with swill, etc. It is the same with the teeth. To put the mouth in good condition for a child who has no habits of dental cleanliness would be ill-advised charity, and before we can help this class they must be taught their own duty to themselves. This, then, means a course in oral hygiene by means of text-books or lectures. While lectures are productive of much good, they only reach a comparatively small part of the population, whereas a course in oral hygiene would permanently affect the entire generation.

The want of a suitable text-book, however, makes us rather timid about approaching school authorities, and it seems to me that this can only be rectified in the following manner:

Perhaps the reading of two letters will illustrate my plan of campaign. As a member of the Oral Hygiene Committee I have written to a number of authors of the physiologies and text-books on hygiene used in the public schools of this country the following letter:

Dear Sir,—As there is at the present time no hygiene or physiology used in our schools or colleges which contains a chapter on oral hygiene, I am writing to ask if you would be willing to have incorporated in your book, ————, a chapter on oral hygiene, compiled and copyrighted by the National Dental Association. We are endeavoring to have oral hygiene taught in every public school in the Union, and this seems to be the only way to obtain a uniform course of instruction. I should be glad if you would make any suggestions in regard to the same.

Sincerely yours,

PAUL G. WHITE.

A reply from Seneca Egbert, one of the leading hygienists of this country, reads in part:

Shortly after receiving your letter I consulted my publisher as to the advisability of your proposal, and found that he was quite willing to consider it seriously. He suggested that it might be well to ask you to send on the manuscript of the proposed chapter, so that we might judge not only of its subject-matter, but also as to how much space it would take. As I understood it, there is not much likelihood of there being another edition of my book issued this year, but the publisher suggested that your chapter might go in as an insert in copies not yet bound just before the index, together with an explanatory paragraph or two.

Yours sincerely,

(Signed) SENECA EGBERT.

Do not these letters bring out the way to introduce oral hygiene all over this

country in the shortest possible time, and
without the objection by school boards,
boards of education, legislatures, etc., on
account of expense? I therefore wish
to ask that the National Dental Association vote authority to the Oral Hygiene
Committee to prepare this chapter, and
to give them power in the name of the
National Dental Association to carry out
this plan.

As Dr. Osler says, there is nothing
more important to the public in the
whole range of hygiene than oral hygiene,
and it is the most important work the
National Association can ever attempt.
The suggestion of Dr. Corley made last
year that the state associations create
standing committees to act as subcom-
mittees to the National committee, with
such changes and modifications as may
be thought best to meet the needs of
their special field, and that they submit
an annual report to the National committee, is an absolutely necessary one to
further the work of the association; for
without such co-operation of what real
use is a National Dental Association?

Some people are as afraid of a new
idea as a tramp is of soap. They will
not look it squarely in the face until
they are compelled to, and then will
search heaven and earth to find a reason
why it is not so. Some people use a
gold pen and only write in mud. I
would gladly use a steel pen and send
out words of living fire—words which
would stir to flame the ashes upon many
a dead heart.

Do you realize that the National Dental Association should stand for all that
is uplifting, ennobling, and glorifying
in our profession? Can you name a calling which is more beneficial to humanity?

Are you interested in measures to sup-
press the great white plague, killing annually 132,000 of our brothers in the
United States alone? Do you want your
voice to be heard on this question? Are
the facts of society, state, and nation of
interest to you? Are you on the side of
right in the movements for the abolition
of disease?

Do you say that the rule of quacks
shall end? Are you down upon frauds
in politics, religion, and medicine? Are
you ready to put a little muscle behind
the wheels of progress? Do you really
want to make the world a little better
because you have lived?

If you say, Yes; yes; yes, to all of
these questions, then I say, Your place
is where there is a practical, permanent
organization working to accomplish results. We must do things. There must
not be one single lazy man in the National Dental Association. We are going
to enjoy heartily the atmosphere of accomplishment. Do *you* want to catch
the contagion of success? Then let those
that are not members of the National
Dental Association join the ranks now,
for we are on the march and cannot
stop for anyone!

Discussion.

Dr. W. E. WALKER, New Orleans, La.
I did not expect to be called upon to discuss this subject of oral hygiene, and I
therefore apologize in advance for any
remarks that may ill become our National
body. But the subject is of so much importance that I cannot decline, even
though I am tempted to do so.

I must take exception to the statement
that the text-books of the public schools
contain nothing on the subject of oral
hygiene and prophylaxis. Krone's Hygiene contains a very much better chapter on this subject than I expected to

find, judging from other school books. There are some errors in that chapter, to be sure, but the book should at least be given credit for offering a chapter on this subject. I must also say, and more forcibly than the essayist did, that we need lectures a great deal more than we need a chapter on oral hygiene. Contrary to his statement, I have found by asking children attending schools in which Krone's Hygiene is used, that they seldom studied the entire book during the school year, and that they rarely saw the chapter on oral hygiene at all. They almost always skipped the chapter on oral hygiene, not thinking it an important subject. I would therefore say that simply having such a chapter in the book is not sufficient. Lectures to stimulate interest in this subject are of more importance than a chapter in the school books. I have reference, of course, to the right kind of lecture, properly delivered.

Dr. G. V. I. Brown, Milwaukee, Wis. I would regret the fact that I have had no opportunity to prepare for the discussion of this paper, had not the essayist in my opinion covered the subject so fully that he has left very little necessity for any preparation. In discussing the prevention and cure of oral diseases, we quite unconsciously limit ourselves as a rule to a few underlying fundamental principles that are constantly observed when we look into the oral cavity. We all know that these principles represent a very small proportion of our responsibility, but ordinarily we fail to convey the idea that we are aware of having a greater obligation to all who come to us for consultation. Those who will ultimately settle this question will probably not be doctors or dentists, but the great masses of .people whom the essayist has termed the laity. When we succeed in making the people themselves appreciate the importance of oral surgery and understand what we can do for them and what they can do for themselves, then the problem will be solved.

I was pleased to note that the essayist called attention to the fact that questions which pertain to better breathing, better oxygenation, and better general health have much to do with prophylaxis as we understand it; he has also pointed out the merely germicidal action of drugs used in the mouth or of methods pursued in cleaning the teeth. While I do not wish to decry the latter view of the question, it is, after all, secondary to the other very great principles that we should try to put forward.

I congratulate Dr. Johnston upon having presented the subject in so useful a form. Undoubtedly, there is unanimity of opinion at this meeting as to the desirability of carrying forward this work. The only question is, How shall we do it? I believe that great good can come from wide dissemination of this knowledge, no matter how it may be done, and in my opinion that is the sum and substance of what we are to consider tonight.

Dr. Wm. Conrad, St. Louis, Mo. I wish to compliment the chairman of the committee, and also the gentlemen who prepared the papers, upon the quality of their remarks.

As long as many dentists clean teeth at prices ranging from twenty-five to fifty cents, and oftentimes for nothing, the dental profession has to be educated first, before they are capable of educating the people. It is a fact that there is a result which never fails the conscientious follower of oral and dental hygiene, and that is, that perfect, positive, and continued immunity from the ravages of caries can be prevented forever. But to do that, the intelligent dentist must have charge of the patient from the time of the eruption of the first tooth until the time of the death of the patient. This is a serious fact, because the ordinary as well as the unusually talented and intelligent person is unable to take proper care of the teeth without the assistance of some capable dentist. Therefore, I claim that the first thing to do is to educate the members of the National Dental Association.

One gentleman spoke of the poor care that people take of themselves. I am, however, very happy to say that the people of the United States take better care of their teeth and of their persons today than they ever did. It is the pride of good intelligent people to take care of themselves, and consequently of their teeth. They like to do so and wish to know how, and they are perfectly willing to follow our advice. I do not believe much in infection caused by food particles left in the mouth. I do not think that the human system is very much injured by these particles, because many of you will remember children and women and men who only brush their teeth on Christmas-day, and are perfectly healthy.

One gentleman spoke of the twenty millions of children in this country who need attention. With very little trouble and with but little care, supervised by a corps of intelligent working dentists, these twenty million children could be protected from dental caries, as I said before, forever.

One of the essayists remarked that the dentist should have the care of the teeth from the sixth to the sixteenth year. The dentist, however, should have care of the patient from the eruption of the first tooth until the end of life, not from the sixth to the sixteenth year. At the Chicago Odontographic meeting held in January last, one of the questions asked in the discussion on operative dentistry was what the essayist would do if a case like the following presented: A patient, eight years of age, presents the first permanent molar tooth decayed almost if not entirely to the pulp. I told them that I thought such a question to be entirely out of order; that no respectable dentist should ever be called upon to treat a tooth of that character in a patient of that age.

Another essayist, if I understood him correctly, made the remark that it was impossible to educate old men and old women as to how to take care of their teeth. I do not believe a word of this. A person is never too old nor too young to be taught cleanliness and healthfulness.

There is another point that I wish to speak of, and that is the question of refraining from extraction, which comes under the general head of oral and dental hygiene. I hope to see the day when no tooth will ever be extracted by a reputable or non-reputable dentist, unless the tooth can be removed with the thumb and finger. The greatest crime that the dentist has perpetrated upon the human race is the extraction of teeth. No matter whether you extract one tooth or six teeth from the mouth of any patient, that mouth is crippled for life, and many times the face of an otherwise beautiful woman is marred for life. Therefore I wish to raise a loud protest that "no extraction" should be the motto of the members of the dental profession and of the members of the National Dental Association.

In regard to the second and last point upon this subject generally, it has been in my power in the past to bankrupt many of the most distinguished and celebrated orthodontists in this country. This is a subject that must be considered by the general practitioner, by the practitioners of any of our specialties, and more particularly by the practitioners of the specialty of orthodontia, namely, the decay of the teeth following and accompanying the practice of orthodontia. I have been unfortunate enough to see patients coming cured as far as the correction of irregularities was concerned, from the hands of one of the most distinguished and celebrated orthodontists in the world, but by actual count I found fifty areas of caries in one single mouth. There is not one orthodontist today who does not have caries accompanying and following his work, and from now on let him beware of me! I will no longer lie to patients when they ask me if such caries is not due to carelessness and to the filthy character of their mouths when they were under the care of the orthodontist. It is possible to finish the operation of regulating any set of teeth, no matter whether the time necessary is one month or six months or ten years, with the teeth coming from the hands of the orthodontist more perfect, and with the mouth in a more healthy condition after the completion of the operation than before the orthodontist began.

The Chairman then announced as the next order of business the reading of a paper by Dr. L. C. TAYLOR, Hartford, Conn., entitled, "Dentistry, Past and Present, as Seen by a Modern Hygienist."

Dr. Charles McManus, Hartford, Conn., read Dr. Taylor's paper, which here follows:

Dentistry, Past and Present, as Seen by a Modern Hygienist.

By L. C. TAYLOR.

It is not my purpose to discuss this subject farther back than my personal recollections go.

In the early sixties, I well remember a friend who studied dentistry, such as it was then looked upon, for three months, and served for three months more as an assistant to his preceptor. During another three months he opened an office in a small country town, where he made more money than I did, which gave me the impression that dentistry must be a lucrative business, and I determined that there must be my opportunity. Being of a slow nature and persuaded by my preceptor that I should spend more time, I devoted eighteen months to study before I went forth as a high-class practitioner. To clean a set of teeth and receive fifty cents was considered but little better than highway robbery by the public, and as it was done in those days, I am inclined to think that the public was judging correctly. It is my opinion, based upon long experience, that you can depend upon the common people to judge well of our teachings. The dentist is a teacher, and the value of his service will depend upon his ability to teach and demonstrate. To simply tell a patient that he needs a filling here or there, or to tell him that he must clean his teeth and use some particular mouth-wash, is of very little value, because the whole proposition is vague and carries but little meaning to the mind of the patient.

Rubber plate work · was at that time considered *par excellence,* as the exquisite gold-plate workers were going off the stage of action. Filling teeth in those days was of but little consequence, as most fillings would be in the scrap-heap in from six to eighteen months, and the man who could not make from six to ten fillings in an hour was considered too slow. An occasional soft foil filling that had remained in the mouth for thirty years was considered proof of their being the proper fillings, although usually the environment had been changed so that the filling had little to do with the preservation of the tooth.

The foregoing is a graphic picture and a fair one of what existed in the early sixties; but before 1870 a marked change set in. The treatment of septic teeth was much discussed, and there seemed to commence a progress in the healing art that will, in time we hope, relegate the turnkey and the forceps to the railmaker, as the public becomes better educated in some of the health problems of which dentistry, with its advanced meaning, seems to be the keynote.

During the seventies, I well remember how we all listened to that famous teacher and scholar, Dr. Atkinson; how vigorously he combated the then quite common V-shaped separations advocated by Dr. Arthur, which had left such favorable impressions upon the minds of many as producing a better sanitary environment.

The above, coupled with the extraction of first molars as taught by Dr. Riggs, was considered by many to be a most excellent sanitary treatment. When we consider that these men had no engines and very few instruments to open up septic roots, we must be very considerate in our censure, as all teaching up to that time consisted in instruction as to how to fill roots with medicated cotton, which was forcibly impressed upon young men by our famous and much-beloved Dr. Flagg.

Dr. Atkinson's exceptions to all these teachings caused him to be sought to teach in all New England conventions. While he was even more erratic than any of our teachers before or since, he taught that thorough disinfection should be followed by complete filling of roots with an insoluble substance, and the restoration of the full contour of the tooth-form by a gold filling. In the Connecticut Valley Dental Society, when Dr. Atkinson was advocating the building up of a full gold crown on a molar root, he was asked if he could get pay for such work. His answer was: "Five times in my life I have charged as high as seven hundred and twenty dollars for a single filling." Gold caps soon came to our relief, and the necessity for such fees was obviated. Gold caps, during the eighties, led up to a system of bridge work which has gratified the ambition of many mechanics even to this late day. The question of sanitary environment and bridges has differed according to the teachings received by the different practitioners. That most bridge work is unsanitary all will probably agree, and while in some cases it is of benefit to the patient when well cared for, I believe that nine out of every ten pieces have been a curse rather than a blessing. If our schools would spend three-fourths of the time devoted to bridge work in teaching oral hygiene and prophylaxis, we believe they would be serving the profession and the public much better. When young men, college graduates of four or five years ago, say that they never heard the terms oral hygiene or prophylaxis used in the whole three years of their school life, it is useless to claim that the schools are doing their whole duty.

There is no doubt that the teachings of 1890 to 1900 are producing better methods of practice along the line of oral hygiene, as oral hygiene is not only reaching the dental profession, but is also marking a special chapter in the history of the medical profession as well.

Dr. Tracy, the famous gynecologist, says: "The surgeon who considers the welfare of his patients must examine most thoroughly every part of the body before undertaking any operation. In following out my work along these lines, I am impressed more and more each day with the lack of regard the average patient has for the condition of the teeth and the cleanliness of the mouth. That such a condition exists is due to lack of education in this direction, and the people largely responsible for this state of affairs are the dentist and the clinician. . . . . The dentist is looked upon by the public in general as a man who fills teeth, extracts teeth, and makes artificial teeth. In other words, he is looked upon as a mechanic who has no part in the practice of medicine. And I regret to state, judging by the superficial, careless manner in which many dentists do their work, it is evident they consider themselves in the same light. When the dentist realizes that he is a specialist in one of the most important branches in the practice of medicine, combines this principle with his mechanical ingenuity, impresses upon his patients the importance of thorough dentistry and of oral prophylaxis, then will he be practicing his profession as he should, and will be

regarded by the community at his true value. . . . The person who is really responsible for the terrible condition in which we find the mouths of many patients is the clinician. . . . That infection of the mouth may play an important part in the production of disease in the gastro-intestinal tract or in other parts of the body has largely escaped the medical profession. . . . Dr. D. D. Smith read a paper before the Philadelphia County Medical Society some six years ago in which he calls attention most forcibly to infections of the mouth as a cause of disease in the gastro-intestinal tract. . . . Dr. Smith stated he had seen disturbances of digestion, nervousness, irritation of the kidneys, and many other abnormal conditions cured by no treatment other than disinfection of the mouth. . . . Dr. Register states that he has seen many cases of gastric catarrh associated with pyorrhea alveolaris cured by thorough surgical treatment of the mouth."

Dr. Tracy further says: "Who could wish for a more rational explanation for a gastro-intestinal disturbance than a constant infection from a purulent mouth? The more attention I give my patients as regards the condition of the mouth, the more I am in accord with the position taken by Smith, Register, and other writers upon this subject. . . . The risk of operating upon such a patient is greater than if the mouth were in a healthy condition. . . . A patient whose mouth is in the condition already described will absorb a certain amount of toxins, which will lessen the resistance of the tissues, change the chemical composition of the blood, and will predispose the subject to many diseases."

That Dr. Tracy has reached a sane and rational conclusion, I do believe. That the alimentary tract from the gums onward is affected by septic deposits on the teeth has been clearly demonstrated in my own practice of many years. While the green stain found on young people's teeth is very pernicious to the health of the child, it is usually visible and easily removed by the exclusive use of hand instruments, and health is restored almost within three days, while an attempt to restore health by the use of a germicide is of long duration, and even then of doubtful results. When we see the festoons of the gingivæ slightly elongated, the teeth comparatively clean, the soft palate red and angry, we may know that the trouble lies under the festoons, and after removing the coating and stirring up the gums to a healthy action we will see the redness of the soft parts disappearing, and in a year's time the patient will probably tell us that his rheumatism is better. One lady in my practice remarked that she thought it very strange that she had doctored eight years for rheumatism, and then went to a dentist and had it cured. The cause lay in the mouth, and no amount of medicine would ever have cured the case, whether administered to the stomach or used as a mouth-wash. There were within that mouth the poisons that caused derangement of the stomach, and until these had been removed no cure was possible. Germicides and mouth-washes do not reach the seat of trouble; something more than prescribing this or that remedy is called for. Nervous dyspepsia can be cured in almost every instance by reasonable treatment of the mouth without medicine.

The natural tooth-brush is the tongue, but owing to the use of soft foods the tongue becomes inactive, and in many instances patients seem to have lost control of the tongue. Not only have they lost control as far as cleaning the teeth and stirring up the friction on the soft parts are concerned, but also in regard to articulation. Will you tell me what has become of the orators of thirty years ago? Many men and women spend large sums of money to be able to write a fine essay that will read most beautifully, but when they are asked to deliver it before a public gathering, their address or sermon is remunerated by a sleepy audience because their mouth has become so inactive from neglect.

Irregularities are a source of ill conditions that is much to be regretted. Many of our present orthodontists are rendering good service, and the constant treatment of the mouth for the correction of irregularities so massages and hardens the mouth that the patient is greatly benefited. I sometimes think that the manipulation which a child receives in such cases is almost as beneficial as the correction of the deformity present.

I once heard it said: "As a man's head is, so will his body be," and from careful observation I am inclined to believe in the truth of this remark. Observe how every man who breathes naturally through the nose has a normal occlusion of the teeth without any irritating factors, and a well-balanced brain: and see if you do not find a healthy body in every such instance.

I may seem to be wandering a little from my subject, but dentistry of today must not be limited to mechanical changes that may be made on the teeth alone. It must be considered as reaching well up into the field occupied and supposed to be monopolized by the rhinologist, and in some instances it must even prevent the necessity of further operations.

Why is it that so many eminent and learned men are called scientists who spend some years with the microscope studying the nature of and naming the millions of germs in the mouth, and then tell us that we must use their particular mouth-wash—which is soon captured by a business man who heralds it from ocean to ocean? Has any one of them ever been successful in restoring the mouth to health? That the hypnotic suggestion has caused many to begin a course of cleanliness that has resulted in good, no one doubts, but it was the massage and the hardening of the mouth that caused the betterment, and not the therapeutics. That filthy mouths are loaded with millions of germs no man will deny, and under such conditions the mouth is soft and tender. The hardening of the oral soft tissues will produce a change and clear the mouth of germs, or in other words, the germs will not linger in a mouth that is subjected to strenuous usage.

The filling of teeth, executed well or badly, has occupied the time of the majority of dentists, and today is looked upon by some as being more remunerative than modern prophylaxis. The reason for this is that most practitioners clean off the teeth a little, prescribe their favorite mouth-wash, and call it practicing prophylaxis, while in reality their prophylactic treatment usually produces only partial results.

The modern hygienic filling is another step in advance. By this I mean cement with gold built into it while it is still soft, allowing the cement to form the joint clear to the enamel edge, the gold being a protection to the cement. These fillings will do more toward the preservation of teeth than almost any other method of filling that is in use to-

day, as they are practicable everywhere, which cannot be said of inlays, whether porcelain or gold, both of which depend on the cement for the saving of a tooth. The adaptation of the inlay requires so much waste of tooth structure that it is rendered impracticable, except where there is open access. I believe that inlays are desirable in many instances, but the proportionate number of such cases is only about one to ten as compared with the hygienic filling. The effort to save teeth with gold or amalgam alone is being abandoned by all conscientious and progressive practitioners.

The age of preventive treatment is ours, and he who has spent his life patching up waste already consummated is not the one whom the public holds in requisition. Preventive treatment, both in medicine and dentistry, is sought on every hand, and if we do not heed the call, our friends will.

Discussion.

Dr. N. S. HOFF, Ann Arbor, Mich. Dr. Taylor has given us a very brief glimpse into the past of dental practice, showing that it has been largely confined to efforts to repair the ravages of diseases which have attacked and crippled the masticatory organs, and he asserts that something more is expected from the profession of the present century. He intimates that oral hygiene has not been given the serious attention that it should have received, and that we have cultivated the technical to the exclusion of the more essential and promising hygienic fields of research and practice.

Undoubtedly, much time and effort has been spent in developing methods of mere technical repair, but it is also true that thoughtful men all along the line of progress have sought to know the

14

cause of dental caries, for instance, and a grand record of research as well as result has accumulated, from which we are today profiting and upon which we are building our methods of hygiene. The essayist makes a very true and wise observation in the statement that orthodontic interference in the formation periods is contributing largely to the better hygienic possibilities. We are very certain that he has struck in a too feeble manner the keynote upon which a grand symphony could be constructed that would quickly occupy its place as one of the classics in our professional archives. If we are to hope for a diversion of our profession from its present intense striving for excellence and supremacy in technical achievement, it must necessarily be made possible by the development of a grade of tissue with a higher resistance to infective invasion. It would seem logical that greater immunity should follow a typically normal development of tooth tissue and the ideal arrangement of the teeth in true anatomic form and relations. This ideal is the inevitable conclusion of every follower of the new school of oral prophylaxis, and one comes to feel that restorative achievement only, while of the greatest value and service when needed, can never satisfy the higher conceptions of duty to humanity. It has come to be almost a passion with the practitioners of true oral prophylaxis, not only to eradicate all disease from the oral cavity, but to replace in typical form and physiologic function all damaged and lost dental organs. How much more satisfactory would it be if we could save every tooth in full integrity and in true anatomic relation. Such an ideal may seem impracticable, and an impossible task, but none can say that it is unworthy. May it not

therefore be worth while for us to keep this ideal before us as a kind of laudable ambition, even though it may seem impracticable of realization? We should like to have a number of the younger practitioners, who have the opportunity as far as time is concerned, select a limited number of children whose parents are willing to place the welfare of their children's teeth in their charge, and let them undertake to demonstrate the fact that the teeth should not be appreciably affected by caries until they have reached the usual age of immunity. We confidently believe that children can be carried to the age of say twenty-one years without the loss of a permanent tooth or without appreciable disintegration from caries, or permanent disease of the gums, simply by the intelligent practice of orthodontia and oral prophylaxis. Orthodontic interference may not always be necessary, but practically every mouth that has been left to mature without some such assistance is likely to present some slight malposition that serves to invite detrimental deposits or provide vulnerable points of attack for carious agencies. Consequently there is a fundamental necessity for early orthodontic surveillance, at any rate.

The essayist makes the statement that a healthy body is accompanied by normal occlusion of the teeth and a capacity and habit of normal respiration. This is of course an observation that may in general be true, but it will be difficult to substantiate it scientifically without some extraordinary form of research that up to now has not been made. If, however, we are to place confidence in the statements of Mr. Horace Fletcher and Dr. D. D. Smith, we will be forced to conclude that various systemic disorders have been restored to normal function by thorough mastication of food and oral prophylaxis treatment when medicinal and other remedial agencies have failed after long and faithful application. We ourselves have some convincing data on this matter, of such a character that we are sanguinely hoping for greater evidence after further experience. In fact, it is this evidence that has been so convincing in the treatment of somewhat desperate conditions of the gum environment of the teeth in pyorrhea alveolaris that makes us so certain in the conviction that by a right preventive treatment practically no teeth should be lost either by caries or alveolar pyorrhea.

We wish also to commend another statement of the essayist, namely: "The future dental practitioner must become a teacher in fact rather than a quoter of hygienic precepts." The essayist makes this statement in connection with a reference to the prescribing of mouthwashes and tooth-powders empirically. We have all found that no single treatment will serve all, even similar, conditions to the best advantage. We must study the mouth toilet with a view to adapting it individually, and much effort and time, if need be, must be given to instructing each and every patient as to his individual needs. This will involve a much more frequent inspection of our patients than is now customary, and necessarily it will enlarge our responsibilities. But we confidently believe that it will redound to the honor and glory of our profession and conserve the health of our patients.

Dr. M. L. RHEIN, New York, N. Y. Judging from the interest evinced in this paper the principle of preventive dentistry has undoubtedly taken a firm hold on the profession at this time. It has been said on a number of occasions dur-

ing the past few years that the future province of the real doctor will be to prevent disease instead of curing it, and it is one of the philanthropic acts that our specialty can boast of, that for a number of years we have been preaching this doctrine. It is true that for a long time seeds have been sown in soil that has not been very well cultivated, but the fruits of it are showing more and more as the years go on. While a few years ago the men who were practicing this special work and endeavoring to instil the importance of it in the minds of the public were in danger of meeting with pronounced opposition from members of the profession, at the present day it is safe to say that it would be a very injudicious man who would attempt to deny the benefit of prophylaxis as understood by us at the present time. It is wise, however, that we as a profession in dealing with this subject should handle it with due regard for scientific truth. There have been a great many remarks made about the obliteration of bacteria in the mouth, and we recognize the fact that it is an impossibility to obliterate the bacteria that invade the oral cavity. We may get rid of them for a moment, but they reappear very rapidly. In other words, it is not a question of removing the bacteria, which is a physical impossibility, but of leaving the oral cavity in such a condition that the bacteria have no place to lodge and to exert their injurious effects. In educating the public this subject should be presented to them in an effective manner. When urging upon them that by keeping their mouths clean they will be less liable to possible disease, I usually compare the condition in the oral cavity to the bottom of a boat left unclean, saying, "If you will consider the boat with its aggregation of barnacles on the bottom, you will get a fair comparison of the condition that the enamel of the teeth assume if these bacteria, which are not visible to the naked eye, have had an opportunity to plaster themselves and glue themselves upon the surfaces, millions upon millions, until finally they assume a corporate existence in the aggregate, and we can see them with the naked eye." In this way I believe I am able to give the layman a more correct idea of what the bacteria are able to accomplish when left to themselves in the ordinary unhygienic mouth. This comparison of the barnacles on the boat to the bacterial plaques is one that generally appeals to the intelligence of the layman, and it is along lines of this kind that I feel the appeal should be made to the profession. We should be careful not to make statements that the scientific facts will not corroborate.

It has been truthfully said in the last essay that mouth-washes and preparations of that nature are of very little value in prophylaxis. They are just an aid to keep the surfaces of the teeth in the condition in which the operator has left them until he can again see the patient, and the time that should elapse between these visits varies in different cases. There are mouths whose conditions are of such nature that the self-protecting and self-cleansing properties permit a longer interval of time to elapse. Again, there are people who will heed the advice given to them and devote the necessary time with the brush manipulated in the proper way, so that every surface of every tooth and the gum over the roots of the teeth are massaged and brushed so carefully that they can allow a greater interval to elapse. We must have patience with the class of people whom it takes time to educate

in regard to the necessity of time and care that they themselves must spend. I feel that in this respect we have been lax in our instruction, and have not emphasized enough the amount of co-operation which the patients themselves must give to the operator in this respect.

I do not feel that I should take any more time in discussing this subject, which is very near and dear to my heart. It is a great pleasure for me to see the public interest manifested here tonight in this subject. We know what prophylaxis means for the future welfare of the teeth of humanity, and if we will use our individual efforts in the education of the public, they will soon realize the futility of dental operations performed in an unclean mouth.

Dr. J. D. PATTERSON, Kansas City, Mo. The association at its meeting last year authorized the publication of the pamphlet a copy of which I hold in my hand, and which many have seen. This pamphlet was rapidly carried to completion and is ready for distribution. As chairman of the committee I have had it published in the dental journals, together with information in regard to how it could be secured. The action we took last year is certainly an entering wedge, and if each individual member of the association will provide himself with a sufficient number of copies for his patients and for distribution in the proper places in the bailiwick in which he lives, it will help that wedge along. For myself I have distributed in our city some three hundred copies, two hundred to one kindergarten school and the others among my patients; and if you will do the same, you will help to promote this good cause just a little further.

I wish to make the motion that this association place into the hands of the Committee on Oral Hygiene five thousand copies of this little pamphlet for distribution at the expense of the association, in communities where they think it will do the most good, and I trust that the motion will be carried.

The motion was seconded and carried.

Dr. W. G. EBERSOLE, Cleveland, Ohio. For a number of years I have been endeavoring to obtain some power in the state of Ohio whereby we could have examinations made in the schools of the condition of the pupils' mouths. Within the past few months the chamber of commerce of Cleveland has become interested in this work. The board of health and the school board of Cleveland had been at loggerheads on this question for a number of years, and were unable to do anything. The hygiene committee of the chamber of commerce took the matter up, however, and became interested to know the oral conditions of the school children. In order to learn the oral conditions existing, it became necessary for the district physicians to make examinations of the children. The head of the board of health commissioned the district physicians to make these examinations, which were made in this way: The school children were lined up in a row and marched past the examining physician, who glanced into each mouth, first at the upper and then at the lower portion of the mouth, and in this way they were able to examine hundreds in a short time. It was most striking that even upon such a superficial examination over seventy-five per cent. of the mouths of the children in our schools in Cleveland were marked bad, many diseased. With the data secured in that way the board was able to go before the chamber of commerce showing the absolute necessity for action. I wish to say, however, that what we have secured in Ohio is not due to the efforts of the dental or the medical profession directly, but to those of the committee on hygiene of the chamber of commerce of Cleveland. With the data secured, the two antagonizing boards, the board of health and the school board, have been brought together, and within the past two weeks we have been able to pass a law, which is not as we want it, but the best that we could obtain under the circumstances, a copy of which I herewith submit:

(Senate Bill No. 120.)

AN ACT to supplement Section 4018 of the Revised Statutes of Ohio, relating to general duties of teachers, by a section to be numbered 4018A providing for the health of pupils of public schools.

Be it enacted by the General Assembly of the State of Ohio:

SECTION 1. That section 4018 of the Revised Statutes of Ohio be supplemented as follows:

SEC. 4018A. Any board of education in a city school district may provide for the medical inspection of pupils attending the public schools, and for that purpose may employ competent physicians and nurses and provide for and pay all expenses incident thereto from the public school funds, or may by agreement with the board of health or other board or officers performing the functions of a board of health for such city, provide for medical and sanitary supervision and inspection of the schools which are under the control of such board of education and of the pupils attending such schools, by a competent physician selected by the parent or guardian of the child, but in case of failure upon the part of the parent or guardian, then by the district physicians and other employees to be appointed by such board of health, and any board of education in a city school district making such agreement shall have power to provide and pay compensation of the employees of the board of health, in addition to that provided by the city.

Passed March 12, 1909. Approved March 15, 1909.

JUDSON HARMON, *Governor.*
FRANCIS W. TREADWAY,
President of the Senate.
GRANVILLE W. MOONEY,
Speaker of the House.

Nothing is said in this law with regard to dentistry, but the sole purpose of having it passed as it is was to establish a condition permitting inspection to be made, and this law permits the school board to act in the matter.

I wish to emphasize that people outside of the dental and medical professions are taking this matter up, and it is high time that we do something ourselves in that work.

Dr. J. Y. CRAWFORD, Nashville, Tenn. So much has been said of the presence of bacteria in the mouth, and on the subject of infection, that the public when they come into your office and are asked if they believe in the germ theory of disease, will say, "Oh, yes." When you ask the next question, "Do you understand and appreciate the fact that whenever there is disease by infection there must be a port of entry?" they will answer, "No, I do not understand that." Neither medicine nor dentistry nor the laity recognize the following fact—which I wish to impress upon you: It is strange that the dental surgeon, who has been looking for these centers of infection around the third molars, or the medical man, who has searched for them in various throat troubles, has never stopped to think that in a child's mouth from the eruption of the first tooth until that of the last tooth of the first set, covering a period of eighteen or twenty months, there are twenty openings in the mouth for the introduction of germ life. That in my judgment is the port of entry that more frequently admits dangerous infectious diseases of childhood than any other portion of the organism. With this thought in mind, I have for the past twenty years offered a chromo to any physician who would bring to me a case of diphtheria or scarlet fever in any edentulous child's mouth, and I have not seen one yet. Every member of a family where there is one child with an edentulous mouth may have scarlet fever or diphtheria, but that edentulous child will not contract it. I would not say that there has never been such a case, nor that the mouth is the only avenue of infection, but it certainly is the principal avenue. This fact has impressed the importance of this subject more forcibly upon me than any other observation that I have made in my life.

Dr. HERBERT L. WHEELER, New York, N. Y. The fact that the National Dental Association has taken up the question of dental hygiene is a most encouraging sign. They are beginning to take the proper position, starting at the fundamentals. The experience that we have had in New York leads me to believe that there are not enough dentists in America to attend to the carious teeth in the city of New York alone, and unless we arrive at the point where it will be possible to prevent some of this trouble, the situation is hopeless. The only way of successfully coping with the situation, as has been said here tonight, is to educate the people to the necessity of having a clean mouth if they would have a healthy mouth, although I am quite sure that the present knowledge of what causes the destruction of the human teeth is not sufficient for any dentist to say that it is possible to have in every mouth absolutely clean teeth, which I do not believe. In practicing exclusively among people who are able to pay dental bills without regard to expense, and who take all the care possible of their mouths and teeth, I find that the children, although surrounded by every necessary appliance and by servants to insist upon proper oral care, exhibit a great deal of caries.

The filling of these carious teeth takes a great deal of time. The placing in the books of the schools rules and regulations in regard to the care of the teeth does not sufficiently impress the student or the teacher. It is a well-known fact that at the present time every state has laws requiring that hygiene be taught for a certain number of hours each week, but no text-book is so much neglected as are the books on hygiene.

In New York city, where I took the pains to find out the actual conditions, the board of health and the department of hygiene are attempting by actual comparative methods to find out whether with clean mouths the children show better health and better mental conditions. These experiments are being carried out in the following way: A certain number of children from some of the schools are sent to the dental clinics, and their mouths are and will be kept in order for four or five years; others living in the same community under the same conditions, but without dental care, will be kept under observation for the same length of time, and at the end of that time we shall be able to decide whether those who have received the attention of the dentist, the nose specialist, and the ear specialist are in better condition than those who have not received this attention. Then we shall be able to speak of facts. At the present time the facts are not known, as statements made here have shown.

A most remarkable condition was shown by the examination of 172,000 school children in New York, namely, that ninety-five per cent. need dental care, and that seventy-five per cent. have never been in a dental office. Dental clinics have been established in the Bellevue Hospital, in three other hospitals, and in several of the schools, and furnished with the best equipment; the city is bearing the expense and would establish many more clinics if it were possible to secure dentists to attend those clinics. A most remarkable fact in connection with this work of establishing dental clinics in New York city is that not one of them has been brought about by the dentists. Personally, I have struggled for three years to induce the dentists to take up this work, but it has only been done in a desultory way. What has been accomplished in New York has been done by charitable organizations and through men who have been interested in social settlements and in the physical development and welfare of the people, and the education carried on in this way has aroused the public to such an extent that they are beginning to criticize the dentist, many times unjustly of course, because he has to be educated as the public is educated. The dentist must therefore take heed of this work unless he wishes to pay the penalty of his neglect, and it is my opinion that unless the local organizations take up this work in a practical way, work on an intelligent basis, and bring their results before the National Association, time, energy and money will be wasted. The National Association cannot carry on this work without having obtained practical facts by practical experience. The Dental Hygiene Council of Massachusetts—and I am surprised that Dr. White did not mention their work in his paper—has accomplished some work in oral hygiene, distributing circulars similar to those issued by the National committee. Many of the men in Massachusetts and in some parts of Connecticut are working in harmony with the school committees, with the charity organizations, and with public institutions such as boards of health, and I assure you it is up-hill work. All that has been accomplished is the examination of the mouths of the children of a few schools in Boston, carried on under Dr. Potter, who found that in Brookline, the wealthiest town in America, seventy per cent. of the school children need dental service. Just think what the condition must be in New York, where so many of the people are too poor to buy sufficient clothing! Just think under what difficulties we shall have to labor, and what an enormous amount of labor is involved, if we are to accomplish anything for these children. In one of the clinics in New York the work was taken up by the dentists last October, and has been carried on to the present time, but two dentists working every afternoon five times a week have only succeeded in completing the work in a few hundred children. Look at what we have to face, if we are to do anything for these 172,000 children that have been examined, who represent hardly a quarter of the public school children that need attention in New York city. I merely bring this to your attention to show both sides of the question.

Again let me emphasize that we must get to work on this question in a practical way. Let us first demonstrate how much time will be necessary to carry on this reparative work, and then we must set about to find some way of carrying on preventive dentistry rather than reparative dentistry, and we must educate the public to assist us through their organizations, or else we can do practically nothing.

Dr. WHITE (closing the discussion on his paper). I believe it was Dr. Oliver Wendell Holmes who made the remark that a child's education should commence with his grandfather, and in my opinion we should commence with the children and not with the old men and old women. As has been suggested, when people once have acquired habits of neglect and filth, they are not going to mend their ways after reaching old age. My suggestion of introducing a chapter on oral hygiene in the text-books used in the public schools throughout this country would not cost the National Dental Association nor the publishers of the text-books one cent. While such a chapter would not at the start be productive of as much good as a course of lectures might be, the teachers of oral hygiene in the schools could be made to have the children read the chapter on oral hygiene as well as any other chapters. If the books are laid aside it is not the fault of the books, and it is against the laws of most states, and that could be rectified in the different cities and states where dentists live. I cannot see any harm in adopting the suggestion that this chapter be submitted to various authors of text-books in the United States and be incorporated in the books. It would insure that a uniform course of instruction in oral hygiene would be given in the public schools of our country.

Dr. JOHNSTON (closing the discussion on his paper). Some statements have been made by one or two of the gentlemen in the discussion which I think were rather iconoclastic in their nature. The first was that infected teeth would not poison the system. We cannot take one or two cases to prove anything, but we have all, no doubt, in our clinical experience seen people who had very poor teeth, and who had called upon the physician very frequently without benefit; these same patients after the decayed teeth had been removed have immediately gained in weight and improved in general health. We who live in country districts have seen numbers of cases where there was no doubt that infected teeth poisoned the entire system. As stated in the paper, we do not believe that oral hygiene and oral prophylaxis is the panacea for all ills, but we do know that it is for some of them.

The statement which I made with reference to old people I think to be a true one. There are exceptions to all rules, but old people do not as a rule take up new things. You cannot get people who have lived to the age of fifty years without the use of the tooth-brush to do very much in that line. We must look to the younger generation.

I was misunderstood in what I said as to the care of the teeth from the ages of six to sixteen. I said that many people, dentists, physicians, and laymen, are going through life with a crippled mouth, having lost important, probably the most important, teeth in the mouth, because they have not had the proper teaching at the proper time. I did not intend to lead you to believe that the ages of from six to sixteen are the only periods when care should be devoted to the teeth, but the teaching of the proper care of the teeth in those years would have probably precluded a great number of these mistakes.

One point that I tried to specially accentuate in the paper is that oral hygiene does not mean the saving of the teeth only, but that there are many conditions of the human system that depend more on the care of the oral cavity than is generally believed.

There being no further business before the section, Section III adjourned until the fourteenth annual meeting of the association, 1910.

THE CLINICS.

Notice.—Owing to the unfortunate illness of the chairman of the Committee on Clinics at the time of the meeting it has been found impracticable to present in the Transactions any report of the interesting series of chair and table clinics presented at the thirteenth annual meeting of the Association.

APPENDIX.

Organization of the N. D. A.

OFFICERS, 1909-10.

President—BURTON LEE THORPE, 3605 Lindell boulevard, St. Louis, Mo.
Vice-president—West—W. T. CHAMBERS, California bldg., Denver, Colo.
"   "   —East—C. W. RODGERS, 165 Harvard st., Dorchester, Mass.
"   "   —South—T. P. HINMAN, Fourth Nat'l Bank bldg., Atlanta, Ga.
Corresponding Secretary—H. C. BROWN, 185 E. State st., Columbus, Ohio.
Recording Secretary—CHARLES S. BUTLER, 267 Elmwood ave., Buffalo, N. Y.
Treasurer—A. R. MELENDY, Deaderick bldg., Knoxville, Tenn.

EXECUTIVE COUNCIL.

Chairman—H. J. BURKHART, Batavia, N. Y.

A. H. PECK, 92 State st., Chicago, Ill.
B. HOLLY SMITH, 1007 Madison ave., Baltimore, Md.
W. E. BOARDMAN, 419 Boylston st., Boston, Mass.
C. L. ALEXANDER, 203 S. Tryon st., Charlotte, N. C.
BURTON LEE THORPE, C. S. BUTLER (*ex-officio* members).

EXECUTIVE COMMITTEE.

Chairman—J. D. PATTERSON, Keith and Perry bldg., Kansas City, Mo.

FIRST DIVISION—Committee on Arrangements.

J. D. PATTERSON [*1911], Keith and Perry bldg., Kansas City, Mo.
C. M. WORK [*1912], Ottumwa, Iowa.
W. G. MASON [*1912], Tampa, Fla.

SECOND DIVISION—Committee on Credentials and Auditing.

V. H. JACKSON [*1912], 240 Lenox ave., New York, N. Y.
H. B. McFADDEN [*1911], 3505 Hamilton st., Philadelphia, Pa.
M. F. FINLEY [*1910], 1928 "I" st., N. W., Washington, D. C.

* Term expires.

THIRD DIVISION—Committee on Voluntary Essays.

L. Meisburger [*1910], 85 North Pearl st., Buffalo, N. Y.
F. B. Kremer [*1910], Masonic Temple, Minneapolis, Minn.
C. J. Grieves [*1911], Park ave. and Madison st., Baltimore, Md.

* Term expires.

ORGANIZATION OF SECTIONS.

SECTION I: Prosthetic Dentistry, Crown and Bridge Work, Orthodontia, Metallurgy, Chemistry, and Allied Subjects.

Geo. H. Wilson, *Chairman*, Schofield bldg., Cleveland, Ohio.
Stanley L. Rich, *Vice-chairman*, Jackson bldg., Nashville, Tenn.
B. Frank Gray, *Secretary*, 1003 Security bldg., Los Angeles, Cal.

SECTION II: Operative Dentistry, Nomenclature, Literature, Dental Education, and Allied Subjects.

L. L. Barber, *Chairman*, 718 Spitzer bldg., Toledo, Ohio.
Frank I. Shaw, *Vice-chairman*, 624 Burke bldg., Seattle, Wash.
F. L. Platt, *Secretary*, Elkan Gunst bldg., San Francisco, Cal.

SECTION III: Oral Surgery, Anatomy, Physiology, Histology, Pathology, Etiology, Hygiene, Prophylaxis, Materia Medica, and Allied Subjects.

Wm. Carr, *Chairman*, 35 West 46th st., New York city.
L. F. Luckie, *Vice-chairman*, Birmingham, Ala.
Richard Summa, *Secretary*, 410 Metropolitan bldg., St. Louis, Mo.

COMMITTEES.

Committee on History.

Charles McManus, *Chairman*, 80 Pratt st., Hartford, Conn.
E. C. Kirk, *Vice-chairman*, P. O. Box 1615. Philadelphia, Pa.
Burton Lee Thorpe, *Secretary*, 3605 Lindell boulevard, St. Louis, Mo.
H. L. Ambler, 176 Euclid ave., Cleveland, Ohio.
James McManus, 80 Pratt st., Hartford, Conn.
Wm. H. Trueman, 900 Spruce st., Philadelphia, Pa.

S. A. Freeman, 262 Jersey st., Buffalo, N. Y.
B. J. Cigrand, North and Milwaukee aves., Chicago, Ill.
C. J. Grieves, Madison and Park aves., Baltimore, Md.
J. Y. Crawford, Jackson bldg., Nashville, Tenn.
C. S. Butler, 267 Elmwood ave., Buffalo, N. Y.
W. E. Boardman, 419 Boylston st., Boston, Mass.
W. R. Wright, 324 Capital st., Jackson, Miss.

Committee on State and Local Societies.

H. C. BROWN, *Chairman*, 185 East State st., Columbus, Ohio.

J. W. HULL, *Vice-chairman*, Altman bldg., Kansas City, Mo.

A. J. COTTRELL, *Secretary*, Deaderick bldg., Knoxville, Tenn.

R. W. CARROLL, Beaumont, Tex.

J. C. WATKINS, Winston Salem, N. C.

VICTOR C. JONES, Bethlehem, Pa.

T. T. MOORE, JR., Columbia. S. C.

H. W. CAMPBELL, Suffolk, Va.

C. V. WATTS, Des Moines, Ia.

O. H. SIMPSON, Dodge City, Kans.

MAX EBLE, Louisville, Ky.

J. D. EBY, Atlanta, Ga.

J. Q. BYRAM, Indianapolis, Ind.

W. W. WESTMORELAND, Columbus, Miss.

Committee on Dental Journal.

H. L. WHEELER, *Chairman*, 12 West 46th st., New York city.

W. B. DUNNING, *Secretary*, 140 West 57th st., New York city.

C. S. BUTLER, 267 Elmwood ave., Buffalo, N. Y.

F. T. TAYLOR, 419 Boylston st., Boston, Mass.

F. W. STIFF, 600 East Grace st., Richmond, Va.

J. Y. CRAWFORD, Jackson bldg., Nashville, Tenn.

D. O. M. LeCRON, Missouri Trust bldg., St. Louis, Mo.

Committee on National Dental Museum and Library.

G. W. BOYNTON, *Chairman*, 817 14th st., N. W., Washington, D. C.

C. A. HAWLEY, *Vice-chairman*, The Rochambeau, Washington, D. C.

M. F. FINLEY, *Secretary*, 1928 "I" st., N. W., Washington, D. C.

H. W. MORGAN. 211 Sixth ave., N., Nashville, Tenn.

E. G. LINK, Cutler bldg., Rochester, N. Y.

H. T. SMITH, 116 Garfield Place, Cincinnati, Ohio.

B. D. BRABSON, Knoxville, Tenn.

J. V. CONZETT, Dubuque, Ia.

J. W. DAVID, Corsicana, Tex.

E. P. BEADLES, Danville, Va.

Committee on Oral Hygiene.

W. G. EBERSOLE, *Chairman*, Schofield bldg., Cleveland, Ohio.

E. P. DAMERSON, *Vice-chairman*, DeMenil bldg., St. Louis, Mo.

RICHARD GRADY, *Secretary*, Annapolis Naval Academy, Annapolis, Md.

J. P. CORLEY, Sewanee, Tenn.

W. A. WHITE, Phelps, N. Y.

H. C. THOMPSON, 1113 Pennsylvania ave., Washington, D. C.

PAUL G. WHITE, 419 Boylston st., Boston, Mass.

Committee on Necrology.

WILBUR F. LITCH, *Chairman*, 1500 Locust st., Philadelphia, Pa.

L. P. DOTTERER, *Vice-chairman*, Charleston, S. C.

C. N. THOMPSON, *Secretary*, 3017 Michigan ave., Chicago, Ill.

G. S. VANN, Gadsden, Ala.

JAMES McMANUS, 80 Pratt st., Hartford, Conn.

Committee on Legislation.

WM. CRENSHAW, *Chairman*, Grant bldg., Atlanta, Ga.

W. H. DEFORD, *Vice-chairman*, Des Moines, Ia.

C. W. RODGERS, *Secretary*, Dorchester, Mass.

W. T. CHAMBERS, Denver, Col.

T. P. HINMAN, Atlanta, Ga.

H. C. BROWN, Columbus, Ohio.

C. S. BUTLER, Buffalo, N. Y.

E. A. BRYANT, Washington, D. C.

Committee on Scientific Research.

H. C. FERRIS, *Chairman*, 1166 Dean st., Brooklyn. N. Y.

L. E. CUSTER, *Vice-chairman*, Dayton, Ohio.

CHAS. CHANNING ALLEN, *Secretary*, Kansas City, Mo.

JOSEPH HEAD, Philadelphia, Pa.

H. C. REGISTER, Philadelphia, Pa.

M. C. SMITH, Lynn, Mass.

Committee on Publication.

C. S. BUTLER, *Chairman*, Buffalo, N. Y.

W. R. CLACK, Clear Lake, Ia.

F. W. LOW, Buffalo, N. Y.

Committee on Clinics.

F. O. HETRICK, *Chairman*, Ottawa, Kan.

HOWARD S. SEIP, *Vice-chairman*, Allentown. Pa.

L. A. CRUMLEY, *Secretary*, Birmingham, Ala.

J. E. CHACE, Ocala, Fla.

GEORGE E. SAVAGE, Worcester, Mass.

J. J. SARRAZIN, New Orleans, La.

H. H. SULLIVAN, Kansas City, Mo.

A. O. ROSS, Columbus, Ohio.

J. D. TOWNER, Memphis, Tenn.

J. B. HOWELL, Paducah, Ky.

L. B. McLAURIN, Natchez, Miss.

J. H. LORENZ, Atlanta, Ga.

F. L. HUNT, Ashville, N. C.

J. G. FIFE, Dallas, Tex.

W. G. DALRYMPLE, Ogden, Utah.

R. D. ROBINSON, Los Angeles, Cal.

C. S. IRWIN, Vancouver, Wash.

F. R. HENSHAW, Indianapolis, Ind.

F. L. WRIGHT, Wheeling, W. Va.

R. L. SIMPSON, Richmond, Va.

A. P. BURKHART, Buffalo, N. Y.

S. W. BOWLES, Washington, D. C.

T. M. HAMPTON, Helena, Mont.

J. BRUCE PERRIN, Des Moines, Ia.

Local Committee of Arrangements.

E. R. WARNER, *Chairman*, 401 California bldg.. Denver, Col.

H. A. FYNN, *Vice-chairman*, 500 California bldg.. Denver, Col.

W. A. BRIERLEY, 36 Barth Block, Denver, Col.

W. P. SMEDLEY, 604 California bldg., Denver, Col.

W. W. FLORA, Colorado Springs, Col.

W. T. CHAMBERS (*ex-officio*), California bldg., Denver, Col.

Committee on Pharmacopeial Convention.

M. F. FINLEY, *Chairman*, 1928 "I" st., Washington, D. C.

A. H. PECK, 92 State st., Chicago, Ill.

JOSEPH HEAD, 1500 Locust st., Philadelphia, Pa.

LIST OF MEMBERS.

* *Indicates*—Members of Southern Branch.

*ADAIR, R. B., 502 Lowndes bldg., Atlanta, Ga.

*ADAIR, ROBIN, 502 Lowndes bldg., Atlanta, Ga.

AINSWORTH, GEO. C., 220 Clarendon st., Boston, Mass.

ALBRECHT, MAURICE, 61 Ingalls block, Indianapolis, Ind.

*ALEXANDER, C. L., 203 S. Tryon st., Charlotte, N. C.

ALLEN, C. C., 507 Rialto bldg., Kansas City, Mo.

ALLEN, GEO. S., 51 W. 37th st., New York, N. Y.

*ALLEN, H. JEROME, Colorado bldg., Washington, D. C.

*ALLEN, T. M., Tampa, Fla.

ALLIS, D. HURLBUT, Masonic Temple, Springfield, Mass.

AMBLER, H. L., 746 Euclid ave., Cleveland, Ohio.

AMES, W. V-B., 151 Wabash ave., Chicago, Ill.

ANDREWS, G. F., 820 Germania Life bldg., St. Paul, Minn.

*ARCHINARD, L. D., 830 Macheca bldg., New Orleans, La.

ARGETSINGER, E. H., Pipestone, Minn.

ARGUE, J. E., Red Lake Falls, Minn.

ARTHUR, H. W., Pittsburg Life bldg., Pittsburg. Pa.

*ASKEW, J. B., Vicksburg, Miss.

*ATKINSON, D. D., Brunswick, Ga.

BACON, D. C., 103 State st., Chicago, Ill.

BAILEY, C. M., 807 Pillsbury bldg., Minneapolis, Minn.

BAKE, LOUIS E., 631 43d st., Chicago, Ill.

*BAKER, C. B., Houston, Miss.

BAKER, C. R., 200 Whitaker bldg., Davenport, Iowa.

BAKER, G. T., 149A Tremont st., Boston, Mass.

BALL, F. E., Fargo, N. D.

BALLACHEY, F. A., 450 Elmwood ave., Buffalo, N. Y.

BANDY, R. S., City Hall bldg., Tipton, Iowa.

BANZET, GEO. T., 31 Washington st., Chicago, Ill.

BANZHAF, H. L., Wells bldg., Milwaukee, Wis.

BARBER, L. L., 718 Spitzer st., Toledo, Ohio.

BARKER, J. T., Simpson bldg., Wallingford, Conn.

BARNES, HENRY, 1415 New England bldg., Cleveland, Ohio.

*BARNETT, A., Memphis, Tenn.

*BARNETT, D. G., Arcadia, Fla.

*BARNWELL, C. M., Grant bldg., Atlanta, Ga.

BARRETT, T. J., Worcester, Mass.

BAYLIS, C. F., Oneonta, N. Y.

BEACH, J. W., 52 N. Pearl st., Buffalo, N. Y.

BEACH, LOUIS L., Bristol, Conn.

*BEADLES, E. P., Danville, Va.

*BEALL, M. E., Jeffersonville, Ga.

BEATTY, C. H., 206 Bond bldg., Washington, D. C.

BEECROFT, W. G., 101 N. Hamilton st., Madison, Wis.

BEISE, H. C., Windom, Minn.

BELLCHAMBER, C. E., Effingham, Ill.

BENTLEY, CHAS. E., 100 State st., Chicago, Ill.

BERRY, C. W., 258 Elm st., Somerville, Mass.

BERTHEL, R. W., 240 Lowry Arcade, St. Paul, Minn.

BIBBER, W. R., Grady bldg., Eastport, Me.

BIDDLE, J. F., 517 Arch st., Pittsburg, Pa.

BLACK, ARTHUR D., 31 Washington st., Chicago, Ill.

BLACK, G. V., Madison and Franklin sts., Chicago, Ill.

BLAIR, E. K., Waverly, Ill.

BLAISDELL, E. C., 3 Market st., Portsmouth, N. H.

*BLALOCK. L. F., Ocala, Fla.

*BLAND, C. A., 21 N. Tryon st., Charlotte, N. C.

BOARDMAN, WALDO E., 419 Boylston st., Boston, Mass.

*BOGER, C. F., Natchez, Miss.

*BOGLE, R. BOYD, 719 Russell st., Nashville, Tenn.

BOGUE, E. A., 63 W. 48th st., New York, N. Y.

BOLLINGER, P. L., Ludlow Arcade, Dayton, Ohio.

BOND, SCIPIO, Anoka, Minn.

BOOKER, F. D., Rochester, Minn.

*BOWLES, S. W., 1315 New York ave., Washington, D. C.

*BOYD, H. T., Sweetwater, Tenn.

*BOYD, J. J., Covington, Tenn.

BOYNTON, G. W., 817 14th st., N. W., Washington, D. C.

*BRABSON, B. D., Wilcox bldg., Knoxville, Tenn.

BRADSHAW, C. A., 156 E. Ferry st., Buffalo, N. Y.

*BRANDT, O. L., Thibodeaux, La.

BRATT, C. B., Westinghouse bldg., Alleghany, Pa.

BREEN, J. M., 115 E. 17th st., New York, N. Y.

BREENE, F. T., 105 Washington st., Iowa City, Iowa.

BRIGGS, E. C., 129 Marlboro st., Boston, Mass.

BRIGHAM, W. I., So. Framingham, Mass.

*BROCKETT, C. T., "The Grand," Atlanta, Ga.

BROCKET, HOLLY V., 1204 Broadway, Kansas City, Mo.

*BROOKS, J. H., Burlington, N. C.

BROPHY, TRUMAN W., 6 E. Madison st., Chicago, Ill.

BROWER, E. D., Le Mars, Iowa.

BROWN, ARTHUR I., 1115 New England bldg., Cleveland, Ohio.

BROWN, C. E., Emerson, Neb.

BROWN, G. V. I., 445 Milwaukee st., Milwaukee, Wis.

BROWN, H. C., 185 E. State st., Columbus, Ohio.

BROWN, IRA W., 1114 New England bldg., Columbus, Ohio.

*BRUNSON, J. F., Meridian, Miss.

BRUSH, F. C., 1183 Broadway, New York, N. Y.

BRUZELIUS, AXEL N., Black block, Lima, Ohio.

BRYANT, E. A., "The Burlington," Washington, D. C.

BRYANT, E. R., 972 Chapel st., New Haven, Conn.

*BUCK, F. E., Jacksonville, Fla.

*BUGG, W. E., Madison, Ga.

BURKHART, A. P., 333 Franklin st., Buffalo, N. Y.

BURKHART, H. J., Batavia, N. Y.

BURRILL, C. L., Heron Lake, Minn.

BUTLER, C. S., 267 Elmwood ave., Buffalo, N. Y.

BYRAM, J. Q., 131 E. Ohio st., Indianapolis, Ind.

CALLAHAN, J. R., 25 Garfield Place, Cincinnati, Ohio.

*CAMPBELL, H. W., Suffolk, Va.

*CAMPBELL, J. T., Okolona, Miss.

CANADAY, J. W., 383 State st., Albany, N. Y.

CARD, W. H., Pillsbury bldg., Minneapolis, Minn.

*CARLISLE, JNO. P., Greenville, S. C.

CARR, ELLEN R., 68 Pratt st., Hartford, Conn.

*CARR, G. A., Durham, N. C.

*CARR, I. N., Durham, N. C.

CARR, WM., 35 W. 46th st., New York, N. Y.

CARRABINE, OSCAR, 542 5th ave., New York, N. Y.

*CARROLL, R. W., Beaumont, Texas.

CASE, CALVIN S., 1120 Stewart bldg., Chicago, Ill.

*CASON, W. L., Cartersville, Ga.

*CASSIDY, J. S., Covington, Ky.

CATTELL, D. M., 177 Union ave., Memphis, Tenn.

*CHACE, J. E., Ocala, Fla.

CHAMBERS, W. H., Surgeon-general's office, Washington, D. C.

CHAMBERS, W. T., 504 California bldg., Denver, Col.

*CHESTNUTT, O. LEE, Tifton, Ga.

CHILCOTT, L. S., Bangor, Maine.

*CHIPPS, H. D., Corinth, Miss.

*CHISHOLM, W. W., Anderson, S. C.

CIGRAND, B. J., 1242 Milwaukee ave., Chicago, Ill.

CLACK, W. R., Clear Lake, Iowa.

CLAPP, HOWARD, 238 Newbury st., Boston, Mass.

*CLARK, G. K., Russellville, Ky.

*CLIFTON, W. R., Waco, Texas.

COBB, F. E., 307 Masonic Temple, Minneapolis, Minn.

COCHRAN, VICTOR, 15th and Walnut sts., Philadelphia, Pa.

CODMAN, B. H., 126 Massachusetts ave., Boston, Mass.

COGAN, W. N., "The Sherman," Washington, D. C.

COLDING, H. S., 117 W. 70th st., New York, N. Y.

CONLEY, C. E., LeSueur, Minn.

CONRAD, WM., 3666 Olive st., St. Louis, Mo.

CONZETT, J. V., 256 13th st., Dubuque, Iowa.

COOK, GEO. W., 47th st. and Kenwood ave., Chicago, Ill.

COOK, HENRY P., 503 Main st., Worcester, Mass.

*COOK, S. B., Loveman bldg., Chattanooga, Tenn.

COOKE, W. P., 330 Dartmouth st., Boston, Mass.

CORCORAN, J. C., 270 Lowry Arcade, St. Paul, Minn.

COREY, F. G., Council Grove, Kansas.

*CORLEY, J. P., Greensboro, Ala.

*COTTRELL, A. J., Deaderick bldg., Knoxville, Tenn.

COX, N. J., 606 Masonic Temple, Minneapolis, Minn.

*CRAVEN, F. W., Clearwater, Fla.

*CRAWFORD, J. Y., Jackson bldg., Nashville, Tenn.

*CRENSHAW, THOS., 621 Grant bldg., Atlanta, Ga.

*CRENSHAW, WM., 621 Grant bldg., Atlanta, Ga.

CRESS, G. T., Sac City, Iowa.

*CROSSLAND, J. H., Montgomery, Ala.

CROUSE, J. N., 2231 Prairie ave., Chicago, Ill.

CROW, McF., Versailles, Ky.

*CRUMLEY, L. A., Birmingham, Ala.

CRUTTENDEN, H. L., Bank block, Northfield, Minn.

CRUZEN, E. E., Professional bldg., Baltimore, Md.

CRYER, M. H., 1623 Walnut st., Philadelphia, Pa.

CULVER, M. B., 1529 Locust st., Philadelphia, Pa.

*CUMMINGS, W. G., Harriman, Tenn.

CUMMINS, J. T., Odd Fellows' Temple, Metropolis, Ill.

CURRIE, A. W., 626 Lexington ave., New York, N. Y.

CUSTER, L. E., 28 N. Ludlow st., Dayton, Ohio.

CUTHBERTSON, C. W., 309 7th st., N. W., Washington, D. C.

CUTLER, E. V., Osage, Iowa.

CUTTING, A. J., Southington, Conn.

DAILEY, WILBER M., 19 E. 69th st., New York, N. Y.

*DALE, JAS. A., 217½ N. Summer st., Nashville, Tenn.

DALRYMPLE, W. G., Ogden, Utah.

DAMERON, E. P., 58 DeMenil bldg., St. Louis, Mo.

DAMSON, H. D., Colorado bldg., Washington, D. C.

DANA, A. W., 23 Parsons block, Burlington, Iowa.

DANFORTH, J. S., Gas Co. bldg., Sheboygan, Wis.

DARBY, E. T., 1631 Walnut st., Philadelphia, Pa.

*DASHWOOD, P. T., 613 Grant bldg., Atlanta, Ga.

DAVENPORT, I. B., 30 Avenue de l'Opera, Paris, France.

*DAVIDSON, H. M., Hubbard, Tex.

*DAVIDSON, S. K., Hickman, Ky.

*DAVIS, C. P., Americus, Ga.

*DAVIS, J. W., Corsicana, Texas.

DAVIS, L. F., 1108 New York ave., N. W., Washington, D. C.

DAVIS, SHELDON G., 729 15th st., Washington, D. C.

DAVIS, W. CLYDE, 206 Richards block, Lincoln, Neb.

*DEAN, W. A., Tampa, Fla.

DEANE, W. C., 616 Madison ave., New York, N. Y.

DeFORD, W. H., 515 W. Locust st., Des Moines, Iowa.

DEMO, W. A., Blue Earth City, Minn.

DENTON, H. B., Eveleth, Minn.

*DICK, G. W., Sumter, S. C.

DIEDEL, CHAS., 1120 Vermont ave., Washington, D. C.

DONELAN, T. P., Odd Fellows Hall, Springfield, Ill.

*DONNALLY, WMS., 1018 14th st., N. W., Washington, D. C.

DORR, P. P., Fort Dodge, Iowa.

*DOTTERER, L. P., 102 Broad st., Charleston, S. C.

DOUBLEDAY, ARTHUR W., 313 Marlborough st., Boston, Mass.

DOWSLEY, J. F., 175 Tremont st., Boston, Mass.

*DUBOSE, J. A., Anniston, Ala.

*DUCASSE, A. LOUIS, 204 Camp st., New Orleans, La.

DUNN, J. AUSTIN, 901 Marshall Field bldg., Chicago, Ill.

DUNNING, W. B., 140 W. 57th st., New York.

*DYER, A. A., Galveston, Tex.

EBERLE, EDWARD, Sage-Allen bldg., Hartford, Conn.

EBERSOLE, W. G., 800 Schofield bldg., Cleveland, Ohio.

*EBLE, W. M., Equitable bldg., Louisville, Ky.

*EBY, J. D., Fourth Nat'l Bank bldg., Atlanta, Ga.

EDDY, FORREST G., 21 Butler Exchange, Providence, R. I.

*ELKINS, L. C., St. Augustine, Fla.

ESHLEMAN, G. W., Brummer block, Cherokee, Iowa.

*EUBANK, G. E., Birmingham, Ala.

*EVANS, PAUL W., Bond bldg., Washington, D. C.

*EWALD, W. H., Portsmouth, Va.

EXLEY, F. C., 202 Liberty st., Savannah, Ga.

FARRAR, J. N., Broadway and 32d st., New York, N. Y.

FAUGHT, L. ASHLEY, 1430 Spruce st., Philadelphia, Pa.

*FAWLKES, B. C., Selma, Ala.

*FELTUS, H. J., Raymond bldg., Baton Rouge, La.

*FERGUSON, FRANK, Greenville, S. C.

*FERRELL, W. C., Brundidge, Ala.

FERRIS, H. C., 1166 Dean st., Brooklyn, N. Y.

FICKES, WM. L., 6200 Penn. ave., Pittsburg, Pa.

*FIFE, J. G., 736 Wilson bldg., Dallas, Texas.

*FINLEY, M. F., 1928 "I" st., N. W.. Washington, D. C.

*FINNEY, W. B., 813 Hamilton Terrace, Baltimore, Md.

FISHER, W. C., 373 Fifth ave., New York, N. Y.

FLANAGAN, A. J., 352 Main st., Springfield, Mass.

FOGG, W. S., Cornish, Maine.

FONES, A. C., 521 State st., Bridgeport, Conn.

FOOTE, C. P., 679 E. 3d st., St. Paul, Minn.

FOSSUME, F. L., 616 Madison ave., New York, N. Y.

*FOSTER, S. W., 100 N. Butler st., Atlanta, Ga.

*FRANKLAND, W. S., 1329 "F" st., N. W., Washington, D. C.

FRANZ, HUGO, 31 Washington st., Chicago, Ill.

FRAZEE, O. L., Springfield, Ill.

FREDERICH, V. H., 3263 Jefferson st., St. Louis, Mo.

FREEMAN, S., 965 Madison ave., New York, N. Y.

FREEMAN, S. A., 262 Jersey st., Buffalo, N. Y.

*FRIEDRICHS, A. G., 641 St. Charles st., New Orleans, La.

FRIESELL, H. E., 6120 Center ave., Pittsburg, Pa.

*FRINK, C. H., Jacksonville, Fla.

FRUTH, O. J., 3066 Hawthorne Boulevard, St. Louis, Mo.

FULLER, D. A., 151 Clinton st., Brooklyn, N. Y.

FUNDENBERG, W. H., 508 Lewis block, Pittsburg, Pa.

FYNN, H. A., 500 California bldg., Denver, Col.

GALLAGHER, J. W. S., Winona, Minn.

GALLIE, DON M., 100 State st., Chicago, Ill.

GARDINER, F. D., 1516 Locust st., Philadelphia, Pa.

GAYLORD, E. S., 63 Trumbull st., New Haven, Conn.

GERECKE, F. T., 202 Pillsbury bldg., Minneapolis, Minn.

GETHRO, F. W., 901 Marshall Field bldg., Chicago, Ill.

GILLETT, HENRY W., 140 W. 57th st., New York, N. Y.

GILMAN, W. F., 11 Pleasant st., Worcester, Mass.

GILMER, T. L., 923 Marshall Field bldg., Chicago, Ill.

GINGRICH, C. M., 608 St. Paul st., Baltimore, Md.

GODSOE, FRANK A., 74 King st., St. John, N. B.

*GOLDBERG, E. A., Bennettsville, S. C.

GOOD, ROBERT, 126 State st., Chicago, Ill.

GOODE, GLADSTONE, 29 W. 37th st., New York, N. Y. *

GOODNOW, M. S., Hutchinson, Minn.

GOODWIN, N. J., 783 Main st., Hartford, Conn.

*GORMAN, J. A., Maison Blanche, New Orleans, La.

GOSLEE, H. J., 92 State st., Chicago, Ill.

GRADY, RICHARD, Naval Academy, Annapolis, Md.

*GRANT, W. E., 419 W. Chestnut st., Louisville, Ky.

*GRAY, J. P., 9th ave., S., Nashville, Tenn.

. GREENBAUM, LEO, 741 Fifth ave., New York.

GREENE, F. A., Geneva, N. Y.

GREGORY, F. G., 7 W. Park st., Newark, N. J.

*GRIEVES, C. J., Madison and Park aves., Baltimore, Md.

GRISWOLD, E. R.. Dansville, N. Y.

*GROSJEAN, S. S., New Orleans, La.

GROSS, O. J., 4 S. Church st., Schenectady, N. Y.

GUILFORD, DUDLEY, 1631 Walnut st., Philadelphia, Pa.

GUILFORD, S. H., 1631 Walnut st., Philadelphia, Pa.

*GUNN, C. L., Gadsden, Ala.

HACKER, THOS. S., 50 Willoughby bldg., Indianapolis, Ind.

HADLEY, AMOS I., 125 Marlboro st., Boston, Mass.

*HAIR, GEO. F., Ramburg, S. C.

*HAIR, H. B., Union, S. C.

*HALL, D. M., Macon, Ga.

HALL, E. L., 904 New St. Nat'l Bank bldg., Columbus, Ohio.

*HALL, J. A., S. Birmingham, Ala.

*HALL, WILMER S., Pensacola, Fla.

HALLEY, G. K., 816 15th st., N. W., Washington, D. C.

*HARDIN, J. FELTUS, Tuscaloosa, Ala.

HARDY, C. S., Summit, N. J.

*HARDY, GEO. E., Madison and Franklin sts., Baltimore, Md.

HARPER, W. E., 3441 Michigan ave., Chicago, Ill.

HARRISON, A. M.. 412 Masonic Temple, Rockford, Ill.

HARTZELL, T. B., 512 Nicollet ave., Minneapolis, Minn.

*HASSELL, H. C., Tuscaloosa, Ala.

HAWES, EARL P., 268 Weybosset st., Providence, R. I.

HAWLEY. C. A., "The Rochambeau," Washington, D. C.

HAYWARD. T. T., Excelsior, Lake Minnetonka, Minn.

HEAD, JOS., 1500 Locust st., Philadelphia, Pa.

HECKARD, W. A., 489 Fifth ave., New York, N. Y.

HENDERSON, G. H., 70 Franklin bldg., Springfield, Ill.

HERRICK, B. A., Red Wing, Minn.

HERT, B. S.. 713 Chamber of Commerce, Rochester, N. Y.

HERTZ, J. C.. 111 S. Fourth st., Easton, Pa.

HETRICK, F. O., Ottowa, Kansas.

HINKINS, J. E., 131 53d st., Chicago, Ill.

*HINMAN, THOS. P., Fourth Nat'l Bank bldg.. Atlanta, Ga.

HIPPLE. A. H., 200 Bee bldg., Omaha, Neb.

HITCH, D. M., 1621 Chestnut st., Philadelphia. Pa.

HITCH, GAYL A., Laurel, Del.

HOCKING, W. E., Devils Lake, N. D.

HOFF, N. S.. 603 S. State st., Ann Arbor, Mich.

HOFHEINZ, R. H., 815 Chamber of Commerce, Rochester, N: Y.

*HOLLAND, FRANK, Grant bldg., Atlanta, Ga.

*HOLLOWAY, B. L., Brookhaven, Miss.

HOLMBERG, J. L., St. Peter, Minn.

*HOOD, E. DOUGLASS, Tupelo, Miss.

HOPKINS, S. A., 235 Marlboro st., Boston, Mass.

*HOPPING, J. G., Birmingham, Ala.

HOSLEY, H. EVERTON, Phoenix bldg., Springfield, Mass.

HOURN, G. E., Lanesboro, Minn.

HOW, W. STORER, 1431 Mt. Vernon st., Philadelphia, Pa.

HOWE, HORACE L., 196 Marlboro st., Boston, Mass.

*HOWELL, I. B., Columbia bldg., Paducah. Ky.

HUEY, ROBT., 330 S. 15th st., Philadelphia, Pa.

*HUFF, M. D., Grant bldg., Atlanta, Ga.

HULICK, W. O., 807 Union Trust bldg., Cincinnati, Ohio.

HULL, H. A., Box 74, New Brunswick, N. J.

HULL, J. W., 607 Commerce bldg., Kansas City, Mo.

HUMPHREY, W. T., 13th and "O" sts., Lincoln, Neb.

HUNGERFORD, C. L., 306 Rialto bldg., Kansas City, Mo.

HUNT, F. G., 1705 Lawrence st., Denver, Col.

*HUNT, F. L., Asheville, N. C.

HUNT, GEO. E., 131 E. Ohio st., Indianapolis, Ind.

*HUNT, W. J., Memphis, Tenn.

HUTCHINSON, T. C., Decorah, Iowa.

IRWIN, ALPHONSO, 425 Cooper st., Camden, N. J.

JACKMAN, W. T., 809 Schofield bldg., Cleveland, Ohio.

*JACKSON, A. M., Macon, Ga.

JACKSON, H. H., 317 Jefferson ave., Detroit, Mich.

JACKSON, VICTOR H., 240 Lenox ave., New York, N. Y.

JACKSON, WALTER H., 126 S. Main st., Ann Arbor, Mich.

JAMES, F. S., Winona, Minn.

JAMESON, G. L. S., 1429 Spruce st., Philadelphia, Pa.

JARVIE, WM., 105 Clinton st., Brooklyn, N. Y.

JEFFERIS, C. R., New Century bldg., Wilmington, Del.

JENKINS, H. E., Ironton, Ohio.

JERNIGAN, F. L., 61 W. 56th st., New York, N. Y.

JEWELL, ALBERT B., 429 Center st., Newton, Mass.

JOHNSON, C. N., Marshall Field bldg., Chicago, Ill.

*JOHNSON, E. A., Holly Springs, Miss.

*JOHNSON, H. H., Macon, Ga.

*JOHNSTON, F. A., Sheffield, Ala.

JONES, C. F., 110 Madison ave., Elizabeth, N. J.

JONES, C. W., 713 Germania Life bldg., St. Paul, Minn.

JONES, J. A., 987 Locust st., Dubuque, Iowa.

*JONES, R. H., Winston, N. C.

JONES, VICTOR S., Bethlehem, Pa.

JUNKERMAN, G. S., 231 W. Court st., Cincinnati, Ohio.

*KELLEY, A. B., Yazoo City, Miss.

KELLEY, HENRY A., 727 Congress st., Portland, Maine.

KELSEY, HARRY E., Commonwealth Bank bldg., Baltimore, Md.

*KEMP, C. F., Key West, Fla.

KENNERLY, J. H., 2645 Locust st., St. Louis, Mo.

KENT, EDWIN N., 222 Washington st., Brookline, Mass.

*KETTIG, E. M., 318 W. Walnut st., Louisville, Ky.

KIMBALL, C. O., 27 W. 38th st., New York, N. Y.

*KING, W. C., 212 N. Spruce st., Nashville, Tenn.

KINKEAD, C. J., 66 Spring Garden rd., Wilmington, Del.

KINSMAN, EDWARD O., P. O. bldg., Cambridge, Mass.

KIRK, EDWARD C., Lock Box 1615, Philadelphia, Pa.

*KNAPP, J. ROLLO, 122 Baronne st., New Orleans, La.

KNIGHT, EUGENE W., Bellows Falls, Vt.

KOCH, C. R. E., 87 Lake st., Chicago, Ill.

KREMER, F. B., 407 Masonic Temple, Minneapolis, Minn.

KREPPEL, C. F., 10 Hyde Park, Forest Hills, Mass.

KRUPP, P. C., First Nat'l Bank bldg., Houston, Texas.

LAND, C. H., 64 Elizabeth st. W., Detroit, Mich.

*LAW, E. A., Bartow, Fla.

*LAWSON, A., Greenboro, Ala.

LAYTON, ROBERT E., 1311 Wisconsin ave., Washington, D. C.

LEAK, W. H., Watertown, N. Y.

LeCRON, D. O. M., 501 Missouri Trust bldg., St. Louis, Mo.

LEE, ALFRED P., 1728 Chestnut st., Philadelphia, Pa.

*LEONARD, N. C., 140 N. 8th ave., Nashville, Tenn.

LeROY, L. C., 47 W. 50th st., New York, N. Y.

LEWIS, A. M., Austin, Minn.

LEWIS, O. G. L., 1529 Locust st., Philadelphia, Pa.

*LEYDEN. F. C.. Anniston, Ala.

LIBBEY, J. A., 635 Fulton bldg., Pittsburg, Pa.

LINDSTROM, CARL R., 419 Boylston st., Boston, Mass.

LINK, E. G., 226 Cutler bldg., Rochester, N. Y.

LINTON, CHAS. C., 12 W. 46th st., New York, N. Y.

LIPPINCOTT, J. THOS., 1433 Walnut st., Philadelphia, Pa.

LISCHER, B. E., 504 Humboldt bldg., St. Louis, Mo.

LITCH, W. F., 1500 Locust st., Philadelphia, Pa.

LITTIG, M. D., 419 Boylston st., Boston, Mass.

LITTLE, J. B., 696 Endicott bldg., St. Paul, Minn.

LOEFFLER, EGBERT T., Ann Arbor, Mich.

LOGAN, W. H. G., 5606 Winthrop ave., Chicago, Ill.

*LONDON, JNO. H., 1115 "G" st., N. W., Washington, D. C.

*LORENZ, J. H., Fourth Nat'l Bank bldg., Atlanta, Ga.

*LOVELACE, G. R., Waycross, Ga.

LOVELAND, T. O., 196 Marlboro st., Boston, Mass.

*LOVETT, W. A., Brewton, Ala.

LOW, F. W., 52 N. Pearl st., Buffalo, N. Y.

LOWE, M. F., Buffalo, Minn.

LUCKEY, B. F., 88 Broadway, Paterson, N. J.

*LUCKIE, L. F., 830 S. 20th st., Birmingham, Ala.

*LUCKIE, R. K., Holly Springs, Miss.

LUCKIE, S. B., Chester, Pa.

*LUNDY, W. E., Memphis, Tenn.

LYON, HARRY D., 612 Masonic Temple, Minneapolis, Minn.

LYONS, JAS. W., People's Nat'l Bank bldg., Jackson, Mich.

MACKAY, GORDON R., 333 Commonwealth ave., Boston, Mass.

*McAFEE, S. H., Maison Blanche, New Orleans, La.

*McANNALLY, F. H., Jasper, Ala.

McCALL, J. O., 92 Chenango st., Binghamton, N. Y.

McCLANAHAN, W. B., Iowa Falls, Iowa.

McCLENAHAN, J. T., 926 Farragut sq., Washington, D. C.

McCREA, J. F., 221 Medical block, Minneapolis, Minn.

McFADDEN, H. B., 3505 Hamilton st., Philadelphia, Pa.

McGEHEE, W. H. O., University College of Medicine, Richmond, Va.

*McLAURIN, L. B., Natchez, Miss.

McMANUS, CHAS., 80 Pratt st., Hartford, Conn.

McMANUS, HENRY, 80 Pratt st., Hartford, Conn.

McMANUS, JAS., 80 Pratt st., Hartford, Conn.

McMILLEN, D. J., 11th and Locust sts., Kansas City, Mo.

*McNEIL, D. H., Athens, Ga.

MANN, W. W., 174½ Purchase st., New Bedford, Mass.

*MARLOWE, SEARCY, Tuscaloosa, Ala.

MARSH, J. W., Keokuk, Iowa.

MARSHALL, F. L., 39 Fairfield st., Boston, Mass.

MARSHALL, J. S., U. S. Presidio, San Francisco, Cal.

MARSHALL, M. C., 610 Chemical bldg., St. Louis, Mo.

MARSTON, H. F., 204 Medical block, Minneapolis, Minn.

MARVEL, W. W., 257 N. Main st., Fall River, Mass.

*MASON, J. M., Macon, Ga.

*MASON, R. HOLMES, Macon, Ga.

*MASON, R. M., Sanford, Fla.

*MASON, W. G., Tampa, Fla.

*MASSEY, D. L., Birmingham, Ala.

*MEADORS, JOS. T., 625½ Church st., Nashville, Tenn.

MEISBURGER, LOUIS, 85 N. Pearl st., Buffalo, N. Y.

*MELENDY, A. R., 1 Deaderick bldg., Knoxville, Tenn.

*MERCHANT, M. S., 310 Mason bldg., Houston, Texas.

MERNER, DANIEL, Cedar Falls, Iowa.

*MERRILL, C. A., Birmingham, Ala.

MERRIMAN, A. F., JR., 1065 Washington st., Oakland, Cal.

MERRITT, A. H., 59 W. 46th st., New York, N. Y.

MESSERSCHMITT, FREDERICK, 1023 Granite bldg., Rochester, N. Y.

MEYER, F. S., 413 Medical bldg., Minneapolis, Minn.

MEYER, J. H., 167 W. 71st st., New York, N. Y.

MILLER, F. E., Cedar Rapids, Iowa.

MILLER, HERBERT C., 15th and Couch sts., Portland, Ore.

*MILLER, W. C., Augusta, Ga.

MILLS, EDWARD C., 16 S. 3d st., Columbus, Ohio.

*MILNOR, G. A., Aiken, S. C.

MITCHELL, G. E., 25 Merrimack st., Haverhill, Mass.

*MOCK, J. H., Pensacola, Fla.

*MONROE, W. D., 3104 "N" st., N. W., Washington, D. C.

MONSON, G. S., 304 Baltimore block, St. Paul, Minn.

MOORE, G. T., Mt. Morris, N. Y.

*MOORE, T. T., Columbia, S. C.

*MOORE, T. T., JR., Columbia, S. C.

*MORGAN, HENRY W., 211 N. High st., Nashville, Tenn.

MOSKAU, GILBERT, Mayville, N. D.

*MURDAUGH, L. E., Celeste, Tex.

MURRAY, W. N., 601 Medical bldg., Minneapolis, Minn.

MYERS, CHAS. W., Montpelier, Ohio.

*NANCE, C. L., Tampa, Fla.

NELSON, J. J., 330 S. 15th st., Philadelphia, Pa.

NEWKIRK, GARRETT, 501 Slavin bldg., Pasadena, Cal.

NICKSON, H. E., Forest City, Iowa.

*NISBET, L. G., Aberdeen, Miss.

*NOEL, L. G., 527½ Church st., Nashville, Tenn.

NONES, R. H., 1708 Chestnut st., Philadelphia, Pa.

NORRIS, F. M., Winona, Minn.

NORRIS, G. W., Tracy, Minn.

NOYES, EDMUND, 1108 Stewart bldg., Chicago, Ill.

NOYES, FRED B., 1104 Stewart bldg., Chicago, Ill.

NYCE, J. E., 1001 Witherspoon bldg., Philadelphia, Pa.

NYMAN, J. E., Venetian bldg., Chicago, Ill.

*OHME, B. H., Alexander City, Ala.

OLIVER, R. T., Surgeon-general's office, Washington, D. C.

ORR, A. W., West Newton, Pa.

ORR, G. O., Jordan, Minn.

*ORR, J. M., Union Springs, Ala.

ORR, R. B., New Prague, Minn.

ORTON, F. H., 683 Endicott Arcade, St. Paul, Minn.

OTTOLENGUI, R., 80 W. 40th st., New York.

OWENS, F. M., 416 New York Life bldg., St. Paul, Minn.

*OWENS, H. D., Umatilla, La.

OWRE, ÆNEAS R., 502 Pillsbury bldg., Minneapolis, Minn.

OWRE, ALFRED, 1700 Portland ave., Minneapolis, Minn.

OXNER, WARREN C., Halifax, Nova Scotia.

PAGE, W. E., 38 W. Newton st., Boston, Mass.

PALMER, G. B., 571 Fifth ave., New York.

PALMER, STEPHEN, 272 Mills st., Poughkeepsie, N. Y.

PARKER, RALPH W., 6249 Kimbark ave., Chicago, Ill.

PARKHURST, C. E., 79 Walnut st., Somerville, Mass.

PARROTT, C. E., Perham, Minn.

PARSONS, STARR, 1309 "L" st., N. W., Washington, D. C.

PATTERSON, J. D., Keith & Perry bldg., Kansas City, Mo.

*PATTON, A. W., Tuscaloosa, Ala.

PAUL, JOSEPH L., 3 Park st., Boston, Mass.

PEARSON, J. A., Barton, Vt.

PECK, A. H., 92 State st., Chicago, Ill.

PEESO, FRED A., 4251 Regent st., Philadelphia, Pa.

*PEETE, J. W., Memphis Trust bldg., Memphis, Tenn.

PEMBERTHY, J. W., 301 Medical block, Minneapolis, Minn.

PENDLETON, I. E., 129 Lisbon st., Lewiston, Me.

PEREGRINE, H. G., 217 Globe block, Seattle, Wash.

PERRY, S. G., 130 W. 57th st., New York, N. Y.

*PETERSON, J. A., Tifton, Ga.

PFEIFER, JOSEPHINE D., 1007 Masonic Temple, Chicago, Ill.

*PHILLIPS, J. H., Meridian, Miss.

PIPER, J. R., 179 Newberry st., Boston, Mass.

POTTER, W. H., 16 Arlington st., Boston, Mass.

*POUND, E. H., Jacksonville, Fla.

POWELL, C. B., Jacksonville, Ill.

POWER, J. E., 248 Butler Exchange, Providence, R. I.

PRENTISS, C. C., 926 Main st., Hartford, Conn.

*PRICE, L. B., Corinth, Miss.

PROSEUS, F. W., 38 Monroe ave., Rochester, N. Y.

PROSSER, A. J., 3901 Westminster Place, St. Louis, Mo.

PRUYN, C. P., 92 State st., Chicago, Ill.
PULLEN, H. A., 722 Main st., Buffalo, N. Y.

*QUATTLEBAUM, E. G., Columbia, S. C.
*QUATTLEBAUM, J. M., Columbia, S. C.

*RAMAGE, L. J., Decatur, Ala.
*RAY, H. J., Aiken, S. C.
RAYMOND, H. C., 1134 Majestic bldg., Detroit, Mich.
*REABEN, W. H., McComb City, Miss.
*REEVES, A. T., Selma, Ala.
REEVES, W. T., 1421 Masonic Temple, Chicago, Ill.
*REGAN, C. W., Laurinburg, N. C.
REGISTER, H. C., 1907 Chestnut st., Philadelphia, Pa.
*REID, J. G., Marion, N. C.
REITZ, R. B., 38 E. 61st st., New York, N. Y.
*REMBERT, G. W., New Orleans, La.
REMINGTON, F. A., 57 W. 49th st., New York.
*RENALDS, W. R., Salem, Va.
RHEIN, MEYER L., 38 E. 61st st., New York, N. Y.
RICE, S. K., Northwood, Iowa.
*RICH, CELIA, Jackson bldg., Nashville, Tenn.
RICH, E. L., Savannah, Ga.
*RICH, S. L., Jackson bldg., Nashville, Tenn.
*RICHARDSON, W. C., New Orleans, La.
RICHTER, R. G., 128 Wisconsin st., Milwaukee, Wis.
ROACH, F. E., 67 Wabash ave., Chicago, Ill.
ROAN, H. ACTON, 824 Andrus bldg., Minneapolis, Minn.
ROBERTS, H. E., 1516 Locust st., Philadelphia, Pa.
ROBERTS, NORMAN J., "The Gables," Waukegan, Ill.
ROBINSON, C. H., Wabasha, Minn.
RODGERS, CHAS. W., 165 Harvard st., Dorchester, Mass.
ROE, F. A., Tama bldg., Burlington, Iowa.
ROE, W. J., 1210 Locust st., Philadelphia, Pa.
*ROSE, E. D., Bowling Green, Ky.
ROSE, J. E., Vinton, Iowa.
ROSENQUIST, A. C., St. Peter, Minn.
ROSS, A. O., 807 N. High st., Columbus, Ohio.
ROSSTEUSCHER, C. F., Yankton, S. D.
*ROUX, R. H., Savannah, Ga.
RUGGLES, S. D., 81 W. 2d st., Portsmouth, Ohio.
*RUST, D. N., 1408 "L" st., N. W., Washington, D. C.

RUST, THOS. L., 1408 "L" st., N. W., Washington, D. C.
*RUTLEDGE, B., Lock Box 45, Florence, S. C.

*SALIBA, G. M., Savannah, Ga.
*SANDERSON, E. M., Jacksonville, Fla.
SANDY, BENJAMIN A., 829 Andrus bldg., Minneapolis, Minn.
SANGER, R. M., 34 Harrison st., East Orange, N. J.
*SARRAZIN, J. J., Godchaux bldg., New Orleans, La.
SAVAGE, G. E., 14 Knowles bldg., Worcester, Mass.
SCHAMBERG, MORRIS I., 57 W. 58th st., New York, N. Y.
SCHMIDT, J. A., 1195 Dean st., Brooklyn, N. Y.
SCHUHMANN, HENRY H., 1312 Columbus Memorial bldg., Chicago, Ill.
SEARLES, C. S., 100 State st., Chicago, Ill.
SEIP, HOWARD S., 721 Walnut st., Allentown, Pa.
SEMANS, H. M., 106 E. Broad st., Columbus, Ohio.
SEMSRUDE, ERIC A., Buffalo Center, Iowa.
SHARP, JAS. G., 3049 Washington st., San Francisco, Cal.
*SHARP, S. P., Deaderick bldg., Knoxville, Tenn.
SHAW, F. I., 624 Burke bldg., Seattle, Wash.
SHEPARD, L. D., 330 Dartmouth st., Boston, Mass.
SHIELDS, NELSON T., 61 W. 56th st., New York, N. Y.
SHOREY, E. A., Stafford Bank bldg., Dover, N. H.
SHRYOCK, WM. W., 129 W. Berry st., Ft. Wayne, Ind.
SHUMAN, HARRY B., 131 Newbury st., Boston, Mass.
*SIMMONS, J. J., Kirbyville, Tex.
*SIMPSON, R. L., 1 S. Third st., Richmond, Va.
*SIMS, B. I., Cedartown, Ga.
*SLATER, W. K., Empire bldg., Knoxville, Tenn.
*SLAUGHTER, N. G., Athens, Ga.
SMEDLEY, W. P., 604 California bldg., Denver, Col.
*SMITH, B. HOLLY, 1007 Madison ave., Baltimore, Md.
*SMITH, C. L., Pensacola, Fla.
SMITH, D. D., 1629 Walnut st., Philadelphia.

Smith, E. E., Plainview, Minn.

Smith, Eugene H., 283 Dartmouth st., Boston, Mass.

Smith, G. Marshall, 1009 Madison ave., Baltimore, Md.

*Smith, G. W. B., Gaffney, S. C.

Smith, H. A., 116 Garfield Place, Cincinnati, Ohio.

Smith, H. T., 116 Garfield Place, Cincinnati, Ohio.

Smith, J. Allen, 232 N. Tryon st., Colorado Springs, Col.

*Smith, J. M., Houston, Miss.

*Smith, J. P., Martinsville, Va.

Smith, Karl C., 34 E. 53d st., New York, N. Y.

*Smith, L. A., Port Gibson, Miss.

Smith, M. C., 3 Lee Hall, Lynn, Mass.

*Smith, R. A., Charleston, S. C.

Smith, W. T., Geneva, Neb.

Smith, W. W., 63 East ave., Rochester, N. Y.

Southwell, Chas. C., 409 Goldsmith bldg., Milwaukee, Wis.

*Spurgeon, J. S., Hillsboro, N. C.

Stanley, Ned A., 3 Pleasant st., New Bedford, Mass.

Starr, A. R., 8 E. 92d st., New York, N. Y.

Steeves, Alice M., 355 Boylston st., Boston, Mass.

Stellwagen, Thos. C., 1119 Spruce st., Philadelphia, Pa.

Stephen, Jno. F., 1402 New England bldg., Cleveland, Ohio.

Stephenson, W. H., Lebanon, Ind.

Stern, David, 108 Garfield Place, Cincinnati, Ohio.

*Stewart, H. T., Memphis Trust bldg., Memphis, Tenn.

*Stiff, F. W., 600 E. Grace st., Richmond, Va.

Sting, E. H., Tiffin, Ohio.

Stockton, C. S., 22 Central ave., Newark, N. J.

Straight, M. B., 80 W. Huron st., Buffalo, N. Y.

Strang, C. W., Sanford bldg., Bridgeport, Conn.

*Strickland, A. C., Anderson, S. C.

Stutenroth, C. E., Room 6, Anderson block, Redfield, S. D.

Sullivan, H. H., 420 Altman bldg., Kansas City, Mo.

Summa, Richard, 410 Metropolitan bldg., St. Louis, Mo.

Sweeney, E. S., Osakis, Minn.

Swift, A. L., 140 W. 57th st., New York, N. Y.

Swift, Thos. C., 1 Park ave., Mt. Vernon, N. Y.

Swing, R. H. D., 1623 Walnut st., Philadelphia, Pa.

*Talbot, W. O., Biloxi, Miss.

Talbott, R. W., 1410 "H" st., N. W., Washington, D. C.

*Taylor, C. H., 52 N. 2d st., Memphis, Tenn.

Taylor, F. E., Malone, N. Y.

Taylor, F. T., 419 Boylston st., Boston, Mass.

Taylor, L. C., 68 Pratt st., Hartford, Conn.

*Taylor, R. P., Jacksonville, Fla.

Teague, B. H., Aiken, S. C.

*Tench, J. D. L., Gainesville, Fla.

Thatcher, C. A., 30 Center st., Ashtabula, Ohio.

Thomas, J. D., 1126 Spruce st., Philadelphia. Pa.

Thompson, C. N., 3017 Michigan ave., Chicago, Ill.

Thompson, H. C., 1113 Pennsylvania ave., Washington, D. C.

*Thompson, J. W., Humboldt, Tenn.

Thomson, G. K., Halifax, Nova Scotia.

Thorpe, Burton Lee, 3605 Lindell Boulevard, St. Louis, Mo.

Tibbetts, T. E., Rockland, Maine.

Tift, W. J., Glencoe, Minn.

*Tignor, G. S., Century bldg., Atlanta, Ga.

Tileston, H. B., 314 Equitable bldg, Louisville, Ky.

Tinker, E. L., Wheatland, Iowa.

*Tison, G. B., Gainsville, Fla.

Todd, G. S., Lake City, Minn.

Topliff, C. L., Decorah, Iowa.

*Towner, J. D., Memphis Trust bldg., Memphis, Tenn.

Townsend, A. F., 11 Pleasant st., Worcester, Mass.

Tracy, M. C., 46 W. 51st st., New York, N. Y.

Tracy, W. D., 46 W. 51st st., New York, N. Y.

Trueman, W. H., 900 Spruce st., Philadelphia, Pa.

Truman, James, 4505 Chester ave., Philadelphia, Pa.

*Tucker, E. J., Roxboro, N. C.

TURNER, C. R., 1500 Locust st., Philadelphia, Pa.
*TURNER, M. E., 719 Grant bldg., Atlanta, Ga.
TURNER, T. E., 606 Chemical bldg., St. Louis, Mo.
°TURNER, V. E., Raleigh, N. C.
*TUTTLE, M. H., Montgomery, Ala.

VAN BUSKIRK, W. L., 107 Wyoming ave., Scranton, Pa.
*VANN, G. S., Gadsden, Ala.
VANN, N. N., Attala, Ala.
VAN STRATUM, F. G., Hurley, Wis.   .
VAN VLECK, CHAS. K., 536 Warren st., Hudson, N. Y.
*VIGNES, C. V., Macheca bldg., New Orleans, La.

WADDELL, R. W., U. S. Army Dental Corps, Ft. Slocum, N. Y.
*WAHL, J. P., New Orleans, La.
WALKER, A. J., 33 Main st., Bridgeton, Me.
*WALKER, H. W., Macon, Ga.
*WALKER, J. L., 505 Taylor bldg., Norfolk, Va.
°WALKER, J. R., Gadsden, Ala.
*WALKER, R. H., 231 Main st., Norfolk, Va.
*WALKER, W. E., 157 Baronne st., New Orleans, La.
WALKER, W. W., 58 N. 50th st., New York, N. Y.
WALLS, J. M., 905 Pioneer Press bldg., St. Paul, Minn.
WALTON, J. ROLAND, 700 10th st., N. W., Washington, D. C.
WARD, MARCUS L., 703 University ave., Ann Arbor, Mich.
*WARDLAW, A. B., Greenville, S. C.
WARNER, E. R., 401 California bldg., Denver, Col.
WARNER, G. R., 417 N. 7th st., Grand Junction, Col.
WARREN, HORACE, Missouri Valley, Iowa.
WATERS, T. S., 756 Eutaw st., Baltimore, Md.
*WATKINS, J. C., Winston, N. C.
WATTS, CLARENCE V., Good block, Des Moines, Iowa.
WEAVER, MARSHALL, 726 Rose bldg., Cleveland, Ohio.
WEBER, A. G., 1 Corales, Havana, Cuba.
WEBSTER, F. S., Carthage, Mo.

WEDELSTAEDT, E. K., 204 New York Life bldg., St. Paul, Minn.
*WEICHSELBAUM, WM., Savannah, Ga.
*WEINBERG, A., Camden, S. C.
*WELCH, F. J., Pensacola, Fla.
WELCH, G. B., 1344 "G" St., N. W., Washington, D. C.
WELLS, F. P., Clarinda, Iowa.
*WELLS, W. D., Macon, Ga.
WELSH, J. D., New Hampton, Iowa.
WENDELL, W. C., 708 Goldsmith bldg., Milwaukee, Wis.
WEST, G. N., 100 State st., Chicago, Ill.
*WESTMORELAND, W. W., Columbus, Miss.
WHEELER, HERBERT L., 12 W. 46th st., New York, N. Y.
*WHEELER, J. H., Greensboro, Ala.
WHITE, EDWARD P., 1654 Massachusetts ave., Cambridge, Mass.
WHITE, F. D., 804 Masonic Temple, Minneapolis, Minn.
WHITE, GORDON, 610½ Church st., Nashville, Tenn.
WHITE, PAUL G., 419 Boylston st., Boston, Mass.
WHITE, W. A., Phelps, N. Y.
*WHITMAN, C. B., Orlando, Fla.
WHITMORE, Y. E., 23–25 Mann bldg., Little Rock, Ark.
WHITSLAR, W. H., 700 Schofield bldg., Cleveland, Ohio.
*WILLIAMSON, N. A., Prince st., Knoxville, Tenn.
°WILSON, F. C., 114½ Jones st., Savannah, Ga.
WILSON, GEO. H., 701 Schofield bldg., Cleveland, Ohio.
WIRT, W. N., Rockville, Ind.
WOLD, W. W., Jackson, Minn.
*WOMACK, C. T., Box 234, Martinsville, Va.
*WOOD, F. L., Roanoke, Va.
WOODBURY, FRANK, 137 Hollis st., Halifax, Nova Scotia.
*WOODBURY, G. M., Augusta, Ga.
WOODWARD, MARION L., 2 Commonwealth ave., Boston, Mass.
WORK, C. M., Ottumwa, Iowa.
WRIGHT, C. D., 57 W. 50th st., New York. N. Y.
*WRIGHT, P. H., Oxford, Miss.
*WRIGHT, T. B., Hattiesburg, Miss.
*WRIGHT, W. R., 32½ Capital st., Jackson, Miss.
*WYATT, T. M., Bentonville, Ark.

YEAGER, F. S., 403 Germania Life bldg., St. Paul, Minn.

YERKE, F. J., Owatonna, Minn.

YOUNG, D. H., Attica, N. Y.

YOUNG, J. LOWE, 571 Fifth ave., New York, N. Y.

YOUNG L. A., 4633 Maryland ave., St. Louis, Mo.

ZIRKLE, W. M., English-American bldg., Atlanta, Ga.

PERMANENT MEMBERS WITHOUT DUES.

The following members are "permanent without payment of dues," under Standing Resolution No. 10, by virtue of having been in reputable practice for a period of fifty years:

CHASE, EMMA EAMES, 3334 Washington ave., St. Louis, Mo.

FIELD, GEO. L., 4 Adams ave., W., Detroit, Mich.

HOLMES, E. S., 8 New Aldrich bldg., Grand Rapids, Mich.

LYMAN, A. E., Melbourne, Fla.

PALMER, CORYDON, Warren, Ohio.

RICH, JOHN B., New York, N. Y.

TURNER, V. E., Raleigh, N. C.

Surviving Charter Members of the Southern Dental Association.

The following surviving charter members of the Southern Dental Association are also "permanent members without dues":

AUGSPATH, LOUIS, Little Rock, Ark.

BROWN, J. P. H., Augusta, Ga.

CARPENTER, L. D., Atlanta, Ga.

COLE, W. T., Newman, Ga.

COOKE, W. H., Denton, Texas.

FRIEDRICHS, G. J., 641 St. Charles ave., New Orleans, La.

GORGAS, F. J. S., 259 N. Eutaw st., Baltimore, Md.

LOWRANCE, H. A., Athens, Ga.

MARSHALL, E. B., Rome, Ga.

McDONALD, R. H., Griffin, Ga.

RAMBO, SAMUEL, Montgomery, Ala.

PAST PRESIDING OFFICERS.

I. PRIOR TO CONSOLIDATION.

Ex-Presidents American Dental Association.

1859. *W. W. ALLPORT, Chicago, Ill.
First meeting, for organization.
1860. *W. H. ATKINSON, Cleveland, Ohio.
1861. (No meeting.)
1862. *GEORGE WATT, Xenia, Ohio.
1863. *W. H. ALLEN, New York, N. Y.
1864. *J. H. McQUILLEN, Philadelphia, Pa.
1865. *C. W. SPALDING, St. Louis, Mo.
1866. *C. P. FITCH, New York, N. Y.
1867. *A. LAWRENCE, Lowell, Mass.
1868. *JONATHAN TAFT, Cincinnati, Ohio.
1869. *HOMER JUDD, St. Louis, Mo.
Owing to a change in the constitution, officers elected at this and the sessions following served at the annual meeting subsequent to their election.
1870. *W. H. MORGAN, Nashville, Tenn.
1871. *GEO. H. CUSHING, Chicago, Ill.
1872. *P. G. C. HUNT, Indianapolis, Ind.
1873. *T. L. BUCKINGHAM, Philadelphia, Pa.
1874. *M. S. DEAN, Chicago, Ill.
1875. *A. L. NORTHROP, New York, N. Y.
1876. *GEO. W. KEELEY, Oxford, Ohio.

1877. *F. H. REHWINKEL, Chillicothe, Ohio.
1878. *H. J. McKELLOPS, St. Louis, Mo.
1879. L. D. SHEPARD, Boston, Mass.
1880. *C. N. PEIRCE, Philadelphia, Pa.
1881. H. A. SMITH, Cincinnati, Ohio.
1882. *W. H. GODDARD, Louisville, Ky.
1883. E. T. DARBY, Philadelphia, Pa.
1884. J. N. CROUSE, Chicago, Ill.
1885. *W. C. BARRETT, Buffalo, N. Y.
1886. *W. W. ALLPORT, Chicago, Ill.
1887. *FRANK ABBOTT, New York, N. Y.
1888. C. R. BUTLER, Cleveland, Ohio.
1889. M. W. FOSTER, Baltimore, Md.
1890. *A. W. HARLAN, Chicago, Ill.
1891. W. W. WALKER, New York, N. Y.
1892. J. D. PATTERSON, Kansas City, Mo.
1893. (Formal session only, owing to the holding of the World's Columbian Dental Congress; officers elected in 1892 holding over until 1894.)
1894. J. Y. CRAWFORD, Nashville, Tenn.
1895. J. Y. CRAWFORD, Nashville, Tenn.
1896. JAMES TRUMAN, Philadelphia, Pa.

Ex-Presidents Southern Dental Association.

1869. *W. T. ARRINGTON, Memphis, Tenn.
First meeting, for organization; Jas. S. Knapp being chairman pro tem.
1870. *W. T. ARRINGTON, Memphis, Tenn.
1871. *JAS. S. KNAPP, New Orleans, La.
1872. *F. Y. CLARK, Savannah, Ga.
1873. *H. M. GRANT, Abingdon, Va.
1874. *ROBERT ARTHUR, Baltimore, Md.
1875. *J. R. WALKER, New Orleans, La.
1876. *W. T. ARRINGTON, Memphis, Tenn.
1877. *W. G. REDMUND, Louisville, Ky.
1878. S. J. COBB, Nashville, Tenn.
1879. F. J. S. GORGAS, Baltimore, Md.
1880. *J. B. PATRICK, Charleston, S. C.
1881. V. E. TURNER, Raleigh, N. C.
1882. E. S. CHISHOLM, Atlanta, Ga.

1883. L. D. CARPENTER, Atlanta, Ga.
1884. *H. J. McKELLOPS, St. Louis, Mo.
1885. *A. O. RAWLS, Lexington, Ky.
1886. *W. C. WARDLAW, Augusta, Ga.
1887. *W. W. H. THACKSTON, Farmville, Va.
1888. *B. H. CATCHING, Atlanta, Ga.
1889. J. Y. CRAWFORD, Nashville, Tenn.
1890. *JOHN C. STOREY, Dallas, Tex.
1891. G. F. S. WRIGHT, Georgetown, S. C.
1892. GORDON WHITE, Nashville, Tenn.
1893. B. HOLLY SMITH, Baltimore, Md.
1894. (Same officers held over.)
1895. *H. E. BEACH, Clarksville, Tenn.
1896. JOHN S. THOMPSON, Atlanta, Ga.
1897. W. H. RICHARDS, Knoxville, Tenn.

* Deceased.

II. SINCE CONSOLIDATION.

Ex-Presidents National Dental Association.

1897. *THOMAS FILLEBROWN, Boston, Mass.
1898. HARVEY J. BURKHART, Batavia, N. Y.
1899. B. HOLLY SMITH, Baltimore, Md.
1900. G. V. BLACK, Chicago, Ill.
1901. J. A. LIBBEY, Pittsburg, Pa.
1902. L. G. NOEL, Nashville, Tenn.

1903. *C. C. CHITTENDEN, Milwaukee, Wis.
1904. WALDO E. BOARDMAN, Boston, Mass.
1905. M. F. FINLEY, Washington, D. C.
1906. A. H. PECK, Chicago, Ill.
1907. WILLIAM CARR, New York, N. Y.
1908. V. E. TURNER, Raleigh, N. C.

* Deceased.

Constitution of the National Dental Association.

PREAMBLE.

WE, the members of the American Dental Association and of the Southern Dental Association, do declare ourselves a Society to cultivate the Science of Dentistry, and have adopted the following Constitution and Rules of Order for our government:

CONSTITUTION.

(Adopted at Old Point Comfort, August 5, 1897. Revised and amended at Asheville, N. C., August 1903.)

ARTICLE I.

NAME.

This organization shall be known by the name of the NATIONAL DENTAL ASSOCIATION.

ARTICLE II.

OBJECT.

The object of this Association shall be to cultivate the science and art of dentistry and all its collateral branches, to elevate and sustain the professional character of dentists, to promote among them a mutual improvement, social intercourse and good feeling, and collectively to represent and have cognizance of the common interests of the dental profession.

ARTICLE III.

MEMBERS TO BE OF THREE CLASSES.

SECTION 1. The members of this Association shall be of three clases, viz, permanent, delegate, and honorary members; the two former classes having equal rights and privileges, except that none but permanent members shall be eligible to office.

PERMANENT MEMBERS.

SEC. 2. Permanent members shall consist of those who, coming as delegates and complying with the requirements of the Association, shall sign a statement in a book to be kept for that purpose, signifying to the Treasurer a desire for permanent membership.

DELEGATE MEMBERS.

SEC. 3. All members shall be practitioners of dentistry. They shall be received only from permanently organized state dental societies. They shall be elected by ballot at some regular meeting of their society, and shall be members who have done some meritorious work for the profession; but no person shall be received as a delegate who is in arrears for dues to this Association.

SEC. 4. Honorary members shall consist of prominent, worthy members of the dental profession residing in foreign countries, who shall be elected by ballot.

SEC. 5. It is hereby specially provided that all persons at present permanent members of the American Dental Association and of the Southern Dental Association are permanent members of this Association, and entitled to all the privileges of the class to which they belong, without further action, and the Treasurer is hereby directed to transcribe their names upon the roll of membership of this Association.

ARTICLE IV.

DELEGATES FROM STATE SOCIETIES.

SECTION 1. That delegates may be received from any state society, district society, or local society affiliated with the state society, upon the certificate of the president and secretary of the state society, and that these delegates may become members by sending their certificate together with the fee to the Treasurer of the National Dental Association.

SEC. 2. Each delegate shall present credentials which shall be approved by the Executive Committee.

SEC. 3. If the Committee on Credentials has knowledge that any applicants for membership are violating the Code of Ethics, said applicants shall not be received, but shall be referred by the committee to the societies whose delegates they are, and in no case shall this Association be compelled to treat with violations of the Code except the violator is a member of this body and has no membership in any local body.

SEC. 4. This Association will receive no delegates who, since August 1875, shall have entered the profession without having first graduated at some reputable dental or medical college.

ARTICLE V.

SIGNING CONSTITUTION.

SECTION 1. Each new member, before voting or speaking on any subject before the meeting, shall sign this Constitution, inscribing his name and the title of the society from which he receives his appointment. It is expressly agreed by each member in signing this Constitution that he will accept the discipline of a two-thirds vote of this Association.

DUES.

SEC. 2. The annual dues in this Association shall be five dollars.

DUES TO BE PAID.

SEC. 3. No member is eligible to office, nor can he speak or vote in this Association, in any of its sections, or in any of its branches, until his annual dues are paid.

DUES—IF UNPAID.

SEC. 4. If the dues of any member remain unpaid for two years his name shall be erased from the list of members of this Association.

CONDUCT OF MEMBERS.

SEC. 5. Any act of special immorality or unprofessional conduct committed by a member of this Association shall be referred to the Executive Committee, whose duty it shall be to thoroughly examine into the case, and if the charges be sustained, to report to the Executive Council during the annual session at which the charges are preferred. Whereupon by a vote of the Council the offending member may be reprimanded or expelled, a two-thirds vote being required for expulsion, a majority being sufficient for reprimand.

EXPELLED MEMBERS.

SEC. 6. Any member of this Association being expelled or suspended from his local society, shall from that date cease to be a member of this body.

RESIGNATION OF MEMBERS.

SEC. 7. Any member not in arrears may offer his resignation, upon the acceptance of which by the Council his membership shall cease; but the Council may at any time thereafter reinstate such member by unanimous consent. In case a member is dropped for non-payment of dues, two years' dues must be paid before reinstatement; nor shall he represent his society as a delegate until the two years' back dues are paid.

ARTICLE VI.

OFFICERS.

SECTION 1. The officers of this Association shall be a President, three Vice-presidents, Corresponding Secretary, Recording Secretary, Treasurer, an Executive Committee consisting of nine members, an Executive Council consisting of the President, Secretary, and five members, three Chairmen and three Secretaries of Sections, to be elected as hereinafter provided.

SEC. 2. Each officer, except as otherwise provided, shall hold his appointment for one year, or until another is elected and qualified to succeed him.

SEC. 3. The President shall be chosen from the division in which the next annual session is to be held, and one of the Vice-presidents shall be chosen from each division. (See Article XII.)

SEC. 4. At the first election three members of the Executive Committee shall be elected from each division of the country, who shall hold office for one, two, and three years, respectively; afterward but one member shall be elected each year from each division, and hold office for three years.

SEC. 5. One member of the Council shall be elected each year from the division in which the newly elected President resides, and two members from each of the others.

SEC. 6. At the first election after this amendment goes into effect, one Chairman and one senior and one junior Past Chairman for each section shall be elected. Thereafter one Chairman and one Secretary of Sections shall be elected each year from each division, and each Chairman of Sections shall be known as Junior Past Chairman for the first year and as Senior Past Chairman for the second year after the expiration of his time as Chairman.

SEC. 7. The names of places for holding the next annual session and the candidates for office shall be nominated by informal ballot of the Association. The three names that are highest, or in case of tie, four names having the greatest number of votes, shall be the sole nominee. A formal ballot shall then be taken in which a majority of the ballots cast shall be necessary to a choice. If a choice be not made on the second formal ballot the name of the candidate receiving the fewest votes shall be dropped on the third formal ballot. The informal ballot may be made a formal ballot by a three-fourths vote of the Association. Provided that for the re-election of Recording Secretary, Corresponding Secretary, Treasurer, and Secretaries of Sections a motion, seconded, that the Recording Secretary, or Treasurer, shall cast the ballot, shall be entertained, but if this fails to carry, nominations shall be made as hereinbefore specified.

ARTICLE VII—DUTIES OF OFFICERS.

DUTIES OF PRESIDENT.

SECTION 1. The President shall preside according to parliamentary usage as laid down in "Robert's Rules of Order" and the Rules of Order adopted by this Association, and shall present an annual address.

DUTIES OF VICE-PRESIDENT.

SEC. 2. In the absence of the President, one of the Vice-presidents shall perform the duties of the office, and in absence of these officers a Chairman *pro tem.* shall be appointed by the Executive Council.

DUTIES OF CORRESPONDING SECRETARY.

SEC. 3. The Corresponding Secretary shall attend to the correspondence of the Association with other scientific bodies, when desirable, and with the societies represented in this Association. It shall be his duty to obtain information of and report annually to the Executive Council, and with its approval to this Association, an account of the meetings held, the numbers of the membership and attendance, subjects discussed in papers, essays, or otherwise, by the societies represented in this Association, and such other matters of interest as may be well to incorporate in the proceedings of this body.

DUTIES OF RECORDING SECRETARY.

SEC. 4. The Recording Secretary shall keep accurate minutes of the proceedings of the Association, preserve the archives and unpublished documents, and attend to the other duties that pertain to his office. He shall be *ex officio* Chairman of the Publication Committee, and shall see that due notice is given of the time and place of the annual sessions of the Association. He shall be secretary of the Program Committee, and see to the preparation and printing for this committee and its distribution to the members of all societies represented in this Association, and shall provide each newly elected official with a correct copy of this Constitution.

DUTIES OF TREASURER.

SEC. 5. The Treasurer shall hold all the moneys belonging to the Association, and shall keep an accurate account as between the Association and its members. He shall furnish bonds satisfactory to the Executive Committee. He shall attend the session of the Executive Committee at 9 A.M. on the first day of the annual session to receive dues, and shall attend at roll call to verify the lists of names upon payment of dues within the legal limits, and shall notify all whose names may be erased from the list of membership. He shall pay the drafts of the Secretary, countersigned by the President, and shall report to the Executive Committee, where his accounts shall be audited and by whom his report shall be presented to the Executive Council, together with their own.

SEC. 6. All resolutions appropriating money, except for the legitimate expense of this Association, shall require a two-thirds vote of all the members of the Association present at a general session of an annual session.

ARTICLE VIII.

EXECUTIVE COMMITTEE.

SECTION 1. The Executive Committee shall be the business committee *ad interim* of the Association. They shall report to the Executive Council at each annual session, under the proper head, their doings for the current year.

SUBDIVISION OF THE EXECUTIVE COMMITTEE.

SEC. 2. The Executive Committee shall meet after the election of new members to choose their own chairman and secretary, and to divide themselves into three sub-committees as follows, and for the purpose described:

FIRST DIVISION OF THE EXECUTIVE COMMITTEE.

SEC. 3. The first division of the Executive Committee shall include its chairman. It shall act as the Committee of Arrangements, and shall make suitable preparations for the meetings of the Association, consulting with the Program Committee as to its needs. It shall report to the Executive Council at its first meeting of the annual session and with its approval see to the carrying out of the arrangements during the annual session. It shall provide a book for the registration of members or visitors as they arrive; and it shall be their further duty to secure from the Treasurer a good and sufficient bond.

SECOND DIVISION—CREDENTIALS AND AUDITING COMMITTEE.

SEC. 4. The second division of the Executive Committee shall act as a committee on registration, and shall meet for that purpose at 8 A.M. on the first day of the annual session. They shall examine and verify the qualifications of members, including all violations of the Code of Ethics and the Constitution. They shall register the names of members or visitors as they arrive, with place of their residence and hotel address, and give them all necessary information regarding the arrangements for the meetings, the literary program and arrangements for entertainment, if any. They shall also act as the auditing committee for the year.

THIRD DIVISION—COMMITTEE ON VOLUNTEER ESSAYS.

SEC. 5. It shall be the duty of the third division to examine all essays, papers, or reports that may be referred to it by the Executive Council before presentation to the Association and to report to the Executive Council their approval or disapproval of such essays, papers, or reports in whole or in any particular parts, to the end that the time of the Association may not be occupied by the reading of irrelevant, unimportant, or improper matter.

REPORTS OF SUB-COMMITTEES.

SEC. 6. Each of these Sub-committees shall report from time to time, as may be necessary, to the Executive Committee as a whole, who shall decide upon such report, if possible; but in case of their inability to decide upon any matter, it shall be brought before the Executive Council for its decision.

MEETINGS OF EXECUTIVE COMMITTEE.

SEC. 7. The Executive Committee shall, if possible, meet for consultation and arrangement of their respective duties on the day preceding the annual session of the Association. The Chairman may at his discretion summon the members thereof to a meeting for consultation or making reports, at any suitable hour during the annual session of the Association, and at any other time at the request of five members of the committee.

ARTICLE IX.

EXECUTIVE COUNCIL.

SECTION 1. The Executive Council shall be the business head of the Association during its annual session, and when it deems it necessary have charge of all its business matters whatever; and it will be its duty to take cognizance of the doings of any and all of its officers, see to the smooth working of all of its parts, and attend to all matters referred to it.

Sec. 2. The Executive Council shall meet at nine o'clock on the day of the first meeting of each annual session, to receive reports of committees, and afterward by adjournment or at the call of the presiding officers and committees, for the transaction of other business of the Association.

Sec. 3. All matters not otherwise specially provided for shall be referred to the Executive Council without debate.

Sec. 4. The Executive Council shall report to the Association at each general session the results of their proceedings for ratification or rejection without debate.

Sec. 5. The President and Secretary of this Association shall hold the same positions in the Executive Council as in the Association.

Sec. 6. Five members of the Council shall constitute a quorum for the transaction of business.

Sec. 7. All meetings of the Council shall be public; the time and place for which shall be posted for information of the members. Members may be heard on any matter before the Council.

ARTICLE X.

LOCAL COMMITTEE OF ARRANGEMENTS.

SECTION 1. There shall be appointed by the President, annually, a committee of three, residing at or near the place selected for the next meeting, whose duty it shall be to assist the Executive Committee to procure rooms for meetings, and make such other local arrangements as may be needed for the Association.

VACANCIES.

Sec. 2. In case vacancies occur in the Committees or Officers of this Association by reason of absence from the annual session or otherwise, such vacancies shall be filled by appointment *pro tem.* by the President.

PUBLICATION COMMITTEE—HOW APPOINTED.

Sec. 3. The President shall appoint two members of this Association who shall act in conjunction with the Recording Secretary as the Publication Committee. The Committee shall be authorized to employ a sufficient number of competent reporters to furnish an accurate report of the proceedings of each meeting of sections and of each general session.

ARTICLE XI.

INSTRUCTIONS TO THE PUBLICATION COMMITTEE.

SECTION 1. The Publication Committee shall superintend the publication and distribution of such portions of the transactions as the Executive Council may direct, or the Committee judge to be of sufficient value.

They shall specify in the annual report of this Committee the character and cost of the publications of the Association during the year, to whom they are distributed, and the number of copies still on hand.

Sec. 2. Any report or other paper to be entitled to publication in the volume of Transactions for the year in which it shall be presented to the Association, must be placed in the hands of the Publication Committee in typewritten form within twenty days after the close of the annual session; and must also be so prepared that the proof sheets furnished the authors shall be returned to the Committee without material alteration or addition.

Sec. 3. Every paper received and accepted by this Association, and all plates or other means of illustration, shall be considered the property of the Association, so far as may be necessary for publication in the Transactions of this body.

DISCLAIMER.

Sec. 4. The Publication Committee is hereby instructed to print at the beginning of each volume of the Transactions the following disclaimer, viz: "The National Dental Association, although formally accepting and publishing the reports of the various sections, and the essays read before the Association, holds itself wholly irresponsible for the opinions, theories, or criticisms therein contained, except when otherwise decided by special resolution."

ARTICLE XII.

SECTION 1. For the purpose of this Association, the United States shall be divided into three divisions, to be called the East, the South, and the West.

The East shall include New England, New York, New Jersey, Pennsylvania, Ohio, Indiana, lower peninsula of Michigan, and Ontario.

The South shall include Delaware, Maryland, District of Columbia, Virginia, North Carolina, South Carolina, West Virginia, Georgia, Florida, Alabama, Mississippi, Louisiana, Texas, Kentucky, Tennessee, Arkansas, Oklahoma, and Indian Territory.

The West shall include Illinois, Missouri, Wisconsin, upper peninsula of Michigan, Minnesota, Iowa, North Dakota, South Dakota, Nebraska, Kansas, Montana, Wyoming, Colorado, Idaho, Utah, Washington, Oregon, Nevada, California, Arizona, New Mexico, and Alaska.

PLACE OF MEETING.

SEC. 2. The place of holding the next annual session shall be determined each year by ballot of the Association at its annual session, in the general session of the third day, except that the place of meeting shall be in the West in 1898, in the East in 1899, and in the South in 1900, and thereafter, in the order named, meeting in each section every third year.

ARTICLE XIII.

ORGANIZATION OF SECTIONS.

SECTION 1. This Association shall be divided into three sections as follows:

The First Section shall have charge of prosthetic dentistry, crown and bridge work, orthodontia, metallurgy, chemistry, and allied subjects.

The Second Section shall have charge of operative dentistry, nomenclature, literature, dental education, and allied subjects.

The Third Section shall have charge of oral surgery, anatomy, physiology, histology, pathology, etiology, hygiene, prophylaxis, materia medica, and allied subjects.

SEC. 2. It shall be the duty of each member to identify himself with one or more of the above-named sections, and he shall inform the Recording Secretary of his choice at the time of joining the Association.

SEC. 3. The Secretary shall assign members to the sections in which they are expected to work if they shall fail to make their own choice before the close of the general session of the second day of the annual session.

SEC. 4. It shall be the duty of the Re-

cording Secretary to keep a list of the members of the sections and to furnish copies of the same to the officers of the sections.

SEC. 5. The Chairman of each section shall preside at all of its meetings; shall exercise general supervision over its business, and shall see that the labors of his section are so conducted as to secure the best results. In the absence of the Chairman the senior or junior past Chairman shall preside. (See Article VI, Section 6.)

SEC. 6. The Secretary of each section shall keep full and accurate records of the doings of his section, shall have charge of the stenographic reports, and report the same to the Recording Secretary each day, as soon as possible after their approval by his section.

SEC. 7. For information of all members a list of the names of members of sections shall be published in the Transactions of each year.

ARTICLE XIV.

MEETINGS.

SECTION 1. The meetings of this Association shall be known as annual sessions, general sessions, and meetings of sections.

SEC. 2. The annual sessions shall begin on the first Tuesday in August of each year and continue four days.

SEC. 3. The general sessions shall be meetings of the whole membership in attendance upon the annual session, and shall be held as follows:

The first general session shall convene at 10 o'clock on the first day and shall stand adjourned at 1 P.M., unless adjourned earlier. During this session the functions appropriate to the opening of the annual session may be performed, and the annual address of the President delivered.

On the second, third, and fourth days the Association shall convene in general session at 12 o'clock, noon, and stand adjourned at thirty minutes past one, unless adjourned sooner.

SEC. 4. In the general sessions any member may introduce matters of business, if seconded, which must then be referred to the Executive Council without debate; provided, that any member, opposed to such matter of business or motion, with a second, may call for a vote on such reference. A vote shall then be taken without debate, and if decided in the negative, that shall dispose of the matter for that annual session.

SEC. 5. The general session shall receive reports from the Executive Council as the first order of business after the reading of the minutes, and shall approve or annul any matter of business or motions referred to it by the Executive Council by vote without debate.

SEC. 6. The election of officers of the Association shall be held at the general session of the third day of the annual session, and newly elected officers presiding over the general sessions shall be installed at the close of the general sessions on the fourth day, and those presiding over meetings of each section, at the close of the last meeting of the section during the annual session.

SEC. 7. At the second and fourth general session there may be presented such addresses or reports as may be determined by the Program Committee, with the approval of the Executive Council, but these shall in no case occupy more than one hour of the general session.

SEC. 8. Sections I, II, and III shall each meet in separate rooms at 2.30 o'clock on the first day of the annual session for the reading and discussion of such essays, papers, reports, or for clinics, as may be determined upon by the Program Committee, with the approval of the Executive Council. Thereafter similar meetings of each section shall be held at 9 A.M. and 2.30 P.M. each day of the annual session. Evening meetings of the sections may be held as determined by each section.

SEC. 9. No business of any kind not strictly pertaining to the proper carrying out of the literary, scientific, or clinical work of the sections shall be introduced or considered in the meetings of the sections.

ARTICLE XV.

PROGRAM COMMITTEE.

SECTION 1. The Committee on Program shall consist of the President, Secretary, the Chairmen of sections, and the two last past Chairmen of sections. It shall be the duty of this Program Committee to keep close watch over the progress of dental science and literature, and to arrange with competent persons in the profession who are members of this Association, or with persons of known ability in closely allied subjects in science not members, to prepare and read or to discuss essays, papers, contributions, or perform such clinical demonstrations as will tend to the improvement of dentistry. It shall report to the Chairman of the Executive Committee what special preparations may be needed for carrying out the program that may be arranged or contemplated.

SEC. 2. The senior past Chairman, junior past Chairman, and Chairman of each section shall, subject to the Committee, act as a Sub-committee having especial charge of the program of that section, the responsibility in this work being in the order named.

SEC. 3. The President of the Association shall be President of the Program Committee, or, when present, shall preside over meetings of a Sub-committee. The preparation of the program for the general sessions shall be under his charge. In meetings of the Program Committee, in the absence of the President, the senior past Chairman of sections present shall preside, seniority beginning with the division in which the President resides and following the order of rotation.

SEC. 4. The Recording Secretary shall act as the Secretary of the Program Committee and shall have charge of the preparation, printing, and distribution of the programs. He shall announce at each general session the arrangement of the program for the next general session; and also the program for each of the sections for the next twenty-four hours.

SEC. 5. The Program Committee shall meet for consultation regarding the next year's work as soon as possible after the election of officers, and hold such meetings thereafter on the call of the President or Secretary, as may be deemed necessary to the efficient carrying out of the work.

SEC. 6. The Program Committee shall report to the Executive Council at its first meeting on the morning of the first day of the annual session the program arranged for approval, and thereafter shall hold such meetings as may be necessary to arrange from day to day for the smooth working of the presentation and discussion of the matter of the program in the general sessions and meetings of sections.

ARTICLE XVI.

QUORUM.

Twenty members shall constitute a quorum in this Association.

ARTICLE XVII.

SUSPENSION OF RULES—THREE-FOURTHS TO VOTE.

The regular order of business may be temporarily suspended by a three-fourths vote of all the members present, for the consideration of a specific subject, upon the completion of which the regular order shall be at once resumed.

ARTICLE XVIII.

BRANCHES.

SECTION 1. For the wider diffusion of the benefits of this Association, the members of each division may form themselves into one or more separate bodies, to be styled "Branches."

POWERS AND OBLIGATIONS.

SEC. 2. Branches shall have such powers and privileges, and be subject to such obligations, as shall be determined upon from time to time by the National Association in annual session.

SEC. 3. Each Branch shall be free to hold meetings and to govern itself as its members shall think fit, but no Branch law shall be valid which in the opinion of the National Association may contravene any fundamental law of the Association.

SEC. 4. Each Branch shall pay its own expenses, and no Branch shall be deemed for any purpose the agent of the Association, or have power to incur any obligation in its behalf.

SEC. 5. Each Branch shall furnish a copy of its proceedings, including papers and discussions, for publication with the Transactions of the National Association.

SEC. 6. Each Branch may receive delegates from societies within its division upon the same conditions as the National Association, and such delegates shall have the same standing in the National Association as though admitted directly from state societies.

DUES.

SEC. 7. The annual dues of members attending the Branches shall be paid to the Branch Treasurer. Three-fifths of the dues may be retained for the benefit of the Branch. The remaining two-fifths shall be paid over to the Treasurer of the National Association.

SEC. 8. The annual session of any Branch shall be omitted whenever the annual session of the National Association shall be held in its division.

ORDER OF BUSINESS.

FIRST DAY.

8 A.M.—Meeting of the Executive Committee.

8 A.M.—Meeting of the Program Committee.

9 A.M.—Meeting of the Executive Council.

10 A.M.—Meeting in general session.
Report of Executive Council.
Report on Program for next general session and for each section for next 24 hours.
President's Address.

1 P.M.—Adjournment of general session, unless sooner adjourned.

2.30 P.M.—Meetings of sections for literary and scientific work.

8 P.M.—Meetings of sections for literary and scientific work.

SECOND DAY.

9 A.M.—Meetings of sections for literary and scientific work.

12 NOON—Meeting in general session.
Reading of Minutes.
Report of Executive Council.
Report on Program.
Address, or Reports.

2.30 P.M.—Meetings of sections for literary and scientific work.

8 P.M.—Meetings of sections for literary and scientific work.

THIRD DAY.

9 A.M.—Meetings of sections for literary and scientific work.

12 NOON—Meeting in general session.
Reading of Minutes.
Report of Executive Council.
Report on Program.
Selection of next place of meeting.
Election of Officers.

1.30 P.M.—Adjournment, if not adjourned earlier.

2.30 P.M.—Meetings of sections for literary and scientific work.

8 P.M.—Meetings of sections for literary and scientific work.

FOURTH DAY.

9 A.M.—Meetings of sections for literary and scientific work.

12 NOON—Meeting in general session.
Reading of Minutes.
Report of Executive Council.
Address, or Reports.
Installation of Officers.
Appointment of Committees.
Final Reading of Minutes.
Adjournment of the Annual Session.

AMENDMENTS.

The Constitution, Rules of Order and Order of Business of this Association may be altered or amended at any annual session by unanimous consent of the members present, providing notice has been given in writing at a previous meeting of the annual session at which the amendment is proposed; or by a vote of two-thirds of the members present, providing notice of the alteration or amendment has been given in writing at a previous annual session.

STANDING RESOLUTIONS.

THE following standing resolutions are in force at this time:

1. RESOLVED, That a paper presented to the Committee on Voluntary Essays, and by them considered and returned to the writer with notification that the said paper is not accepted, cannot afterward be read before the Association unless it is made the special order by resolution adopted.

2. RESOLVED, That this Association discountenances the giving of banquets, excursions, entertainments, etc., by local professional societies or individuals, either during or at the close of our annual meetings.

3. RESOLVED, That it is unprofessional to use on cards or signs anything except name, title, and address.

4. RESOLVED, That this Association now in session direct that sections belonging thereto shall in the future be prohibited from inviting individuals who are violating the Code of Ethics to hold clinics or to give other exhibitions before this body.

5. RESOLVED, That a standing committee of three be appointed, to be known as the Committee on Terminology, whose duty it shall be to prepare and submit a carefully prepared report at each annual meeting of this Association.

6. RESOLVED, That this Association believes the conferring of honorary degrees in dentistry to be detrimental to the profession of dentistry, and hereby expresses its disapprobation of the practice.

7. RESOLVED, That a committee of three be appointed by the chair to co-operate with the officers in charge of the Army Medical Museum and Library in enriching its store of dental literature and specimens, especially by appealing to dental societies and individual members of the dental profession for assistance.

8. RESOLVED, That the National Dental Association condemns the use of secret preparations known as *"local anesthetics,"* as well as all other secret preparations.

9. RESOLVED, That the secretary or other officer of each society sending delegates to this Association is expected to make a general report of the work done by the society he represents during the year, giving the subjects of the papers read before them and digests of the same, and to send said report to the Secretary of this Association at least three weeks before the date of each annual meeting; the reports to be forwarded to the chairman of the section to which they belong.

10. RESOLVED, That any member of the dental profession who has been in reputable practice for a period of fifty years may be elected to permanent membership in the Association without payment of dues, and any member of this Association who has been in practice for a like period shall have his dues remitted thereafter by presenting the fact to the Treasurer of the Association.

11. RESOLVED, That lists of the ex-presidents of the American Dental Association and of the Southern Dental Association shall be published annually in the Transactions of the National Dental Association, and that all members and officers hold the same relations to the National Dental Association that they did to the former associations.

RULES OF ORDER.

1. On the arrival of the hour of meeting, the President shall take the chair, call to order, and announce that the meeting is open for business.

2. No motion or speech shall be in order until the mover or speaker shall have been recognized and assigned the floor by the chair, nor shall a motion be open for debate until seconded and stated by the chair.

3. No one shall be permitted to address the Association before giving his name and residence, which shall be distinctly announced from the chair; nor shall he speak more than twice, nor longer than fifteen minutes in all, unless by consent of the Association.

4. At the request of any member a motion shall be put in writing.

5. At the request of five members a question shall be divided or the yeas and nays ordered.

6. When a question is under debate no other motion shall be in order, except—1st, to adjourn; 2d, to lay on the table; 3d, the previous question; 4th, to postpone; 5th, to commit; 6th, to amend—and these motions shall take precedence in the order here stated.

7. The previous question and the motions to adjourn, to lay on the table, and to postpone, shall be decided without debate.

8. A motion to adjourn shall always be in order, but no member can make such a motion while another is speaking or while a vote or ballot is being taken.

9. A second amendment to the main question shall not be in order until the first is disposed of, nor shall there be an amendment of an amendment to an amendment.

10. After a motion has been seconded and stated by the chair, it shall not be withdrawn without the consent of the Association.

11. No member shall interrupt another while speaking, except to raise a point of order.

12. When called to order, a member shall sit down until the point of order is decided by the chair, or, in case of appeal, by the Association. If the point of order be sustained, the member can proceed in order by the consent of the Association.

13. Every member shall vote upon a question unless excused by the Association.

14. When any motion, except to adjourn, has been rejected, it shall not be renewed without unanimous consent.

15. Any member who on a question voted in the majority may move a reconsideration of that question; but if that motion shall be lost or laid upon the table, it shall not be renewed without unanimous consent.

16. The President may vote with the members upon all questions, but having so voted, shall not give the casting vote in case of a tie.

17. Motions for filling blanks shall be put in the order in which they are moved.

18. On a division, or in voting by yeas and nays, any member may change his vote before the result is declared.

19. These rules may be suspended by unanimous consent.

Code of Ethics.

ARTICLE I.

THE DUTIES OF THE PROFESSION TO THEIR PATIENTS.

SECTION 1. The dentist should be ever ready to respond to the wants of his patrons, and should fully recognize the obligations involved in the discharge of his duties toward them. As they are in most cases unable to correctly estimate the character of his operations, his own sense of right must guarantee faithfulness in their performance. His manner should be firm, yet kind and sympathizing, so as to gain the respect and confidence of his patients, and even the simplest case committed to his care should receive that attention which is due to operations performed on living, sensitive tissue.

SEC. 2. It is not to be expected that the patient will possess a very extended or a very accurate knowledge of professional matters. The dentist should make due allowance for this, patiently explaining many things which may seem quite clear to himself, thus endeavoring to educate the public mind so that it will properly appreciate the beneficent efforts of our profession. He should encourage no false hopes by promising success when, in the nature of the case, there is uncertainty.

SEC. 3. The dentist should be temperate in all things, keeping both mind and body in the best possible health, that his patients may have the benefit of that clearness of judgment and skill which is their right.

ARTICLE II.

MAINTAINING PROFESSIONAL CHARACTER.

SECTION 1. A member of the dental profession is bound to maintain its honor, and to labor earnestly to extend its sphere of usefulness. He should avoid everything in language and conduct calculated to dishonor his profession, and should ever manifest a due respect for his brethren. The young should show special respect to their seniors; the aged, special encouragement to their juniors.

SEC. 2. It is unprofessional to resort to public advertisment, cards, handbills, posters, or signs, calling attention to peculiar styles of work, lowness of prices, special modes of operating; or to claim superiority over neighboring practitioners; to publish reports of cases or certificates in the public prints, to circulate or recommend nostrums; or to perform any other similar acts. But nothing in this section shall be so construed as to imply that it is unprofessional for dentists to announce in the public prints, or by cards, simply their names, occupation, and place of business, or in the same manner to announce their removal, absence from, or return to business, or to issue to their patients appointment cards having a fee bill for professional services thereon.

SEC. 3. When consulted by the patient of another practitioner the dentist should guard against inquiries or hints disparaging to the family dentist or calculated to weaken the patient's confidence in him; and if the interests of the patient will not be endangered thereby, the case should be temporarily treated, and referred back to the family dentist.

SEC. 4. When general rules shall have been adopted by members of the profession practicing in the same localities in relation to fees, it is unprofessional and dishonorable to depart from those rules, except when variation of circumstances requires it. And it is ever to be regarded as unprofessional to warrant operations as an inducement to patronage.

ARTICLE III.

CONSULTATIONS.

Consultations should be promoted in difficult or protracted cases, as they give rise to confidence, energy, and broader views in practice. In consultations that courtesy and just dealing which is the right of all should be especially observed.

ARTICLE IV.

THE RELATIVE DUTIES OF DENTISTS AND PHYSICIANS.

Dental surgery is a specialty in medical science. Physicians and dentists should both bear this in mind. The dentist is professionally limited to diseases of the dental organs and adjacent parts. With these he should be more familiar than the general practitioner is expected to be; and while he recognizes the broader knowledge of the physician in regard to diseases of the general system, the latter is under equal obligations to respect his higher attainments in his specialty.

ARTICLE V.

THE MUTUAL DUTIES OF THE PROFESSION AND THE PUBLIC.

Dentists are frequent witnesses, and at the same time the best judges of the impositions perpetrated by quacks, and it is their duty to enlighten and warn the public in regard to them. For this and many other benefits conferred by the competent and honorable dentists, the profession is entitled to the confidence and respect of the public, who should always discriminate in favor of the true man of science and integrity against the empiric and impostor. The public has no right to tax the time and talents of the profession in examinations, prescriptions, or in any way without proper remuneration.

Lightning Source UK Ltd.
Milton Keynes UK
UKHW020752220119
335989UK00010B/1035/P